Praise for

The Well-Tuned Brain

"Peter Whybrow combines gripping big themes with an abundance of fascinating stories. The big themes revolve around the collision between our ancient human habits, our human brains often operating on autopilot, and the seductive material success of our modern market economy. You'll find this book as rich and as thought-provoking as it is enjoyable." —JARED DIAMOND,
Pulitzer Prize–winning author of *Guns, Germs, and Steel*;
Collapse; and *The World Until Yesterday*

"As we face the biggest problems civilizations have ever confronted—climate change above all—it's crucial that we understand why our brains are being hijacked in the wrong direction. Peter Whybrow's book does exactly that, making it possible for us to summon the grace and will necessary to do the right thing." —BILL McKIBBEN,
environmental activist and best-selling author of
Eaarth: Making a Life on a Tough New Planet

"Though *The Well-Tuned Brain* is packed with powerful recent research, its punch comes from the philosophical meditation at its core. Peter Whybrow ponders how living our best lives can make the best world. This book is a courageous manifesto about human frailty that delineates the care with which we need to treat ourselves and those around us. We ignore its message at terrible personal and social cost." —ANDREW SOLOMON,
National Book Award–winning author of
The Noonday Demon and *Far from the Tree*

"Psychiatrist and author Peter Whybrow reminds us that the brain's construction is about survival in the wild, not about navigating a land of plenty in food and consumer goods."

—**GEOFFREY RILEY** and **EMILY CURETON,**
Jefferson Public Radio

"Whybrow's knowledge clearly ranges far and wide—the book melds together history, philosophy, anthropology, economics, psychology, and neuroscience. . . . For those who want to see how to put everything together to better understand our nature and make positive social change, they will find the book quite readable, intriguing, and . . . instructive." —**JILL SUTTIE,** *Greater Good*

"By harnessing modern science to better understand the nature of ourselves and by returning to ancient human truths that in our frenzy we now overlook, Whybrow asserts that we can live not only better individual lives, but also build together a thriving future that serves the common good." —*Zen Commuter*

The Well-Tuned Brain

The Well-Tuned Brain

The Remedy for a Manic Society

PETER C. WHYBROW, MD

W. W. NORTON & COMPANY

INDEPENDENT PUBLISHERS SINCE 1923

NEW YORK LONDON

Copyright © 2015 by Peter C. Whybrow, MD

For information about permission to reproduce selections from this book, write to
Permissions, W. W. Norton & Company, Inc., 500 Fifth Avenue, New York, NY 10110

For information about special discounts for bulk purchases, please contact
W. W. Norton Special Sales at specialsales@wwnorton.com or 800-233-4830

Manufacturing by Quad Graphics, Fairfield
Book design by Lovedog Studio
Production managers: Devon Zahn and Ruth Toda

The Library of Congress has cataloged the hardcover edition as follows:

Whybrow, Peter C.
  The well-tuned brain : neuroscience and the life well lived / Peter C. Whybrow,
MD. — First edition.
    pages cm
  Includes bibliographical references and index.
  ISBN 978-0-393-07292-1 (hardcover)
1. Neurosciences—United States. 2. Consumption (Economics)—United States.
I. Title.
  RC338.W46 2015
  612.8—dc23
                    2015000168

ISBN 978-0-393-35304-4 pbk.

W. W. Norton & Company, Inc.
500 Fifth Avenue, New York, N.Y. 10110
www.wwnorton.com

W. W. Norton & Company Ltd.
Castle House, 75/76 Wells Street, London W1T 3QT

1 2 3 4 5 6 7 8 9 0

For Nancy

Why is it, do you suppose, that an Englishman is unhappy
until he has explained America?

E. B. White (1971)

The supreme test of all political institutions and industrial
arrangements shall be the contribution they make to the
all-around growth of every member of society.

John Dewey (1920)

Contents

Preface

I FIRST BEGAN THINKING about the ideas that were to become *The Well-Tuned Brain* in 2008, in the wake of America's ruptured housing bubble and the worldwide financial seizure that it provoked. *American Mania* had been published a couple of years earlier and essentially predicted such a meltdown. But why, I asked myself, had the madness become so pervasive in Western culture? What were we thinking? Looking back, it defies common sense to believe that any economic system, but particularly a globalized market system, could indefinitely sustain itself on debt and speculation.

Amid the wreckage of subprime mortgages, easy money, and shifting weather patterns, I was not alone in my rumination. As the workaday treadmill slowed, and the collective anxiety mounted across Europe and in the United States, the mood was one of angry, confused reflection. In the public forum, perhaps in fright, perhaps in hope, we thrashed about searching for villains and plausible causes. And rogues there were, with the bankers being high on most lists, but *self*-reflection and discussions around the part we each may have played in the economic debacle were remarkably muted. In the main we preferred to find explanation "out there," apart from our personal behavior and our responsibilities as informed citizens.

This intrigued me. The foibles of humankind are no secret but are written large in the history of our species. Nor are our assets obscure when it comes to thinking about who we are. One of the amazing things about modern times is that we have made great strides in understanding the biology of the brain and its role in shaping human culture. And yet when thinking about our social and political organization, we tend to ignore such insights, especially in commanding our own behavior. *The Well-Tuned Brain* is my effort to highlight how knowledge of science can improve self-understanding and how such insights can serve all of us, and the common good, going forward. But that is only one part of my agenda. As intensely social creatures, we have many qualities, some that we are in danger of forgetting, which are essential to living together constructively in the frenetic, information-saturated world that we have created for ourselves. My effort is to bring these diverse elements together, integrating history, psychology and neuroscience with sociocultural insight and economic commentary, to craft a cohesive story upon which to build a balanced future vision.

I am fully aware that this is an ambitious undertaking. As such, I temper my ambition with humility. We still have much to learn about human behavior, and inevitably my analysis falls short. But I have learned over the years that it is easier to criticize than to construct—to look back rather than forward. Hence, while I take full responsibility in attempting this synthesis, I make no apology.

Woodstock, Oxfordshire,
September 2014

The Well-Tuned Brain

In *The Age of Man*:
Progress and Its Pursuit

> ... progress, man's distinctive mark alone,
> Not God's, and not the beasts'.
>
> Robert Browning, "A Death in the Desert" (1864)

WE ARE LIVING in the shadow of our achievements.

Our compelling, technology-rich, supercharged world is one born of explosive economic growth. While over the past half-century the planet's human population has increased, more than doubling since 1950, the global economic output over the same period has multiplied nearly eightfold. In the developed Western nations this unprecedented expansion has led to a massive increase in material goods and in market choice—a shift particularly evident in the consumer society of the United States, the nation that for over a century has been the world's commercial and economic leader.

This invention of the modern world owes much to capital markets and to the spirit of the European Enlightenment, of which America has become the Grand Experiment. The material affluence we now enjoy validates the Enlightenment principle of individual freedom and the conviction that scientific and technical advance is best achieved by harnessing human reason within a competitive marketplace. This grand reimagining of the human condition, one where we strive to control our place in nature and maximize economic growth as the source of personal well-being, we now describe as "progress."

Since the last ice age, some ten thousand years ago, the Earth's climate has been peculiarly stable—a period that geologists call the Holocene—and that constancy has aided the human ascendancy to planetary dominance. However, over the past two or three centuries—indeed since the Enlightenment—we have witnessed a cultural revolution that has been a faster and more profound driver of that dominance than anything in history. Catalyzed by an insatiable curiosity and served by a superior intelligence, we have contrived ways to unleash the power of fossil fuels, temporarily breaking free from the living world's organic-based energy cycle and harvesting to our advantage the Earth's great natural resources.

In this energy-rich modern age health and wealth have never been so abundant: we live longer; the vast majority of our offspring survive childhood; we are largely literate, and in the developed economies many individuals enjoy material comforts that for centuries were beyond the reach of kings. That is not all: as economic growth continues to quicken and material poverty declines, it is the American contemporary ideal of material progress that shapes expectations for China, India, and the rest of the emerging world. As John Stutz of the Tellus Institute has described it, "We are a global consumer society poised on the brink of affluence."

Or perhaps we are courting disaster? We are discovering, in this headlong pursuit, that our material progress has unintended consequences, both personal and environmental. In less than a century we have wrought changes in the Earth's geology and biosphere on a massive scale. It is a dubious testimony to our zeal that the stigmata of some of our most ambitious projects are now easily detectable from an orbiting satellite two hundred miles above the Earth's surface—the disappearing Aral Sea and the vast excavation of the Athabasca tar sands in northern Alberta being but two examples. And then in addition, given our addiction to fossil fuels there is mounting evidence—now reinforced by "superstorms" such as Katrina and Sandy—that human appetites play a significant role in climate change.

In a globalized commercial world, human intervention is suddenly everywhere, monopolizing the ecosystem for our singular benefit and significantly disturbing its balance. Today's world is fundamentally different—a new planet "Eaarth," as Bill McKibben has described it—from the ancestral environment that nurtured the human species. The distinguished biologist E. O. Wilson has calculated that with seven billion of us now living on this planet, the human biomass that the Earth must sustain is roughly one hundred times greater than the biomass of any previous large animal species. Indeed, some scientists suggest that we can no longer study the "natural" world in isolation from human action. They argue—following the lead of the Nobel Prize–winning chemist Paul Crutzen—that we have entered a new geological epoch that is better described as the Anthropocene: this is *The Age of Man*.

The implication that logically follows is that in this *Age of Man* human destiny lies in our own hands. This poses some tough questions. How do we intend to survive as a species on a planet of finite resources when we pursue an economic policy committed to continuous growth? If we persist in maximizing material consumption, how do we hope to live within the means of a delicate and limited biosphere? Such questions not only challenge the sustainability of human "progress" as we currently define it—within a competitive global framework of continuous economic expansion—but also suggest a denial of our fundamental biology as evolved creatures, dependent for our very existence upon the Earth's habitat.

Our collective behavior, in its disregard of biology and human values, falls short of the Enlightenment principle of rationality. So, for example, while sporadic concern is expressed regarding carbon emissions and potential ecological pitfalls, we have yet to develop serious international intent to combat climate change. Resistant to changing our behavior, we put faith in science and technology in the hope of discovering a panacea. We have begun to explore alternative sources of energy to the Earth's finite supply of fossil fuels; fear of climate change similarly promotes "green" building codes and cleaner transport systems. But in the aggregate our vision of the future is short term and shaped largely by our experience of what has fostered economic "progress" in the immediate past. As a matter of cultural habit, we are attuned to a commercial ethos of material self-interest, consumption, and continued economic growth, with only marginal concern for the human and environmental impact of such policies. This is a world where personal and corporate reward is myopically focused upon competition and immediate advantage, with little regard for the healthy ecological and social infrastructure upon which all markets depend over the long term.

A similar myopia and adherence to habit is evident in our personal lives. Thus, rather than accepting that in the face of plentiful supplies of food we eat too much, and mostly the wrong stuff, we turn to the medical profession, hoping for a quick fix to our growing obesity, ignoring the sociocultural and economic factors that drive the epidemic. With rising energy costs we feel exploited by the oil companies but do little to address our personal dependence on fossil fuels. When millions of "rationally minded" citizens take on unsustainable debt to buy houses they cannot afford, then later borrow against that assumed equity to sustain consumption beyond their means, we first blame the bankers and the regulatory agents rather than our spendthrift ways and the culture that drives them.

We each want to believe that the crises we face are beyond individual control, perpetuated by government, big business, or the indiscretions of others. But such a mindset does not do justice to our intelligence and to what we know about human behavior. If we are to think seriously about our responsibilities and to make informed choices, both in averting serious health consequences and in shaping a balanced human destiny, it is imperative that we each work to better understand ourselves. Going forward, we must take ownership of our behavior, for it is there that our troubles are rooted.

This is the fundamental premise of *The Well-Tuned Brain*. I argue that the challenges we face *are* open to rational problem solving and to proactive planning, but that first we must accept ourselves for who we are. The major cultural focus of my inquiry is the United States, a country that has been my adopted home for thirty years, but the essence of my argument is broader in range and implication. I suggest it is time to reflect upon what we have learned about the human animal—both positive and negative—from the rise of Western mass-market materialism. By integrating what we now know about the brain from neurobehavioral science with what we have forgotten about ourselves as sociocultural animals, we can reimagine the idea of human progress and bring greater harmony to everyday life. It's important, however, that the steps we take be informed and adaptive to circumstance, for the pitfalls that lie ahead are both ideological *and* physical. If we persist along our chosen path, we are in danger of reducing ourselves to mindless consumers—to the addictive pursuit of a market ideology where profit is the major prize, and where social capital and a sustainable habitat are largely neglected. In practical terms, to reshape the future we need first to better understand and reshape ourselves.

AT THE PRESENT MOMENT there is much in the way we behave to suggest that we are confused. For many ordinary Americans the banking debacle of 2008, which brought the world to the brink of financial implosion, called into question the prevailing mythology that only continuous material growth can maintain the nation's economic vitality and deliver individual happiness. Yet after a few months of angry protest regarding the ethics of the banking industry and anguished self-reflection that the good life may be more than materialism, we quickly returned to our old habits. Blindly we lapsed back into the short-term, helter-skelter pursuit of debt-fueled economic growth. And we persist in doing so despite accumulating evidence that we are fostering social inequity, making ourselves sick, harming other species, and perhaps wrecking the environment that sustains us.

Two simple neurobehavioral questions arise from this puzzling behavior. First, why is it that human beings tend to consume excessively when living in a resource-rich environment, and second, why despite our growing conscious awareness of the challenges we face do we find it so difficult to change our ways? The answers to these questions and an explanation for our self-destructive behavior are to be found in a contemporary mismatch among three cardinal factors—ancient instinctual strivings that seek short-term reward, an efficient habit-driven brain, and the material affluence of contemporary market culture. Succinctly, the human brain is not "well-tuned" to modern-day circumstance.

First our instinctual strivings: the propensity for overconsumption is the relic of a time when individual survival depended upon fierce competition for scarce resources. Achieving affluence has not changed those fundamental biological templates. Indeed, the material abundance we have achieved and our adherence to a model of progress founded on competition and maximizing economic expansion has served only to reveal and reinforce such ancient proclivities. Thus the reward-seeking, short-term focus that is particularly evident in American society today finds its origins in normal mammalian biology. Our acquisitive mania, with all its unintended consequences, has emerged not because we are evil but because in a time of plenty such ancient instinctual strivings no longer serve their original purpose. Strivings for more food, more sex, and more safety were once regulated by scarcity of opportunity. In the consumer society, where enticement and opportunity holds sway, the tables have turned: what was once our greatest asset is becoming a fatal flaw.

Second, that we are creatures of habit confounds our instinctual striving. One reason why we find change and adopting a long-term perspective so difficult is the illusion that we are in full conscious control over the decisions we make and have made in the past: we believe that the enlightened, rational self is dominant in human affairs. In reality, however, what we now know from brain science is that much of what we feel within ourselves and perceive about the day-to-day world is harvested and acted upon preconsciously. In other words, many of the complex brain patterns that shape our day-to-day decisions and drive our behavioral routines function in parallel to, or outside of, immediate conscious awareness. *Habit* is the word most commonly used to describe such routines. These are behaviors that the brain adopts to deal with repetitive circumstance, behaviors that later become so familiar that little conscious attention is required, or is necessary, for their automated execution.

Everyday life would be impossible without habits. Habits are the brain's way of handling the events of a familiar world with speed and efficiency, essentially a personal autopilot that when provided with the appropriate environmental cue knows the routine and takes over to complete the necessary chore. Once you pick up that toothbrush in the morning, the complex muscle activity required to effectively manipulate the brush to successfully clean the teeth follows smoothly and is completed without thought. The routine of dressing is similarly automated, as is driving the car along the familiar route to work. We "think nothing of it" until something unusual occurs, such as a pedestrian unexpectedly stepping out in front of us, which then "catches our attention."

It is through habit that the brain "tunes" itself to optimally engage the world. Some habits we consciously seek to cultivate, such as playing a good tennis game or a better round of golf, while other habits intrude without conscious permission, such as when, under stress at work, we find ourselves craving doughnuts and drinking more coffee. Thus habits can be good and bad, even compulsive, and either way habits are hard to break. While we celebrate the efficiency habits afford, and in these accelerated times we even boast about our capacity to "multitask," we also worry about "poor" habits and their addictive potential, as in the case of consuming too many sodas or repeatedly checking e-mail.

But beyond these mundane examples we each have other habits of which we are much less consciously aware, and yet are crucial to understand if the potentially addictive bondage of consumerism is to be avoided. These are *habits of mind*, patterns of thought, opinion, and social behavior that are informed by instinct and tuned through personal experience. Commonly called *intuition*, these thought habits largely operate preconsciously and complement reasoned choice, profoundly influencing how we feel about things, other people, and ourselves. Intuition, we shall find, has its own distinct brain network and is the brain's fundamental operating system when it comes to efficient thinking. Indeed, probably some 80 percent of our behaviors and actions are managed by the preconscious intuitive mind.

The third element in the mismatch is cultural change. Habits of intuitive thought are profoundly shaped, and given meaning, by the culture into which we are born. And in turn it is the habits of individuals that collectively shape culture. Our early cultural experience exerts a continuous and powerful effect not only upon the language we speak but also on how we characteristically conduct ourselves as adults, including the values we perceive as important and the meaning we attach to them. Think of the intuitive process as a narrative—as a personal story—that is held in the preconscious library of the mind. Over a lifetime we carefully piece together the chapters in the story— our personal patterns of intuitive thought—from the thousands of cultural and social cues that are drawn from our everyday experience. The stories we construct are passed from person to person and across generations, and through these shared habits of mind—in tune with the collective experience—our cultural beliefs are perpetuated. In short, the intuitive personal narrative and its individual expression not only shape culture but also are the glue that holds society together.

Today in the United States and Western nations the master cultural narrative—the way we habitually think about everyday life—is written in the language of the market. Each day we confirm the market narrative at work, at home, and at play. Profit, competition, and wealth creation have become the dominant and recurring theme of the national story. While market exchange is far from a complete expression of the human social values, the drive to maximize market growth is now entrenched and powerful, dominating life's meaning. Commercial product—the brands we buy, the entertainment we choose—increasingly populates the personal narrative. In consequence, we find ourselves rewarded less in the role of concerned citizen than in that of self-seeking consumer. Through habituation, we have grown indifferent to those aspects of human culture that fall outside market reference.

"Happiness," wrote Adam Smith in 1759, "consists in tranquillity and enjoyment," and in America it is happiness that has been the pursuit. But somewhere along the way—conjured from the material success of the Great American Experiment—we have abandoned tranquillity for the convenience of immediate satisfaction and become mesmerized by enticements of our own manufacture. This is the cultural shift that now drives our biology. Our ancestral hunger for short-term reward both serves the global market's need for continuous economic growth and feeds the abiding hope that with "progress" the American Dream, one day, can be made material. Although evidence is accumulating that our fixation on consumption and wealth creation has failed to deliver to the average American family the benefits promised—equal opportunity, upward social mobility, security, and personal well-being, to name a few—as a nation we find it difficult to move beyond the myth of material happiness.

While common sense suggests that any civil society requires more than self-indulgence and shopping to maintain its health and cultural integrity, the merry-go-round that now serves as everyday life distracts us from imagining the rational alternatives. We have created for ourselves a form of trickery, but for the moment the seduction works: and as I shall explain, it's an easy habit to acquire. Thus, driven by the instinctual search for immediate reward, we find ourselves caught up not in the enjoyment of happiness but in a relentless pursuit of its material surrogates. We have fallen out of tune with who we really are, and in consequence the mismatch continues to flourish.

THE WELL-TUNED BRAIN is divided into two complementary parts. In Part I, "Who Do You Think You Are?" I reflect upon the lessons learned about human behavior from our experiment in mass-market materialism. I begin by investigating the growing challenge of obesity as an example of the mismatch that I have just outlined. Using the epidemic as a case history, I explore how, over time, many elements— biological, behavioral, economic, and cultural—have conspired to create this public scourge that is now driving us off balance, both physically and economically. As a physician with expertise in emo- tional and social behavior, and with knowledge of the part such factors play in the development of disease and disability, I illustrate how the personal stressors engendered by a demand-driven consumer culture play upon normal physiology, fostering self-destructive habits that are hard to break. How such habits are formed in the brain and how the neuroscience of habit brings insight to understanding our intuitive thought is the focus of Chapter 2.

Self-interest is the engine of the consumer society, but it is habit and our fascination with novelty that sustains it. To fathom how this came to be, I reach back, in Chapter 3, to the Scottish Enlightenment and to the Age of Reason, a time of insatiable curiosity that gave birth to the Industrial Revolution and provided the philosophical foundation for Western society today. Not surprisingly it was an era that had great respect for science and the manufacturing trades. It is there—in the debates of over two centuries ago—that we unearth the origins of the "rational" self, a concept that has been of seminal importance in the creation of the Western democracies and the cap- italist enterprise. My particular focus will be on the work of Adam

Smith, not only his concept of the free-market society as a balanced self-regulating economic order but also his writings on moral development, an inquiry that offers profound insights regarding today's social challenges, and their potential resolution.

This brings me to how the brain makes choices. I outline from the perspective of behavioral neuroscience how the fundamental free-market operating "principles" of reward, punishment, and the evaluation of risk are reflected in the information-processing mechanisms of the brain. It is through such brain mechanisms that we perceive the world, arrive at decisions, and take action, learning from the results of those actions to refine future behavior. This activity mirrors what is essentially the brain's own "internal market," seeking to find balance through continuous interaction with a complex, ever-changing world. So I ask, is it this proclivity of the brain that makes the give-and-take of the external marketplace so universally compelling? Is this why barter is ubiquitous in human society, from the merchant colonies of Anatolia thirty-five hundred years ago to the globalized megacompanies of today?

In closing Part I, I investigate this possibility and offer another case history—this time comparing the collapse of the competitive Bronze Age empires of the Mediterranean to the cultural circumstances in the United States that led up to, and followed, the global financial meltdown of 2008. How may we understand the behaviors that led to such apparently precipitous self-destruction? I argue that in both instances clues may be found through an understanding of how the brain's internal market is distorted by myopic preoccupation with the short term and by an obsession with continuous growth. In our contemporary experience, I conclude that the 2008 financial crisis, the obesity epidemic and environmental degradation have *a common behavioral root* that is fed by the enticements of affluence, degrading the brain's capacity for self-regulation.

Material achievements, it appears, are just one ingredient of the "happiness" prescription. In America, and generally in the world's rich nations, we have reached a point in our postindustrial experiment where intelligent reflection upon what constitutes human progress is desirable, even imperative. We have discovered that affluence, like poverty, has the power to throw the biology of human behavior off balance, potentially fostering a cultural amnesia that damages character development, encourages self-destructive habits, and fosters neglect of the sustaining environment.

Starting from this premise, Part II of the book, "How to Live?," again poses fundamental questions but goes beyond diagnostic analysis to outline our strengths in constructing a way forward. How may we bridle our short-term instinctual cravings to better focus on long-term environmental and personal challenges? How, in society, can we foster the habits of character in the young that will intuitively guide them to independent choice and self-discipline, which will help them navigate a seductive, debt-fueled consumer culture? In the helter-skelter of modern life, what knowledge about ourselves have we forgotten that we need to learn once more? How may we reinvest in the social skills that served us so well in the past? In sum, how should we live in this *Age of Man*?

The barriers to intelligent reflection are many. Present-day commerce is built on the principle that for the individual having more is better, simply because for most of human existence we lived in scarcity. But now, in the rich countries and in the emerging economies, that circumstance is shifting. For the first time in human history many in Western society are grappling with how to live under an avalanche of information, of material goods, of food, indeed with a surfeit of everything but time. Rather than scarcity we now confront abundance, although for many, including many living in the United States, it is an abundance increasingly poorly distributed.

Social and economic progress are disconnecting from each other. It is the paradox of modernity that as market choice and material prosperity have increased, health, educational achievement, and personal satisfaction have reached a plateau. The compelling Enlightenment vision that science and reason would bring happiness and steady social progress is now tarnished. In America, despite extraordinary economic growth, the quality of everyday life has stagnated for the average citizen while the disparity in wealth between the rich and the poor has grown exponentially. The founding narrative of America as a land of equal opportunity is fading.

Also damaging to the social fabric is that in consumer society intuitive acts of essential human caring—activities that give pleasure to the self and bring happiness to others—have been increasingly removed from their source and placed within the marketplace: the rearing of children, the care of the elderly, and the preparing of a family meal being just three simple examples. Such behaviors co-opted into the gross domestic product are now considered measures of growing economic wealth. In reality, however, such metrics reflect not new wealth but the conversion of natural human caring into commodities and relationships into services. We now pay for things that we once did for each other out of love or gratitude, thus removing not only an important source of personal happiness but also weakening the warp and weft of the social fabric essential to a balanced social order.

It is challenges such as these, lurking in the shadows of our success, that I investigate in Part II of *The Well-Tuned Brain*. In a series of chapters harnessing what we know about ourselves from common sense and the behavioral neurosciences, I explore the development of healthy behaviors that nourish our social order and personal growth—why and how they are essential to the education of our children, to a vibrant habitat, to the food we eat, to the creative process, and to sustaining a human-friendly planet ecology. As will become clear, it is when these elements are knit together in harmony to support individual opportunity, well-being, empathy, and personal responsibility that the social and ecological fabric thrives. It is a reminder that human progress flows primarily not from simply amassing material wealth but from self-awareness and from the wise use of our achievements and our resources to the benefit of ourselves, of others, of future generations, and of the planet.

FINALLY, IN CLOSING this introduction, a word about my title, *The Well-Tuned Brain*. It is a play on Johann Sebastian Bach's collection of keyboard music entitled *The Well-Tempered Clavier*. In 1722, when he was thirty-seven years old, Bach applied for the prestigious position of cantor to the Thomaskirche in Leipzig, a post that he was to hold for twenty-seven years, until his death in 1750. Among the cantor's responsibilities was the teaching of music to a gaggle of students, and *The Well-Tempered Clavier* is essentially the textbook that Bach assembled to fulfill that duty. A collection of preludes and fugues in all the possible keys, Bach described his compositions on the title page as "for the profit and use of musical youth desirous of learning, and especially for the pastime of those already skilled in this study."

So what is the meaning of "well-tempered?" *To temper*, the verb, is "to moderate, to blend, to free from excess," and "to adjust according to need"—in today's language, "to tune." Thus to be well-tempered is to find optimum balance, as in tuning the strings of a keyboard instrument to achieve harmony across the different keys. That may seem of little consequence when considering the modern family piano, which gets tuned once a year to what is called *equal temperament*, where it is arranged that all the notes of the keyboard are the same distance apart in pitch. But as the ancient Greek mathematician Pythagoras determined long ago, this is a contrivance, for in reality the intervals between the notes of the musical scale do not perfectly add up: nature's math is different. Start with the note C on a stringed instrument and progress through the octave, and when you get to the next C, the note has overshot. It sounds out of tune.

This was a big problem in Bach's time, for the clavier—the early harpsichord—was notoriously "temperamental" and in constant need of adjustment. A change in room temperature, or the shifting humidity provoked by a passing rain, would perturb the instrument's delicate balance. To achieve fine performance, the musician and the keyboard are as one: each depends on the other. Thus Bach, in his consummate skill, taught not only the art of expression at the keyboard but also the care and tuning of the harpsichord as an instrument to be respected and loved for its subtle sensitivity. Equal temperament was recognized as a practical tuning method, but it wasn't standard practice. Many musicians of the time preferred tuning to *irregular temperament*, where the intervals between the notes of the octave were tweaked to personal preference, and the instrument could be played in all keys without the necessity of retuning. Bach was in this camp, devoted to the flexibility and sensitivity of his keyboard instruments. That's what his workbook *The Well-Tempered Clavier* is about.

It is a story that offers only a crude analogy when thinking about the interactive sensitivity of the human brain and the subtle beauty of mind, but nonetheless I find it useful and compelling. Just how Bach made the adjustments to "well temper" his clavier is a subject upon which experts continue to disagree, but the writings of his contemporaries suggest it took him little more than fifteen minutes. Here my analogy with the brain stumbles badly, of course. For each of us the care and tuning of the brain—and an understanding of the "music" that is the mind at work—is the commitment of a lifetime, by necessity. As we shall find, when it comes to the human brain, the quick fix, analogous to tuning the family piano to equal temperament, does not serve. Tuning the brain demands knowledge, attention, and hard work. However, there's no investment more worthwhile: striving to be in tune with one's self simultaneously makes common sense and serves the common good. The nurturing of the well-tuned brain offers harmony and hope—to each of us as individuals and to our collective enterprise.

Part I
PROLOGUE

Who Do You Think You Are?

SEARCHING FOR TRUTH about one's self is a perennial human quest. The Greeks found it compelling but challenging. Similarly, Benjamin Franklin, reflecting upon life in his *Poor Richard's Almanack*, considered three things extremely hard, "steel, a diamond and to know one's self." Today in the hope of probing this puzzle further, once the exclusive study of theologians and philosophers, we have conscripted the neuroscientist, the geneticist, the engineer, and the nanotechnologist.

We have turned now toward understanding the self through knowledge of the brain. We are at the point where we can map the living brain, where we can see in real time how those who suffer with depression, Alzheimer's disease, or autism have different brain activity patterns than those of the "normal" brain. We can define the major networks of the brain and copy them using computer-based simulation. Stem cells aided by synthetic scaffolding may soon heal damaged brains and help nerve networks rewire. Neural engineers are designing robotic systems that can operate at the interface of the mind and the machine. All this is amazing. This is science.

But there is another, equally important challenge for science in understanding the behavior of the brain and the self. It is a task more intimately connected with our daily lives and with securing our future. We need to better grasp why and how the mass consumer society, in its abundance, plays on certain hardwired evolutionary drives to remold the brain's neural pathways, guide our choices, and shape our habits, compelling the unwary toward addictive self-gratification. We have discovered that a state of plenty can have unintended consequences. It is the paradox of our times.

Chapter 1

Off Balance:
Surprised by Affluence

> Man with all his noble qualities . . .
> Still bears in his bodily frame the indelible stamp of his
> lowly origin.
>
> Charles Darwin, *The Descent of Man* (1871)

WHEN THIS BOOK was in its infancy, I spent a year working with colleagues at the University of Oxford. We found lodging in Woodstock, a small village just a few miles outside Oxford, where the pastoral landscape is dominated by Blenheim Palace, the large country estate that is the home of the Churchill family. It was there in the early spring that I met Henry, a pheasant who had become a local celebrity.

It's no fun being a pheasant on an English country estate. This was particularly true that year. The winter had been long and hard, the earth was ice- and snow-covered, and the game hunters had taken their toll. On some days three or four hundred brace of birds had fallen to the hunters and their dogs. But not Henry, as he had been fondly named: this rooster was no gullible youngster. Henry was shrewd, with long and shiny leg spurs, suggesting that he was tough and canny enough to have endured a year or two despite the harsh conditions. And he was a handsome fellow, with his copper-colored plumage shining mottled and iridescent in the sunlight; his feathered helmet shimmered a forest green. In his strutting walk and regal bearing, he had the mark of a warrior. This bird was a survivor.

Then that spring came his downfall: Henry fell unexpectedly into affluence. His preferred hangout was a pasture by the lake, close to the neck of an old dam where the water cascaded into the river below. Over the winter the dam had been repaired, and new drainage fields had been built to better control the flow of water during the spring runoff. Late in the project, after the backhoes and trucks had disappeared, the groundskeepers reseeded the meadow. By early March all was complete. As the sun strengthened, daffodils thrust up their heads along the riverbank, the new-sown grass and clover germinated, and the worms and insects multiplied. For a pheasant recovering from a winter of privation, it was a banquet like no other.

When it comes to survival, game pheasants are no dumb birds. They run fast and fly low, and their staccato alarm ensures that most will take cover before you've even seen them. They're cautious in their habits, feeding early in the morning and again late in the afternoon, as the sun begins to wane. During the heat of the day most pheasants retreat to what the hunter calls "loafing" cover—light brush or tall grass that affords protection from predators and a little time for relaxation. Henry, however, in his delight at having discovered nirvana, began to ignore these survival principles. He commandeered the wealth of the newly sown field as his private preserve. There he was to be found each day, even at noon, fully exposed, head down, feeding away. Never was Henry seen to run; rather he strutted with head held high, wattles bobbing red against his purple throat.

Henry grew and grew; no longer sleek but of Pickwickian proportion, he gained notoriety as the largest pheasant many had ever seen. Visitors gathered to watch him feed. He began to rival the water cascade as an attraction to the park. Little boys threw pebbles to provoke him: he hardly noticed, intent on his self-indulgence. No screaming sprint into the thicket for Henry. It was as if he had written those signs around the reseeded field to warn away competitors, "Newly planted area; please keep off." With a long winter behind him and the human predators at bay, Henry had become complacent, addicted to his personal preserve and the affluent life. "He's lost his common sense, has that there bird," advised a local countryman one afternoon as we stood together among a clutch of gawping visitors. "If he don't kill himself, then the fox he will." He was right. Toward the middle of April Henry disappeared. Only a few days later, walking on the hill that overlooks the lake, I found a bloodied carcass and a fine set of wings. It was what was left of Henry; those long shiny spurs were unmistakable.

THE SAGA OF HENRY—how the noble pheasant fell into affluence and lost his common sense—has the makings of a fine fable, one worthy of inclusion in Rudyard Kipling's *Just So Stories*. But also, as do many fables, it offers a cautionary tale. The growing epidemic of obesity across the world, a challenge particularly evident in the United States, suggests that when faced with abundance, we humans may share Henry's insatiable appetite.

So did simple gluttony kill Henry? I think not: rather, Henry had been *surprised* by affluence. At the center of his undoing was a calamitous mismatch between his instinctual drive to take advantage of the moment and the novel, unparalleled plenitude of the seeded meadow. Thrown off-balance by unprecedented opportunity, Henry neglected his long-term self-preservation: here was a bird literally too fat to fly.

On a human scale, a similar challenge is evident today for those living in America and the world's other prosperous nations. We too have been surprised by affluence. Seduced by a compelling, resource-rich culture—one engineered by our own material success to offer a paralyzing plethora of everything desirable—we are on a collision course with our own biology, myopic to the long-term consequences of our immediate behavior. Our growing obesity is just the most obvious marker of a cascade of health problems that have been triggered by the mismatch between our evolved biology and the behavioral challenges of living in a rapidly changing, competitive, commercial culture. It is no accident that type 2 diabetes, vascular disease, anxiety, and depression are found clustered together in their prevalence and distribution with obesity, for they are all unintended consequences of a high-stress society. These predominantly metabolic ills are "ailments of affluence," or more specifically ailments suffered by those among us in the affluent society who, for a variety of reasons, find themselves insecure and continuously challenged.

Affluence—defined as an abundance of choice at ever-decreasing cost—has a seductive potential that is pervasive. When exposed to the pleasurable stimuli and repetitive rewards of today's consumer culture, we are prone to excessive behaviors and addictive habits in many spheres of daily activity. We have come to accept that an "addict" can become habituated to cocaine, heroin, or alcohol just as Henry became "addicted" to the pleasures of his meadow. But what is less understood is that the same neural architecture that in a "normal" person promotes habituation to the double cheeseburger also promotes habituation to credit-card shopping, video games, smartphones, electronic social networks, Internet surfing, stock-option gambling, pornography, and the countless other novel "pleasures" that an affluent society has on offer. In such a world of affluent choice, where the choices play directly to our instinctual drive for pleasure and reward, self-control has become hard to exert and sustain.

The capacity for self-restraint is further eroded by a market culture that not only reinforces such acquisitive behaviors but also has become economically dependent upon them. With the globalization of trade the accepted model of human progress has become one of continuous material growth. Increasingly, commercial success is measured not by the quality but by the *quantity* of product sold. Hence the rich world economies are now focused by necessity upon inducing and encouraging addictionlike behaviors—in America consumer spending accounts for some 70 percent of economic activity. The *amount* we consume has become a measure of a nation's vitality. In today's society the twin drivers of commercial growth are the merchant's discovery that when faced with material abundance the human brain does not effectively self-regulate desire and the classical economist's delusional insistence that it does. As portrayed in the media, this is the American Dream—a world of choice, material abundance, excitement, energy, and self-actualization. But as I shall explore in this introductory chapter, using obesity in America as my illustration, it is also a world where a mismatch of physiological and cultural factors promote insecurity, harmful habits, and the ill health of stress-driven metabolic disorganization.

AMERICANS, WHILE LEADING the world in material wealth, living standards, freedom of choice, and extraordinary technological development, also have the dubious distinction of being among the fattest people on earth. In 2008 the Centers for Disease Control estimated that 68 percent of the U.S. population was overweight and within that group some 33 percent were considered to be obese as measured by a body-mass index (BMI) above 30. To give some perspective, the U.S. statistics for obesity are ten times the rate reported for Japan. Such excessive weight gain reflects physiology out of balance, not only predisposing millions of Americans to type 2 diabetes, cardiovascular disease, and the tragedy of chronic illness but also exposing the nation to a massive public health and economic burden.

Careful analysis suggests that Americans have been slowly gaining weight for several decades, but there's no doubt that beginning sometime in the 1980s the curve began to rise exponentially. This time scale corresponds with a shift in our dietary habits away from home-cooked meals to an increased consumption of preprocessed and energy-dense foods that contain high levels of refined sugar and saturated fats and, most importantly, are readily available, tasty, and cheap.

So why, we must ask, do we find ourselves in this fix? After all, among all the creatures of the earth, are we not the wise ones? Not only are we sentient in thinking, choosing, and acting, but we also take pride in learning from experience. In America we tend to think of obesity as a personal issue. So why, as intelligent creatures, do we behave insatiably in the face of newfound abundance, much as Henry did in the newly sown meadow? What *did* happen to self-restraint: why can't we just say no and keep our eating habits under control?

Unfortunately, as a growing number of citizens have become painfully aware, maintaining a healthy body weight in America today—for reasons that range from the genetic and physiological to the interpersonal and cultural—is just not that easy.

Obesity is now America's number-one problem in public health. To understand its roots a good place to start is with our species's evolutionary history. Simply stated, for the human animal to live with an abundance of cheap, tasty food is a unique experience. In harmony with Henry the fabled pheasant, both metabolically and by instinct, we human beings are designed for survival during times of scarcity rather than times of plenty.

Physiologically the equation underlying weight gain is straightforward: it is the direct result of the body storing excess energy when, over time, the calories available from the food we consume become greater than those required to meet metabolic need. Multiple genes are involved in balancing the energy requirements of the body, and these not only interact with one another but also are responsive to changing environmental conditions. It's an experience familiar to each of us: think of those extra pounds acquired from Thanksgiving and other winter feasts. But for our forebears who struggled repeatedly with inconsistent food supplies, this capacity to store energy supplies through weight gain was a major asset. During periods of famine such conservation could quickly become a life-saving adaptation. Hence people of African or indigenous South American descent have developed a greater metabolic facility to conserve and store energy than have those of European ancestry, where the early adoption of agriculture gave greater stability to the food supply and an opportunity for the genome to adapt accordingly. The body's metabolic programming, however, does not shift easily. Thus when individuals—particularly those with a metabolic propensity to conserve calories—consistently consume a high-calorie diet, and especially when combined with a sedentary lifestyle, significant weight gain and obesity are commonplace and a threat to long-term health.

A celebrated, well-studied example of this interaction between genes and environment is the profound obesity that has emerged in the Pima Indians of Arizona with exposure to an energy-dense "Western" diet. In their ancestral habitat these genetically homogeneous "river people" of Native American migrant heritage survived through hunting, fishing, and subsistence farming. Physiologically and culturally they were well adapted to periods of famine. In the late nineteenth century, however, when American settlers homesteading upstream diverted the Pima people's water supply, the Pima traditions of two thousand years were profoundly disrupted, with accompanying widespread starvation. Within a few short decades the replacement diet provided to these river people by the U.S. government—with its principal ingredients of animal fat, processed sugar, and white flour—coupled with the development of a culturally alien, sedentary lifestyle induced not only weight gain but also type 2 diabetes, which today afflicts some 32 percent of the population.

The plight of the Arizona Pima is in stark contrast to a community of comparable genetic inheritance located several hundred miles south, in the Sierra Madre Mountains of Mexico. Here where the Pima people have preserved their ancestral traditions—including a diet of maize and squash supplemented with small game and fish—the inhabitants of the community have remained of normal weight with a low prevalence of diabetes.

While the Pima experience is in many ways unique, it serves to highlight how the rapid development of an environmental-metabolic mismatch can have powerful and significant consequences. With a sudden shift in culture and diet, a biology that evolved to conserve calories and prevent weight loss under conditions of privation will not only prove ineffective in stabilizing metabolism but will promote pathological weight gain when the calories consumed consistently outpace those expended.

Our instinctual behavior presents similar complications in adapting to affluence. In the course of our evolution not only the genetic control of metabolism but also our instincts have been programmed for scarcity. In an impoverished world the consistent message is to gather and consume whatever is available whenever it's available, for such opportunity may not return. But as I shall explore later, the brain that guides us each day is a jerry-rigged organ of expedience, one that relies for its core operations on a collection of mechanisms that evolved long ago. In the face of affluence this presents a problem. The process of evolution is essentially conservative, sorting through alternative models of adaptation to select the optimum environmental fit for success and survival. Those adaptive mechanisms that have proven valuable are retained from one generation to the next and also across species. Thus when it comes to instinctual behavior, a little of Henry's brain machinery still lurks within each of us.

In the instinctual game of survival, pain and pleasure are the red and green lights that shape our behavior and guide the brain's adaptive strategy. Fear and pain warn of the threat of harm and induce retreat, while pleasure is the reward for success, promoting curiosity and continued exploration. In our evolutionary experience, pain was commonplace and reward hard-won. In foraging for something to eat, self-restraint was rarely required. Our ancestral home in the sub-Sahara yielded little, and what little there was others wanted too. Thus it was privation and competition that controlled our energy intake. When good fortune surprised us—when we stumbled across the abundance of a tree in fruit, or the remains of a large kill—it was etched in the brain's emotional memory, and that excitement seeded the desire to repeat the experience. But such joyous moments were few and transient at best. In self-interest it was essential to take immediate advantage of any opportunity presenting itself. Thus the dopamine-driven, pleasure-generating systems of reward were tuned to the short term: when you were successful in the hunt, you gobbled as fast as you could and hoarded the rest, preferably before some rival appeared to contest the prize.

In today's affluent world, it's a different story. In the last decades of the twentieth century low-cost preprocessed food delivering goodies high in salt and fat, together with soft drinks laced with caffeine and corn syrup, became readily available in America and other rich nations. Such affluence makes us vulnerable. This shift to a cheap, convenient, novel, and high-calorie diet has been difficult to resist. In each of us, rational choice is distorted by novelty and immediate opportunity. So when tempted by such tasty goodies, the brain's ancient reward hardware becomes quickly engaged and dominant, sometimes even to be hijacked into an addictive spiral. When we respond repeatedly to such temptation, then metabolic conservation of the extra calories follows, and weight gain is not far behind. Compounding the situation is that in the short run there is no physiological penalty for such behavior, only reward. So today as in ancient times, when the blood-sugar level drops, threatening the brain's energy supply, the alarm bells ring—we feel faint and hungry; but excessive calorie intake carries no subjective warning, just the feeling of a full belly. It is not like filling the car at the gas pump: there is no physiological shut-off valve for calories. Thus as obesity emerges, high blood-sugar levels, which accompany weight gain and are the harbinger of diabetes, sometimes go undetected for years.

To summarize, today in America, when it comes to what we eat, the opportunities available have shifted dramatically, but our instinctual behavior has not evolved. As a matter of rational choice we may be committed to maintaining a reasonable body weight, but when we are "surprised" by the convenience of fast food, that rational commitment is overwhelmed by the ancient brain's preference for immediate reward. A sedentary lifestyle and reduced physical labor, which accompanies rapid technological advance, complicates the picture. Economic stagnation, especially among growing numbers of middle-class families, further compounds this double jeopardy, driving people toward obtaining the most calories at the lowest cost. In inner-city neighborhoods, where a lack of healthy food choice is commonplace, this third factor, in confluence with the other two, has made obesity in America an illness of the poor rather than of the rich. This is in contrast to past experience, when those most commonly obese were the wealthy and the privileged, in demonstration of their status and special access to food.

BUT PREDISPOSING GENES, ancient cravings, and the opportunities of affluence are only part of this complex story. Although significant in their contribution, these factors alone are an insufficient explanation for America's leadership in the world's obesity tables. While the United States has within its diverse migrant population a significant number of persons of African descent and also many from South America with an ethnically mixed Native American heritage—both populations that are genetically predisposed to calorie conservation and thus predisposed to obesity—individuals of Caucasian, European origin, especially males, also have become significantly overweight. Thus the prevalence of obesity reported in men, as measured by BMI between 1999 and 2010, was 36.2 percent for Caucasian males, 38.8 percent for African-American males, and 37.0 percent for those of Hispanic background, suggesting that in addition to genetics there is a common cultural driver influencing all groups.

Highlighting that cultural factors may be important in promoting obesity are the statistics that although mean body weight increased across most affluent societies in the closing decades of the twentieth century, this rise was not uniform; nor was it correlated with a nation's per capita income. Despite the deep penetration of American-style fast food across the world—evidenced by *The Economist* magazine's use of the price of a McDonald's Big Mac as a comparative index of purchasing power among different countries—when it comes to weight gain in most surveys, it is a cluster of wealthy, English-speaking nations that leads the pack, with America at its head. At the turn of the twenty-first century, the prevalence of obesity in this group—the United States, Britain, Australia, New Zealand, and Canada—was greater than for other rich countries, including many in Scandinavia and several in Europe with comparable per capita incomes.

So what distinguishes these Anglophone nations? One possibility is market philosophy. My colleague Avner Offer, the Emeritus Chichele Professor in Economic History at the University of Oxford, has made this suggestion. Offer noticed in the course of his research on obesity that its exponential increase worldwide corresponded in time not only with the growing promotion of high-calorie preprocessed foods but also with the rapid rise of globalized, deregulated market systems, of which, in the 1980s, the United States and other English-speaking countries had been early and enthusiastic proponents. Together with his Oxford colleagues Rachel Pechey and Stanley Ulijaszek, Avner subsequently conducted a careful analysis of ninety-six surveys measuring body weight, across eleven countries, between 1994 and 2004. The investigation indicated a positive correlation between obesity and the cluster of liberal "Anglo-American" economies when compared to nations with a similar gross domestic product per capita but with a narrower spread of income distribution and a stronger social infrastructure.

Evidence from the American experience provides potential support for this hypothesis. Lengthened work hours, increased competition, and greater financial insecurity—frequently associated with liberal economies—may be inducing pervasive *metabolic stress*, which then becomes a mediating factor in promoting weight gain. Americans work longer hours and take shorter vacations than do their European counterparts. Furthermore, in today's technology-driven society, many of the physical factors that once limited the workday have fallen away. The convenience of the Internet, instantaneous electronic communication, and a revolution in transportation mean that time and distance are no longer barriers to globalized commercial activity. The growth-focused economy fosters a demand-driven "fast new world" that never rests, one where the twenty-four-hour clock increasingly dictates our working life, crowding out family, physical activity, leisure time, and sleep.

So what is metabolic stress? The fundamental biology of the stress response—the coordinated brain-body reaction to uncertainty and threat—is a vital mechanism of adaptation that we share with our evolutionary forebears, just as we share the brain systems of reward. It's another tried-and-true mechanism inherited from our ancestral past. Once triggered, the human reaction is little different from that of the young pheasant when the hawk's shadow falls over the nest. But we are not pheasants. What is different, given our intelligence and capacity for learning, planning, and imagination, is that we perceive stress in ways that are unique to our experience—to the specific social context in which we live, and have lived in the past, and to our individual perception of how much control we have over what's happening to us. *A subjective sense of control is of primary importance to the human mind.* Thus highly competitive work environments—where time pressure is pervasive and repeated confrontations are the norm—are commonly experienced as profoundly stressful. This is especially true for those in subordinate roles, who frequently lack a sense of personal control in the workplace.

Chronic stress takes a toll. Physiologically the stress response is designed to defend us in *acute emergency* when the brain, through activation of the autonomic nervous system, places the body on instant alert. We all have experienced the tingling sensation that runs down the back of the neck when we are surprised. Next the heart beats a little faster and the blood pressure rises: the adrenal glands flood epinephrine into the bloodstream, and subjectively we feel a sense of increased awareness and tension, even anxiety. Secondary systems of bodily defense—the endocrine and the immune systems—are similarly activated to prepare the body for possible trauma in the fight ahead. But, and this is critically important, *in their evolution each of these systems has been tuned to shut down quickly once the danger has passed.* They are not designed to be constantly active and on guard. When called upon to be so, they slowly destabilize the body's vital balance increasing our vulnerability to inflammation and illness.

As a young physician, when I was on call around the clock for seven days a week, it was considered an aberration. But in today's global world—with many yoked electronically to their work 24/7—such exhausting schedules are widespread and frequently accepted as the norm. Faced with serial deadlines, the brain's alarm bells ring repeatedly, and the stress response is continuously in play. In response the immune system, now chronically activated, floods the body with *cytokines*, which are important signaling molecules. When cytokines are produced in excess, they can increase vulnerability to chronic metabolic illness, which includes obesity.

Cytokines are small protein molecules, similar to hormones, that play a role in the metabolism of fat cells; in the obese person they are actively produced by the accumulated fat, stimulating other inflammation in the body. Thus cytokines fall under suspicion as potential mediators between stress and obesity. Indeed, obesity may be considered a deranged metabolic state of overnutrition, which generates its own inflammatory process, helping throw the body's homeostatic mechanisms—its metabolic gyroscope—off balance. Once this vicious cycle is set in place, and the brain-body tuning is lost, the task of reversing the spiral becomes infinitely more difficult, as any overweight person knows only too well.

Those most affected by chronic work stress in America—and among whom obesity is prevalent—are the skilled and semiskilled members of the middle class, both men and women, who toil long hours with marginal financial security, often to the neglect of their families and their own health. Since the 1980s the average American worker has assumed increasing financial risk. Swings in annual income have become greater, and the minimum wage in constant dollars has declined, as has job tenure and those receiving employment-based health insurance. Social inequality—another index of stress and insecurity—is also growing in America, with this same middle-class group being left behind. Since the 1980s the median family income in the United States has been essentially flat, with a growing disparity between the haves and the have-nots. As was reported by the Congressional Budget Office in 2011, the top 1 percent of earners have more than doubled their share of the national wealth since 1980. In parallel, boosted by the recession that followed the financial crisis of 2008, unemployment escalated. Thus for many middle-class citizens workplace competition increased while job security decreased, engendering a rising level of metabolic stress that is frequently expressed as anxiety and weight gain.

Adding further to this stress-driven metabolic burden is a lack of sleep. Most Americans report stealing one to two hours from their natural sleep time every working night, catching up on weekends, which only feeds into the cycle of inflammation and chronic stress. Large population surveys—one including more than a million participants—find a high correlation between less than seven hours of sleep and an increased body-mass index. While it is tempting to consider sleep as merely a suspension of daily activity, in fact it plays a vital restorative function in knitting up the "ravell'd sleeve of care," as Shakespeare poetically described it. And yet in departure from such understanding many Americans now accept a short night's sleep as a necessary evil.

It is a harmful practice. Laboratory evidence is accumulating that sleep loss further feeds the body's pro-inflammatory cytokine response—just as does loss of control and chronic stress—inducing a threefold increase in the genetic messengers that initiate the manufacture of cytokines. Even a period of sleep deprivation as short as one hour can have a significant impact on inflammatory cytokine production and the hormonal regulation of appetite, which helps explain why after disrupted sleep one can awaken hungry with the feeling that a cold is in the offing. In one study of healthy, normal-weight young men, sleep reduction was associated with striking alterations in the body's metabolic functions. In health there is a daily rhythm of hormone production that is synchronized with the cycle of sleep and wakefulness. In the young men deprived of sleep, however, this rhythm was flattened, and the stress hormones such as cortisol were elevated, suggesting a disturbed tuning of the feedback mechanisms that communicate between the body and the brain. The metabolism of sugars was also impaired in these young men. Glucose clearance from the blood following a glucose challenge test was 40 percent slower when the subjects were in a sleep-deprived state than when they were fully rested, a change similar to that found in normal aging and in people during the early stages of diabetes.

Subsequently, the same team of laboratory-based investigators studied the daytime blood profiles of the appetite-controlling hormones *leptin* and *ghrelin*, together with subjective ratings of hunger and food preference. The men in the study were restricted to four hours of sleep for two days and then allowed a "catch-up" sleep of ten hours to simulate real-world working conditions. The sleep restriction time, when compared to the catch-up recovery period, was associated with an 18 percent *reduction in the appetite-suppressing hormone leptin* and a 28 percent *increase in the appetite-enhancing hormone ghrelin*. Interestingly, the young men also reported a 24 percent increase in hunger and a similar increase in appetite, especially for calorie-dense foods with high carbohydrate content. This suggests that the anecdotal reports of increased craving for fast food when sleep deprived—I have experienced it myself after a night on emergency call—may have a metabolic basis. And perhaps even more important in considering the role that the stress of sleep deprivation plays in the genesis of obesity is the finding that the vital balance between the appetite hormones

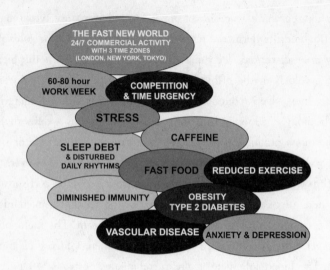

Figure 1.1: A cascade of health consequences: Obesity is the most visible of a cascade of health consequences that flow from the stress-inducing, demand-driven, and time-urgent economic environment that is the consumer society.

ghrelin and leptin becomes persistently impaired in those with chronic insomnia.

These studies highlight the second important insight to be drawn from the obesity story. *We must conclude that obesity is merely the most visible of a cascade of health consequences that flow from the stress-inducing, demand-driven, and time-urgent economic environment that we have created for ourselves.* In tying together the threads of evidence that I have identified, and that I illustrate in Figure 1.1, it becomes clear that the antecedents of America's obesity epidemic and its associated disabilities are best understood as an interconnected whole, one within which evolutionary, biological, *and* cultural elements are interwoven. From the standpoint of public health planning, this is of critical importance. Physiologically, these stress-induced disabilities reflect a dangerous disruption of the homeostatic equilibrium—of the bodily harmony—essential to healthy living. Thus America's obesity pandemic is a warning. Of the health problems plaguing America, many are driven by the choices we make and the maladaptive behaviors that follow. Would we not do well, therefore, to revisit our choice of consumer-driven economic growth and a workplace strategy that demands 24/7 allegiance?

It seems logical enough. So why then do we continue to fall victim to self-harm? I believe the answer lies in the profound cultural shift we have experienced. Under the rubric of progress, we have been discarding, for several generations, the social mores that encourage economic responsibility and self-control in favor of the instant gratification offered by consumerism. Our addictive pursuit has eroded prudent habits and the capacity for objective choice. Of even greater impact, however, is that in our myopia we are neglecting the social institutions that teach such skills to future generations. For families that rarely meet face to face except perhaps in the car, that never eat together around a table, and where the parents both work outside the home, grabbing food on the go, the pattern of life is hardly one well lived and certainly one unlikely to instill the capacity for self-restraint in children. In a culture of excess—where compulsively getting and spending is the norm and where almost the only choices people make are over what items to consume—the opportunity for instant gratification will quickly defeat any conscious effort for self-constraint, be that in appetite, emotion, or impulse.

Thus if we desire to thrive in the novel, light-speed culture that we have created—one that is rapidly running ahead of our capacity to sustain biological, ecological, and economic fitness—we must employ our intelligence, not as a slave to the fulfillment of short-term desire, but as a thoughtful, creative force in the design of social systems that have the capacity to integrate our passions and our rational purpose for longer-term sustainability. This will be particularly important as the digital age continues to unfold and the technologies delivering the addictive novelties—the "electronic cocaine"—of this coming revolution are perfected. We must give ourselves time to think and to understand who we are, for we have much to learn about ourselves from our experiment in mass-market materialism.

Ideally we must return to the time-honored Delphic maxim "know thyself," not in the interest of some abstract philosophy but rather in the practical terms of understanding our propensity for novelty and myopic craving. To do so will inform the choices that we make—both intuitively and consciously—as we grapple with the opportunities and pitfalls of the technology-rich, market-driven culture that now shapes our lives.

While America, together with the other rich English-speaking nations, has been the stalking horse in this growing health crisis, we are no longer alone in the world. As the "emerging" nations deregulate their markets, industrialize, and change their traditional diets, similar problems are becoming wide spread. The World Health Organization documented in a report published in 2000 that morbid obesity is now a global challenge imposing substantial economic burden and a growing threat to personal health not only for those living in the postindustrial nations but also for those in the quickly developing world, particularly the Middle East and China.

Inadvertently, the United States and the consumption-focused English-speaking nations have stumbled upon a new behavioral maxim: the better human society becomes at providing instant gratification, the less capable each individual citizen becomes at self-regulation. We are now visiting upon ourselves the circumstances that in simple form destroyed Henry. It is the very abundance of American society—we produce more, consume more, and throw away more than any other group of people on the planet—that nurtures our consumptive appetites. In America, and increasingly across the rest of the world, we are falling victim to enticements of our own making.

IN JANUARY 2012 new obesity statistics for America were released by the Centers for Disease Control in Atlanta and published in the *Journal of the American Medical Association*. They engendered some excitement. The report summarized data collected over a two-year period between 2009 and 2010 and compared them with those obtained a decade earlier; it suggested that the exponential growth of obesity was leveling off. Prevalence surveys among some six thousand adults and four thousand children indicated that although men had become marginally fatter over the decade—with the average body-mass index up from 27.7 to 28.7—for women it was unchanged at 28.5. While some 78 million people—approximately one in three adult Americans—remained obese, this slowing was comparatively good news, given that the nation's waistline had been expanding steadily for thirty years and exponentially for over ten.

The flattening statistics also suggested that America was slowly emerging from denial and beginning to face its problems. In 2008 the Centers for Disease Control had put the cost of obesity in America at $147 billion, from the escalating bill for the gasoline consumed in hauling around our more ample selves to the increased costs placed against the already overpriced and overburdened health care system. In America money talks, and it was becoming obvious regardless of the personal burden of obesity that as a nation we could no longer afford the self-indulgence of oversized dinner plates and an "all you can eat" culture.

Potential remedies proposed varied from top-down prohibition to bottom-up self-help technologies. The first lady, Michelle Obama, was pushing ahead with her school lunch program—the Healthy, Hunger-Free Kids Act of 2010—and growing vegetables on the White House lawn; Michael Bloomberg, then the mayor of New York City, in a bold gesture proposed a ban on the sale in public places of jumbo-sized sugar-laden soda pops; and a movement to ban soft-drink machines in schools had gained traction across the country. Similarly a report, after fast-food chains were required to post calorie counts, had helped Starbucks customers cut their consumption by 25 percent, suggesting a gentle tilt toward greater self-control, at least in the latte set.

At the other end of the scale, in a blending of technology and self-improvement, health-monitoring applications for the smartphone were rapidly gaining ground. One example, originating in San Francisco, was designed to track appetite, exercise, drinking habits, and sleep with the goal of using the database to "self-quantify" and shape future behavior. Collecting data to measure progress and to refine decision making has been standard practice in organizations for many years, of course, but electronic self-quantification is different. In addition to monitoring short-term behavior against long-term goals, it offers a technological fix in replacing capacities that we have lost, or may never have acquired, such as the mental control of appetite or alcohol consumption. Here a technology that was initially designed to extend human communication had metamorphosed into a prosthetic device.

Given the enormity of the task, however, such efforts represented little more than a Band-Aid for those Americans already struggling with obesity. The harsh reality is that in all probability such individuals will encounter significant ill health in their middle years and even a diminished life span. If over the long term the epidemic is to be curtailed, the focus needs to be on children and youth. Of particular concern in this regard was the evidence that for young Americans obesity was continuing to increase, especially in boys, where between infancy and nineteen years the prevalence of obesity rose from 14 percent in 2000 to 18.6 percent a decade later. In contrast, for girls the statistics remained relatively steady, rising from 13.8 percent to about 15 percent in 2010.

Unfortunately interventions designed to help adolescent children eat healthfully, in the hope of heading off adult diabetes, have had only marginal success and not only in America. A carefully matched yearlong study of an intensive program of nutrition and optional exercise for girls between twelve and fourteen years—implemented across twelve low-income school districts in New South Wales, Australia— failed to show any benefit. At the outset some four in ten children were bordering on obesity, with an average body weight of about 130 pounds. However, only 25 percent of the girls enrolled in the project chose to attend the lunchtime exercise classes, and only one in ten took advantage of the home-based physical activity or nutrition programs. Perhaps not surprisingly, by the end of the year weight gain in the experimental group was similar to that in the matched controls, with an average obesity rate of 33 percent for the school population in general.

The lessons from such studies are painful but valuable. First, changing established eating behavior is not easy because (as I shall explain in Chapter 2) we are creatures of habit: foods healthy or otherwise that we enjoyed as children are those that we continue to prefer later in life. This has long been known to the food industry, of course. That's what McDonald's Happy Meals are all about: giving young children exactly the tasty treats they want and exactly the high-calorie diet that they don't need. Burger King has a similar giveaway program, offering cardboard crowns for kids along with their burgers. Engaging the minds and stomachs of the young is a powerful commercial strategy because it works. While the public health concerns are clear, efforts to limit such marketing of junk food to children meet with fierce industry opposition and also as it happens from the children themselves, especially those who have grown up with the enticement of processed food.

In 2010 there was a student rebellion in the Los Angeles school district, which serves 650,000 meals each day, when healthful foods such as jambalaya, vegetable curry, lentils, and brown rice were substituted for the traditional fast-food fare of the school lunches. Participation plunged 13 percent, as thousands of students dropped out of the lunch program in favor of an underground market for chips, candy, and fast-food burgers. It is further evidence that changing nutrition standards in the face of a culture that is habituated, perhaps addicted, to fast food is difficult, particularly for those families in poorer districts where grocery stores are sparse and preprocessed food predominates.

By adolescence our eating patterns are set, so the second lesson is that in shaping eating preferences it's essential to start early. Contrast, therefore, the L.A. school lunch debacle with a program of *parent training* conducted, again in Los Angeles, by Wendy Slusser, a pediatrician at the Mattel Children's Hospital. This focused seven-week program for young low-income Latino mothers who had overweight children aged between two and four years blended nutrition, physical activity, and parenting advice. Delivered as an interactive and participatory exercise in a clinic setting, where the mothers learned from each other and then practiced their parenting skills at home, the results were highly successful. In stark contrast to the Australian program, a 9 percent reduction in weight was achieved for these younger children in the parent-training group. By comparison, in the matched group of children where the mothers were not counseled, the number becoming overweight and obese increased by 16 percent. This focus on healthy eating in infants and young children may now be paying off. While obesity rates in general in the United States were holding steady, in 2014 the Centers for Disease Control reported a 43 percent drop in the obesity rate among two-to-five-year olds, the first such decline in any group for a decade.

The Mattel study illustrates something that is obvious but easily forgotten: that in our development as unique individuals we are deeply conditioned in our habits through family, culture, education, markets, media, illusion, and much more. Not so obvious is that much of this social habituation is acquired intuitively—below the radar of conscious self-awareness—and that friendships beyond family also have a powerful influence in shaping our behavior. There is substantial evidence, for example, that obesity spreads among friends, much as does the contagion of the common cold. The most intriguing study in this regard comes from Framingham, Massachusetts, where a cadre of families (now a network of more than 12,000 persons) has been followed for over half a century. The project began in 1948 with a focus upon the natural history of cardiovascular disease: in 1971 the offspring of the original 5,000 individuals were inducted, and in 2002 the third-generation children were added to the study, making it one of the most comprehensive longitudinal health assessments in the United States.

In addition to behavioral and physical measures, including body-mass index, the Framingham study offers, over three decades, detailed information documenting the ebb and flow of the social relationships among neighbors, friends, and relatives. Employing this remarkable resource, in 2007 Nicholas Christakis of Harvard and James Fowler of the University of California, San Diego, published an analysis of the spread of obesity in the Framingham community between 1971 and 2003. This time frame is important because it maps almost perfectly onto the growth years of the obesity epidemic in America. The evidence confirms that the company we keep profoundly influences obesity: we learn our habits in the main from those we trust.

Clusters of obese individuals were evident in this densely interconnected social network of 12,067 people at the beginning of the study. The prevalence of obesity in the sample advanced, however, over the subsequent three decades, just as it had done in the nation as a whole. Strikingly, this growth was not random but was defined by the social bonds that held the clustered individuals together. Social ties, particularly those between intimate friends, were much more powerful in predicting the development of obesity than was geographic distance or even kinship. If an individual had a close friend who became obese, the chances that he or she would become similarly overweight increased by 57 percent. Among adult siblings, if one became obese, the chance that the other would follow suit increased by 40 percent, and for a spouse by 37 percent. Although many miles might separate siblings or intimate friends, the influence prevailed. In contrast, the effect was not seen among neighbors in the immediate geographic location who had no special relationship with one another.

Obesity, we may conclude, is contagious among friends. And indeed, subsequent analyses by Nicholas Christakis and colleagues using an infectious-disease model suggest that the spread of obesity through social networks has become a significant factor in sustaining the epidemic. Only 14 percent of the Framingham study participants were obese in 1971, but subsequently that number has risen in step with the rest of the country. "Our analysis suggests that while people have gotten better at gaining weight since 1971, they haven't gotten any better at losing weight," said Alison Hill, the lead researcher. An American adult has a 2 percent chance of becoming obese in any given year, a figure that has increased in recent decades. This number rises by 0.5 percent with each close friend who is obese. Thus having four overweight friends double one's chances of becoming similarly obese. While in today's American culture high stress levels, short sleep, easy access to unhealthy foods, and a lack of exercise continue to be major drivers in gaining weight, living in a tightly knit subculture where such behaviors are the accepted norm also significantly increases the risk of obesity. With two-thirds of the American population already over-weight, such subcultures are now ubiquitous. In our habits we subconsciously conform to the behaviors of those who influence our lives.

In the United States, where we are surrounded by an abundance of food, subtle environmental triggers further promote overeating and weight gain. Brian Wansink, a professor of consumer behavior at Cornell University, has shown that myriad cues powerfully influence and sustain our eating habits and how much we consume throughout the day. In his book *Mindless Eating*, Wansink concludes from a series of studies—conducted both in his laboratory and in homes, restaurants, and movie theaters, indeed wherever people eat—that not only "family and friends [but also] packages and plates, names and numbers, labels and lights, colors and candles, shapes and smells, distractions and distances, cupboards and containers" may profoundly sway appetites and consumption. Seemingly inconsequential factors—such as where we store food, whether it is easily accessible, or how foods are paired and served—can reflexively trigger behavioral habits and have a major influence on what and when we eat. And indeed, I see such idiosyncrasies in my own eating preferences: a cup of morning coffee triggers a powerful craving for doughnuts, and in a throwback to my childhood, I find Marmite a necessity when preparing scrambled eggs on toast.

MUCH OF WHAT WE DO each day is shaped by what we have done before. We call this habit—perseverate patterns of behavior that operate largely outside our conscious awareness. Wansink's studies, the Framingham analyses of friendship networks, and even the pleasures I find in doughnuts and Marmite—all are examples that reflect the brain's habit mechanisms at work. Habits are essential, as I noted in my introduction, for constructively and efficiently managing the activities of the day. But habits can become emotionally charged and maladaptive, especially when they reinforce short-term, instinctual striving. This is illustrated by the obesity scourge and by our response to the novel opportunities and material abundance of the affluent market society. The emotional reaction, rather than being one of pleasure, satisfaction, and contentment, is paradoxically to overconsume, imagining that to have more must be better.

I'm reminded of Cevantes's classical novel *Don Quixote de La Mancha*, written at a time when Spanish society was on the edge of economic chaos. Riding out from his village, Don Quixote seeks to find the preferred world of his imagination—as many ride out today in material pursuit of the American Dream—mistaking hostelries for castles, herds of sheep for armies, and windmills for threatening giants. Cervantes delegates the task of keeping his hero grounded in the real world to the sound habits of Sancho Panza, the good knight's faithful squire. Sancho is the voice of common sense, the stable realist who has come to understand the world in all its mundane complexity.

I believe Cervantes's story still has much to teach us. If we are to reimagine the American Dream in a way that will sustain genuine human progress—where the health of our species and those with which we share the planet will continue to thrive rather than to dangerously decline—we all must seek to know and channel the common sense of our inner Sanchos. Cervantes's story is a reminder that many of the cues that shape and give meaning to our behavior are embedded in the cultural mores and the belief systems that surround us and in the intuitive habits of mind that frame and perpetuate our beliefs and customs. Perhaps most important, Cervantes's story, in today's demand-driven market culture, reminds us—as does the story of Henry—that if we are to better tune our behavior to the opportunities and risks of living and working amid affluence, we must better understand how habit and intuition work. How does the brain respond to the world in which we find ourselves? Why is it that we appear to be insatiable? Could it be that what we often accept as conscious choice is in reality an unconscious reaction of the mind, governed by instinct, by our imagination, and by our conditioning as social animals? Could it be that we are not making as many conscious choices as we believe? It is to that subject that I now turn.

rience, and culturally acquired social practice—of which markets are a prime example—that shapes the behavior of each of us through the choices we make. Within these swirling, surging inner and outer worlds we each seek to find ourselves; from among these elements, through choice, is created the whole of the self. Further, in navigating this complex world, we assume that all choices are deliberate and that we actively control how we behave either by intention or through our ability to respond to changing circumstances. In short, we take pride in the *conscious distinction* of who we are as a person: our likes and dislikes, our assets and our liabilities.

In what is a uniquely human capacity, we consciously string these fragments of self-knowledge together to construct a meaningful life story that tells who we believe ourselves to be: a compassionate mother, a poor tennis player, a recovering alcoholic, a dedicated father, and so on. It only takes a moment of reflection to know that based on this unique story we each have the extraordinary ability to answer an endless assortment of questions about who we are and what we think about the world and our place in it. Every day we use such *reflective*, evidence-based self-understanding to express opinions and to negotiate with others as we engage and embrace the intricacies of human society. This is the *conscious mind* at work: the activity of brain systems that both serve our identity and, more practically, those that we call upon when we must remember a telephone number or find our way in a city.

However, as I explain in this chapter on the self-tuning qualities of mental habit, an ability to recall autobiographical detail on demand and the capacity for conscious problem solving are only the most obvious of the mental mechanisms through which we engage the world and find a healthy level of interaction with it. While in our subjective experience of everyday life we seem to rely on conscious self-knowledge, much of the time, as a growing body of research reveals, a complementary system of *reflexive* perception and action within our brains is robust. This reflexive system, which operates largely in the *preconscious* and *unconscious* realms, is not only vital to our efficient navigation of everyday life but also shapes, through acquired habit, much of what we believe, how we perceive the motives of others, the moral rules we follow, and what we decide in subtle but profound ways, sometimes to our advantage and sometimes not. Think of it, if you will, as the brain's neural network for everyday social behavior, the basic operating system that is not only essential to the personal story that we write but also to the infrastructure that helps hold civil society together through interpersonal exchange. This preconscious network of reflexive self-knowledge is commonly known as *intuition*.

OF COURSE, THAT THE LIFE of the mind is subject to preconscious or unconscious forces is not a new idea. Sigmund Freud, more than any other in recent history, through his exploration of psychoanalysis and the accessible nature of his writings, brought to public attention the power of the unconscious in shaping our worldview. These first stirrings of our contemporary advance in the understanding of unconscious mental life took place against the intellectually vibrant backdrop of turn-of-the-century Vienna. As Eric Kandel, the Nobel Prize–winning neuroscientist, has described in his book *The Age of Insight*, the movement toward self-examination that swept up both artists and scientists in a vigorous dialogue was driven in part by a reaction to the Enlightenment ideal that only through reason would progress be achieved.

The industrial society of the nineteenth century valued discipline, thrift, organization, and faith as the path to human betterment, devaluing in the process human emotion and instinct, which the Victorians saw as "base" and "immoral." Freud's revolutionary writings highlighted what he believed to be the psychic consequences of living in a society that repressed human instinct, particularly sexual desire. And in support of Freud's assertion we would do well to remember that when Igor Stravinsky's *The Rite of Spring*, erotically choreographed by

Nijinsky, was first performed in Paris in 1913, the audience rioted. Thus Freud, in striving through psychoanalysis for a more complex theory of mind, was a pioneer in asserting that in our behavior we are equally as subject to cultural and social influences, and to the passions, as we are influenced by conscious awareness and our ability to use reason.

But the introspective explorations of psychoanalysis are limited when it comes to defining the anatomy of the living brain and dissecting the dynamics of neural communication that may support conscious and unconscious mental life. Although it was first observed in animal experiments in the late nineteenth century that the brain exhibits rhythmic electrical activity, it is only with the advent of modern brain-imaging technology that we have had the capacity to investigate the workings of the human brain in real time. First came the electroencephalograph (EEG), through which the brain's spontaneous electrical discharge can be measured by electrodes placed on the scalp. Despite its simplicity this technology has stood the test of time. Early in my neuropsychiatric career in London I learned the value of a special type of electrode in the diagnosis of complex epileptic seizures in children, a technique that has changed little, even today.

Then in the 1970s came X-ray computed tomography (CT), a technology that permitted observation of brain structures without resorting to surgery. But the true conceptual advance arrived with positron emission tomography (PET), where a rapidly decaying radioisotope injected into a patient's bloodstream made it possible to measure changing levels of regional blood flow in the brain. For the first time, because blood flow is intimately connected to neuronal activity, it became possible to obtain real-time images indicating which anatomical regions became physiologically active when undertaking simple mental tasks.

Within a few years, in a sudden plethora of riches, the methodology of magnetic resonance imaging (MRI) was developed. The technology of MRI is dependent upon the physics of atoms exposed to a powerful magnetic field: many of them behave like little compass needles that then can be made to line up by artful manipulation of the magnet, yielding a detailed anatomical picture without PET's potential hazard of ionizing radiation. Then in the early 1990s a sophisticated elaboration upon MRI technology made it possible, again by the measurement of blood flow, to track the *functional dynamics* of activity in the living brain.

A useful analogy in thinking about functional magnetic resonance imaging (fMRI) is the experience of flying over a modern city at night: the relative activity of the city's districts is reflected in the clustered patterns of light seen below, with the great highways that connect these urban centers snaking between them. It's a crude picture, you might complain, and it is: but for the first time—just as the early cartographers contoured the great continents—fMRI offers the capacity to map the brain's geography and correlate that with how it is functioning physiologically. We can literally map the interactive processes of mind. Objective investigation of the conundrum that so preoccupied Freud and his Viennese colleagues—defining the dynamic relationships among brain, cultural experience, and the conscious and preconscious self—had entered a new era.

MATT LIEBERMAN, A PROFESSOR of psychology and a colleague of mine at the University of California in Los Angeles, is in the forefront of these new research efforts to understand how we think about ourselves. Intrigued since his graduate student days at Harvard, in the early 1990s, by the challenge of social behavior, Matt is a pioneer in the fledgling field of social cognitive neuroscience. This new discipline yokes together the power of the brain-imaging technologies with the proven experimental methods of cognitive neuropsychology to examine the neuronal underpinnings of complex social behavior.

The Social Cognitive Neuroscience Laboratory is based in Franz Hall, the sprawling home of UCLA's preeminent psychology department. Walking north on the campus, beyond the urban density of the medical center where I work, and crossing the Court of Science, you'll discover a venerable portico framed by gnarly olive trees and shaded by giant eucalyptus and pine. It announces the first of Franz Hall's several buildings. Together their architecture chronicles the growth of the university itself, from the mellowed brick and stone facades that reflect an early romance with the academies of northern Italy to a massive 1960s cube of concrete and reflective glass—a structure that in the late afternoon of my visit was splashing generous pools of sunlight into the gardens below.

Matt Lieberman's corner office is on the sixth floor of that cube, a place where a wall of windows looks straight into a canopy of pine. I found him there working on a new book. "It's about how the brain got its social network," he quipped with a smile, rising from his chair. He's a man of easy and comfortable manner, with a square jaw and a close-cropped head of dark hair, now flecked with gray. The room mirrors that comfort. Books tumble from laden shelves onto the floor, mingling there in piles. Titles range widely, from those expected in a psychologist's workplace to others less familiar; sociology, cognitive neuroscience, physiology, anatomy, religion, and evolutionary theory all jostle together. Then there's philosophy, with the usual suspects, but in addition you'll find Fromm, Sartre, Nietzsche—lots of Nietzsche. On the opposite wall, above a massive computer screen displaying a grid of MRI images and the unfolding draft of the book, hangs a large reproduction of Magritte's *Golconde*. The familiar portrait—an urban facade beleaguered by a down-pouring of bowler-hatted men—seems strangely at home.

Intrigued, I asked Matt how he had acquired such eclectic social and philosophical interests. "The philosophy is a legacy from my father," Matt began. "In his youth he had been working toward a Ph.D. in philosophy but changed his plans when children began arriving." In the 1970s no one was hiring philosophy graduates, so Lieberman senior switched to law. "But we still had the books," Matt went on, "and I grew up reading all that I could find. It was my first true passion in the world of ideas."

The interest in cognitive sociology came later. First, as an undergraduate at Rutgers, Matt had been greatly influenced by Bruce Wilshire, the professor who introduced him to Nietzsche, nineteenth-century German philosophy, and the writings of William James. For Wilshire understanding subjective experience was key in the study of social behavior. Then, following these leads as a graduate student at Harvard, Matt discovered brain imaging and began studying with the renowned psychologist Daniel Gilbert, whose popular book *Stumbling on Happiness* has brought wide public recognition to the field of social cognition. "So I was hooked," Matt explained. "A large percentage of our waking lives is spent navigating the social world, and I wanted to know more about how that is coded in the brain."

It was one of Matt Lieberman's early papers, "Intuition: A Social Cognitive Neuroscience Approach," written while he was still at Harvard, that first drew my attention to his research. In it he proposed that intuitive thinking, rather than being mysterious as it is commonly construed, is a brain-information-processing strategy—a habit of mind—that is based on *implicit learning*. As the term is used by psychologists, implicit learning is unintentional, a means whereby facts and cues about the relationships that exist in the world—information that helps us better navigate—are acquired just by going about our daily business. An obvious example is how when we go to live in a foreign country, we pick up some of the local language, customs, and gestures without really trying. Another is when walking in a familiar city, we seem to follow an uncanny sense of direction without much conscious effort. On the flip side, we all have had the experience of feeling that something is not quite right about the "energy" in a conversation with someone without really knowing why, or of being surprised by an unexpected sense of optimism or opportunity for no immediately discernable reason. Perhaps even more intriguing, under such circumstances, in our culture we often find ourselves assuming that these reflexive sensibilities—or "gut feelings"—have greater validity than do conscious attempts at rational analysis of the situation.

It is clear that the brain can initiate us to carry out routine motor behaviors seemingly without bothering the conscious self to consider the details. So why is it not the same for thinking? Why are not some processes of thought similarly triggered automatically? We find no discomfort in accepting that many motor skills and certain mental abilities—catching a ball, skiing, riding a bicycle, learning to read and write—become automatic with practice. It is clear, for example, from watching a baby playing in the crib that the human animal has an inborn facility—perhaps an "instinctual" desire—to reach out and grasp at an object. With countless hours of practice such preprogrammed drives become transformed later in life into an efficient routine of "habitual" behavior—a reflexive, tuned skill—that provides the bedrock for the enjoyment of countless ballgames.

So, Matt Lieberman wondered, does intuition—that is, reflexive self-knowledge based on implicitly learned, social habits of mind—although more nuanced and individual than something such as learning to catch a ball, develop and operate in a similar way to motor habits? And if so, what are the brain mechanisms supporting such reflexive skills? Matt postulated that if intuitive self-knowledge is indeed habit based, then the basal ganglia—the same set of nuclei found deep in the old brain that coordinate the motor programs enabling us to ride a bicycle or swing a baseball bat—are probably also involved in how we acquire and sustain our social relationships, as might be expressed in a preference for particular friends or a detailed knowledge of favored leisure activities.

Subsequently at UCLA, and in keeping with his maxim that theories are only opinions until proven one way or the other, Matt undertook a series of experiments to test whether *reflective* (consciously recalled) and *reflexive* (intuition-based or subconscious) self-knowledge were served by different brain systems. The designs were ingenious. In one significant study he recruited two groups of experienced individuals, one accomplished soccer players and the other improvisational actors (this was Los Angeles after all) and compared them against each other in the way they accessed their knowledge about these two domains of experience—one familiar and one unfamiliar to each group. Matt's reasoning went something like this: those individuals proficient in soccer would have a different "book of life" experience, a more detailed self-knowledge of the game, when it came to soccer than would the professional actors, and vice versa.

Specifically Matt surmised that those individuals intimately familiar with the nuance of being an actor would be able to *reflexively* (intuitively) respond to self-knowledge descriptions pertinent to their profession (for example, is an actor creative, dramatic, quick witted), while those unfamiliar with acting—the soccer players—would need to consciously *reflect* upon each inquiry prior to making a judgment. And of course with descriptors involving soccer, he supposed that the reverse would be true for the two groups. Then if the neuronal architecture responsible for intuitive and conscious processing were distinct, this would be reflected in a variation of the regional blood flow recorded in the fMRI scanner.

The tunnel of an MRI machine is a rather noisy place, and so the participants were fed the descriptive words, interspersed with neutral ones, through a set of fiber optic goggles hooked up to a computer and their responses were recorded by the finger pressing of one of two buttons. It was clear from the results that indeed there are two distinct brain systems supporting self-knowledge. While the *speed* at which the healthy young subjects answered the two sets of questions was not significantly different, the fMRI data clearly demonstrated two distinct yet overlapping neural alliances at work.

When a participant in the study made a judgment regarding the subject she knew most about—*intuitive* or *reflexive* retrieval where little conscious effort was required—she activated a network of brain centers that included the nuclei of two ancient structures, the amygdala, the sentinel of emotion, and the basal ganglia, the home of habit, together with a

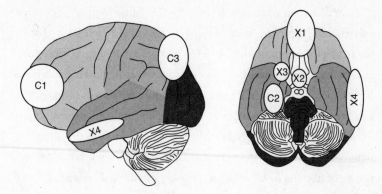

Figure 2.2: The neural alliances active in the brain during reflexive (intuitive) thinking and reflective (conscious) thought. Those regions active during conscious, *reflective* thought include the lateral prefrontal cortex (C1), the hippocampus and medial temporal lobe (C2), and the posterior parietal cortex (C3). Interacting during *reflexive* thinking are the brain regions of the ventromedial prefrontal cortex (X1), the basal ganglia (X2), the amygdala (X3), and the lateral temporal cortex (X4). (Illustration based on the work of Matthew Lieberman and presented here with permission)

section of the new brain known as the ventromedial prefrontal cortex. This alliance equates with the capacity to quickly recall self-knowledge that has been acquired implicitly. In contrast, when a participant had to choose descriptors on a less-known subject, she drew on her *conscious, reflective* ability to remember explicit, evidenced-based learning. In association with doing so were activated the lateral prefrontal cortex (part of the highly evolved "executive" cortex), the hippocampus (the seat of memory formation), and parts of the medial and temporal cortices of the new brain (see Figure 2.2).

MATT LIEBERMAN'S RESEARCH confirms that we are literally of two minds when it comes to knowing ourselves. And his research is not alone. The suspicion that two separate but parallel brain processes are at work in self-knowledge and decision making has been widely discussed in neuropsychology since 1977, when William Schneider and Richard Shiffrin first postulated the activity of such distinct brain mechanisms. Blandly labeled in those early years "Systems 1 and 2," the concept of dual process thinking is now well established. It was brought to wider attention in 2011 by the book *Thinking Fast and Slow* by Daniel Kahneman, the psychologist who won the Nobel Prize for economics a decade earlier. The descriptors of the characteristic behaviors of the twin mechanisms have evolved, but most simply, *reflective conscious reasoning* is slow, controlled, effortful, serial, and rule governed, while *reflexive thinking*—tuned, intuitive habits of mind—is fast, preconscious, emotional, parallel, automatic, and effortless. Think of the notion of "reflecting" actively upon something that needs a decision versus reflexively "catching the drift" of an ongoing conversation, and you will have a sense of the difference.

The mystery that has surrounded the brain's reflexive processing of information thus falls away when we recognize that anatomically the brain structures that are responsible for such intuitive activity are also the brain centers that support familiar habitual motor behaviors, just as Matt Lieberman had predicted. In other words, everything we learn to do well by habit—be that acting, playing soccer, or being considerate to others—is orchestrated and sustained at its core by that area of the brain known as the basal ganglia. Located at the base of the forebrain, this group of brain nuclei—each with a descriptive Latin name designed to tax the sharpest memory—function together as a cohesive unit. Historically these brain centers, of which the corpus striatum (in translation, "striped mass") is the largest aggregation, have been understood as the autopilots of the body's motor activity. It is now accepted, however, that these same automatic brain systems operate in a similar fashion when it comes to managing routine patterns of social engagement and even individual, personal habits. Such patterns of learned behavior, triggered by well-known cues and coordinated by the ganglia's extensive connections to other parts of the brain, are executed reflexively, automatically, smoothly, and without conscious effort. Just as through practice the brain can be tuned to master the game of tennis, so does experience tune social behavior.

What we call intuition is the sudden, conscious experience of this process. The mysterious, almost divine subjective sense of "having a feeling" or "knowing what's right" about something in fact reflects the emergence into awareness of preconsciously held thought patterns, learned long ago. In most instances, however, as with any automatic control system, the presence of the brain's autopilots is barely noticed, until they fail. Such failure is most easily understood—although the principle is the same for social habit—when describing a loss of habitually tuned motor function, as in Parkinson's disease. Among the most important functions of the basal ganglia is the subliminal positioning of the body in space, something that we practice and learn when very young and that later underpins the capacity to walk, run, jump, and play physical games. When the nerve cells supporting these abilities are damaged or degenerate, as they do in Parkinson's disease, the normally unconscious, fluid movements of the limbs and body are replaced by stiffness and slowing. This loss of motor programming—or perhaps more precisely the incapacity to automatically initiate smoothly operating neural habits—is associated with degeneration of the substantia nigra (black substance) of the ganglia, and particularly with a loss of its dopamine-producing cells.

Here the specific brain chemistry is important in understanding how habits are acquired. In Parkinson's disease, where dopamine is deficient, treatment with L-dopa, a dopamine precursor, significantly improves the slowing and stiffness for many sufferers and frequently elevates mood. You will recall that it is the dopamine system—introduced earlier with the story of Henry—that drives the reward pathways. Indeed, dopamine is the molecule of motivation, influencing learning—and the development of habit—through the reinforcement of reward and punishment. When something is perceived and experienced as rewarding and pleasurable, either consciously or preconsciously, we seek to repeat the experience, and during such moments dopamine neurons in the striatum increase their rate of firing. Conversely, when action is met with punishment or pain, or even familiarity and boredom, the striatal dopamine activity diminishes. This is the brain's tuning system at work.

It is true across mammalian species. Thus Ann Graybiel, of the McGovern Institute for Brain Research at the Massachusetts Institute of Technology and a leading figure in habit research, has shown that when rats are trained to run mazes in pursuit of a chocolate reward, neuronal firings in the basal ganglia are particularly strong at the beginning and at the end of the learning process, when reward is imminent. This education of a specific set of neurons through repeated experience enables the brain to store information in useful, habitual patterns that later can be quickly activated when encountering the appropriate environmental cue. Once triggered, that habitual pattern of behavior then runs automatically.

The basal ganglia thus are central to the brain's networks of habitual motor behavior and intuitive, reflexive understanding, connecting as they do the new frontal cortex and the ancient limbic structures in a continuous loop of information processing. Developing and tuning such reflexive behaviors offers a great biological advantage, promoting efficient "autopilot" behaviors and thereby freeing time for conscious appraisal of opportunities and challenges that require careful thought. These habitual patterns are robust and preserved over long periods—witness the capacity to ski or ride a bicycle after many years of abstinence; or the patina of social grace that often is preserved in the early stages of Alzheimer's disease, despite short-term memory deterioration. But these stable habits of the brain can also plague us, as when texting on a mobile device becomes so routine that we attempt it while driving a car, or when an addictive behavior—be it to cocaine, tasty processed food, gambling, sex or the Internet—gets triggered by an established cue. The lesson to be learned is that the brain's tuned patterns of habit and intuitive thinking—both good and bad—take form through trial and error, but once laid down, they are notoriously resistant to change and even more difficult to eradicate.

*   *   *   *

INTUITIVE PATTERNS ARE NOT habits of mind that come pre-assembled as part of the brain's survival kit, as do the essential primary emotions of anger, fear, surprise, and disgust. Rather they are reflexive mental capacities—a compendium of practiced shortcuts usually created under familiar circumstances and available for immediate engagement—that are built incrementally from experience *in association* with the primary emotions. This functional association is evident in the network of anatomical centers that support reflexive self-knowledge—a network of information flow that links the ancient structures of the amygdala and the basal ganglia together with the ventromedial prefrontal cortex, an area of the new brain that (as I shall describe in Chapter 4) is important in shaping reward preference.

So what part does reflexive, intuitive brain tuning play in the complex social interaction and emotional give-and-take that is everyday life? How is it that we can take exception to an individual as "not my type" on first meeting, without even a conversation? Why do we sometimes startle at a stick in the woods, thinking it to be a snake, as happened to a countryman friend of mine while walking through a grove of trees near the U.S. Capitol in Washington? Or experience feelings of nausea at the smell of a particular food as did I when, many years ago, I developed an aversion to bacon and cooked liver. These are all examples of how the brain makes autonomous and preconscious judgments in the face of a perceived threat.

Take my own acquired aversion to cooked liver as an example. When I consciously and deliberately thought through the experience, I was able to associate it with a period in my life when as a young doctor I had been working under considerable stress. As was the tradition in Britain at the time, I was on call every other night and living in the house officer's quarters. We were given room and board including breakfast and dinner. While, at the time, I did not consciously associate the two, I had caught a stomach virus, complete with the usual symptoms of nausea and vomiting. On the evening prior to my falling ill the main dish served had been liver, bacon, and mashed potatoes, an English staple. Although my deliberative self might have considered these events unrelated, the amygdala centers of my brain, which as the sentinels of safety receive sensory information from all parts of the body including the olfactory system, associated the stomach flu with the smell of the meal. The two became paired in my preconscious mind, just as for Pavlov's dog the conditioned stimulus of the bell became paired with being fed. Thereafter this reflexive conditioning became absorbed into my personal narrative. Whenever the smell of liver and bacon was in the air, I received an emotional alert from my preconscious self, consciously registered as a sense of nausea.

Based on noxious experience, my brain "retuned" itself in the (misguided) interest of self-preservation. Only later, reflecting upon the events surrounding my sickness, for I had enjoyed eating liver prior to the episode, did my nausea signal disappear. This, of course, is an example of association that is simple to understand. But the question arises: does social "intuition"—the reflexive capacity to form opinions about those we meet, such as that unexplained aversion to an occasional stranger—rest upon similar, associatively tuned brain templates? And how do such associations influence the life story that we build?

HOMO SAPIENS ARE AN intensely social species and have been so for millennia. Indeed, Robin Dunbar, the British anthropologist and evolutionary psychologist, has provided evidence that the large human forebrain evolved not through improved nutrition, as we once thought, but in response to the competitive challenges of living in social groups. What drove the growth of the human brain was not survival in the natural world but a need to negotiate the social environment. So given that evolution is an exercise in adaptive parsimony, it becomes reasonable to ask whether the capacity for intuitive social understanding shares a common neural platform with other preconscious habit development. This would help explain why it is that as children mature, within approximately the same time frame, they come to understand the feelings of others and develop empathic concern until—in the larger cultural context—they master the capacity for self-control and delayed gratification that is required to work collaboratively in large groups.

Leda Cosmides and John Tooby, from the Center for Evolutionary Psychology at the University of California, Santa Barbara, have suggested that fundamental to our development of such social habits is what they describe as mental "heuristics"—innate rules originally derived from trial-and-error learning that promote rapid and efficient (in their words, "fast and frugal") decision making. Cosmides and Tooby have suggested that in our ancestral past such mental rules evolved through trial and error when we were critically dependent upon one another for safety and survival. This does not mean, they argue, that such social behaviors are ancient and instinctual, as are those of a suckling baby. Rather the notion is that templates of social interaction that facilitate rapid mutual understanding or that warn of potential interpersonal strife have been acquired more recently by natural selection—essentially Cosmides and Tooby consider them behavioral archetypes—that are then later embellished by individual experience.

Here we again glimpse the mechanisms of the brain's preconscious operating systems at work. Building upon evolving mental templates, social intuition becomes for each of us a preconscious, dynamic store of self-knowledge and practical understanding regarding codes of social behavior that is continuously being upgraded through ongoing cultural and personal interaction. Via this *reflexive* preconscious integration, the intuitive mind complements the deliberation of the *reflective* conscious self by facilitating the rapid and efficient assessment of social mismatch, opportunity, and risk. And on occasion, in the process of this deliberative integration, "gut feelings" are generated—

whether the fundamental assessment is right or wrong—that in the moment seem "intuitively" more valid than any conscious reasoning. This helps explain the *reflexive* "not my type" stranger reaction. Only later, upon *reflective* assessment, is it realized that the individual has triggered an intuitive template of mind—let's say he is loud and bombastic in manner—that is a painful reminder of that distant uncle who always teased us at Thanksgiving dinner. In this illustration, reflexive awareness has offered a warning—much as for me as a young doctor, the smell of liver would reflexively turn my stomach.

And broader speculation then arises. Perhaps in human culture such integrative archetypes reach beyond the narrative of immediate personal experience to become the foundation of qualitative judgments—of ethical and moral beliefs—that are handed down across the generations to shape the stories that define the social virtues. The research of Jonathan Haidt, a professor of psychology at the University of Virginia who has made an extensive study of how morality varies across cultures and political ideology, throws light on such musings.

Haidt's comparative studies have involved some 30,000 individuals worldwide, ranging from the United States and Europe to South America and East Asia. The behavioral analyses of this large and varied group of people suggest that there are five universal templates of mind—involving caring, fairness, loyalty, respect, and impurity—upon which every culture builds its own set of virtues. From these data Haidt argues that it is through intuitive social understanding that we *care* for each other and willingly adhere to the concept of *fairness* that nurtures the human social fabric, even within the complex societies of our contemporary world. *Loyalty* to the family, community, and nation and *respect* for tradition and authority also emerge as fundamental concerns, while abhorrence of *impurities*—of what we consider the disgusting actions by others, of contaminated food and of environmental degradation—constitutes the fifth cluster of intuitive emotion that is common across all cultural groups. These foundational systems Haidt considers as intuitive "learning modules" of the evolved mind that during development, comparable to the acquisition of language, help children quickly recognize culturally specific virtues and vices.

Reflexive templates of mind that largely facilitate social cohesion may also help explain why some human practices and institutions endure, to be found in similar form across many different ethnic and cultural groups, while other social systems collapse or are discarded within a few generations. Consider, for example, the barter and exchange of the marketplace, which is a human institution that has endured for thousands of years and is of particular relevance to this discussion. As we struggle with America's infatuation with consumerism, understanding our attraction to market temptations becomes of pivotal importance. Is such infatuation, then, an example of how the conscious mind can become the puppet of our reflexive habits?

Daniel Kahneman, the Nobel laureate, has emphasized that the brain's preconscious system of intuitive learning works with what it observes and that sometimes those observations are inaccurate, explaining why we can behave irrationally and impulsively under familiar circumstances. Thus, as was clearly evident in the financial crisis of 2008—perpetrated by millions of Americans being induced to assume debt they couldn't afford—an intuitive sense of good fortune is not automatically an indicator of accurate judgment. Intuitive insight can be trusted, Kahneman asserts, only when operating under experiential circumstances that are regular, predictable, and stable at the time that the reflexive insight occurs. In the absence of such stable contingencies, he says, intuition is unreliable.

TO KNOW ONE'S SELF is not easy. But it is essential in achieving a well-tuned brain. In seeking such self-understanding we must be prepared to accept that much of what drives our actions is not of our conscious choosing: that in the mature, healthy individual it is the intuitive mind that preconsciously writes our stories and shapes much of our behavior. We are all "strangers to ourselves," as Timothy

Wilson, the Sherrell Aston Professor of Psychology at the University of Virginia and a researcher on self-knowledge, has evocatively described it. This is not inherently a bad thing. The brain's fashioning of a reflexive, intuitive faculty, in complement to the reflective, conscious mind, ensures the necessary means of stability and orientation—as by analogy do the keel and the compass of a sailing vessel—with which to navigate the world with confidence, safety, and efficiency. Ideally in assuming responsibility for the mundane tasks of vigilance and everyday interaction, the intuitive mind preserves the time and focus essential for attention and conscious deliberation, while adding texture and memory to self-awareness. Thus in the ideal world habit shapes character, which in turn shapes the personal narrative of who we are as a unique individual.

But we do not live in an ideal world. While we remain creatures shaped in our biology by evolution, it is largely in our relationships with one another—and the cultural context of those relationships— that we find meaning. To preserve and enjoy certain individual freedoms, we strive to live together in some semblance of harmony. We call this democracy, a social order based upon equality and reason. At one end of the spectrum, in the private realm, we all have freedom to make our own decisions and are responsible for our acts: nobody else has a choice in what we do. At the other end, the legal realm, we are all subject to strict laws designed to ensure the freedom of others. In between lies a vast middle ground of public and social domains where the choices we make and actions we take are not binding but nonetheless interface with those reasoned norms and accepted values essential to the maintenance of the cultural fabric. It is in this vast middle ground that the reflexive, intuitive mind is largely dominant.

So if we believe ourselves to be consciously in control of the decisions we make, while in reality much of our choosing is preconscious and pretuned, dependent upon the accuracy and efficiency of reflexive habit, what are the social implications? One hidden consequence, as Kahneman observed, is that reflexive habit can become distorted and maladaptive, as can any behavior. As is evident in America's obesity epidemic, our habits can feed back and reinforce themselves to create a pathological cycle. This should come as no surprise. Intuition is powerfully tempered by experience and by the culture in which we are reared. And in turn it is our intuitive understanding of the motivation and purpose of others that plays a vital role in sustaining cultural cohesion. Culture and intuition thus form a dynamic, mutually reinforcing whole, which is the glue that holds human societies together—for good or for bad.

So what are the consequences of such self-knowledge when we are striving to understand our love affair with consumerism? In the Western democracies, and especially in the United States, the consumer market is held up as a haven of individual freedom and conscious choice, one where the decisions we make are rational, consciously determined, and designed to achieve maximum personal value. But price and need are not the only factors that influence us. Emotional striving, culture, and habit also profoundly influence our decisions in the market, as I have outlined. When we are confronted by a shifting cultural landscape in an increasingly globalized consumer society—one now dedicated to continuous economic growth, competition, and celebrity—how can we continue to believe that in economic matters we are predominantly rational beings? And when did we first see ourselves as so rationally endowed?

I posed these questions to Matt Lieberman during our discussion on that sunlit afternoon in his office at UCLA. "Yes, in modern times the concept of the self has been changing," agreed Matt. "Over the past two centuries the idea of the self has become qualitatively different from that held by people living in the Middle Ages. Who we think we are is no longer equated in a transparent fashion with inherited social status and the dictates of the church. Despite its many drawbacks the medieval identity was simple and stable. Self-definition—beginning essentially with the Enlightenment—has become complex, even problematic."

By comparison with medieval times, as has been emphasized by the social psychologist Roy Baumeister, personal identity today is considered self-determined and choice-driven. But we conceive of choices as needing to be resolved in a conscious manner. We tend to discount the power of social tuning. Matt had wondered aloud whether this explains, as society becomes ever more challenging, why we find comfort in defining ourselves by "those moments in our past when we were faced with obstacles for which . . . habit . . . could not guarantee safe passage." I found it an interesting notion. Is this why, amid the shifting "culture" of modern consumer society, with its social pressures and relentless promotion of products, we celebrate conscious market choice as the royal road to self-satisfaction? Is this our only perceived locus of control?

Despite mounting evidence that the intuitive mind powerfully influences who we are and what we do in the world, we persist in considering the conscious self to be king. How, during the Age of Reason, this concept first evolved and later became central to the philosophical underpinnings of the market society is the subject of my next chapter.

Chapter 3

Enlightened Experiments: Inventing the Market Society

> Money begets trade . . .
> And trade encreaseth mony.
>
> Thomas Mun, "England's Treasure by
> Forraign Trade" (1664)

> And who are you? said he. . . . Don't puzzle me, said I.
>
> Laurence Sterne, *Tristram Shandy* (1759–67)

DRIVE DOWN THE LEAFY LANES of Oxfordshire, England, on a summer afternoon, heading west from Blenheim Palace in Woodstock, and you will come across the village of Combe. It is clustered on a small knoll, away from the original settlement that once encircled the watermill buildings nestled along the riverbank of the meandering Evenlode. As local folklore would have it, a mill has been at that spot, in one form or another, since before the Domesday survey of 1086. When the villagers moved uphill in the fourteenth century to escape miasma and the Black Death, the mill continued to operate, with waterpower being replaced by steam in the late eighteenth century.

In 2000 Combe Mill was retired from commercial activity, but even today when "in steam"—as when I visited in 2012—the mill's venerable beam engine will hiss and pulse with life, opening a window to the ingenuity and technology that first fired Britain's industrial revolution over two centuries ago.

The Combe engine is of the advanced "beam" design that was first engineered by James Watt and built by the entrepreneurial Matthew Boulton in the 1760s in his factory at Soho, now a Birmingham suburb. Refined steam engines such as these were first developed to pump water from the copper mines of Cornwall. Fed by Britain's prodigious supply of easily accessible coal, these steam engines helped decouple the nation's productivity from the constraining, sun-driven annual cycle of organic growth and initiated our dependence on fossil fuel. This successfully shifted motive power from the horse to machines, driving technical advance in everything from mining, to metallurgy, to textiles, to transport.

Watt and Boulton were both members of the Lunar Society of Birmingham, the name now given to a group of friends who in the 1760s began meeting informally at Boulton's house on the Sunday nearest to the full moon to share ideas, food, and copious drink. Erasmus Darwin—philosopher, inventor, poet, and the grandfather of Charles Darwin—who practiced medicine up the road in Lichfield, was a founding member and close confidant of the ebullient Boulton. Fascinated by the emerging science of the time, novel ideas, and their practical application to society (it was said of Boulton that he never saw a business without conceiving of a way to improve it), the Lunar men ranged widely in their talents and influence. Other regular participants were John Whitehurst, a clock and instrument maker, Josiah Wedgwood, an ambitious young potter and clever businessman, and Joseph Priestley, the radical preacher and chemist who first isolated oxygen and whose house was burned down in 1791 for his outspoken support of the French Revolution.

This colorful cast of characters has long intrigued me. I first became aware of their exploits when, as a newly minted physician working in London, I read Robert Schofield's book *The Lunar Society of Birmingham*, which had been published in 1963. This group of friends, as Schofield captured them, was a "brilliant microcosm of that scattered community of provincial manufacturers and professional men who found England a rural society with an agricultural economy and left it urban and industrial." Subsequently, with the pretensions of youth, a small group of us began to meet regularly at a local pub for "discussions and drink," modeling ourselves on the gatherings of the Lunar men. While never as august or erudite as those who had inspired our gatherings, we nonetheless had some wild evenings and learned much from one another.

Among the things that I learned was that Robert Schofield, the author of the book that had first intrigued me, was an American physicist and historian. This information, which initially surprised the Englishman in me, soon made much sense, for the Lunar Society's connections with America were many. Later, especially after I migrated to the United States in the 1970s, my fascination with the lives of the Lunar men was strengthened by my own curiosity about America, which I came to see as the great social experiment of Enlightenment principles. Benjamin Franklin—who was in England during 1758 as the representative of the Pennsylvania Assembly—had become connected to the "Lunatics" through their common interest in electricity. And later when William Small—who in the early 1760s had taught natural philosophy and mathematics to Thomas Jefferson in Williamsburg—returned to take up a medical practice in Birmingham, he was soon central to the group's intellectual life. The Lunar Society was, in short, a prodigious and broad-based fellowship among clever, merry men—each driven by enviable energy, intense curiosity, and a fascination with experimentation—who came together, as Erasmus Darwin once modestly described it, to indulge informally in "a little philosophical laughing."

But beyond the jocularity of their union, as I shall explain in these next pages, the Lunar men are emblematic of a shifting cultural vision that eventually would define the modern market society. Like other clubmen they drank and joked and argued, but they were also intent upon reforming the culture in which they lived and worked. Importantly they carried forward a passion for material improvement that went beyond philosophy to the marketplace. Together with the leading economic and social theorists of the time—with Smith, Hume, and Locke—they believed the human mind to be malleable, and they nurtured dreams of a better future, one where social benefits would flow from individual talent and the conscious exercise of rational choice. How these Enlightenment ideas evolved to shape the economic system of human relationships we now call capitalism, why the balance of those relationships has shifted in the face of modern-day affluence, and how with insights from neurobehavioral science we may understand why that is so, is the subject of this chapter.

IN THE TIME OF THE Lunar men England was already a thriving commercial nation and Birmingham a fast-growing industrial center with smelting and iron trades, textile manufacture, pottery, and a nascent chemical industry. A century earlier the English Civil War and the political upheavals that followed had increased the influence of men of commerce and of wealthy landowners. With the death of Cromwell, the coronation of Charles II, and the return of the monarchy in 1660, Britain's burgeoning merchant class had been well served. Charles had learned from his exile in the Netherlands—the Dutch were great traders, rivaling England in entrepreneurial flare—and besides Charles needed money to pay off Cromwell's debts and reestablish his royal household. Bankers were courted from across Europe and welcomed to London, property rights were accepted, and private investment was encouraged. In the following decade came some shaky times as Charles sought repeatedly to assert his authority over Parliament. After his death, however, and the abdication of his brother

James II in 1688, an alliance with Holland and William of Orange gave political stability to England and unleashed a revolution in public finance. By the mid-eighteenth century the productive powers of the economy had grown substantially. As England grew in commercial strength, now as a trading nation with a global reach, there was money to be made.

Philosophical and cultural shifts of great magnitude had also occurred: faith in rationality and the power of human effort was ascendant. Of particular significance was the incipient rise of Protestantism and the decline in influence of the Roman Catholic Church, which had been dominant in European culture for a thousand years. In 1704 the armies of the Catholic Sun King, Louis XIV of France, had been defeated by the Duke of Marlborough at the battle of Blenheim—a mighty achievement for which John Churchill was awarded the royal estate in Woodstock, of which Combe Mill remains part—thus finally securing the Protestant cause against Catholicism and French imperialism.

As commerce in Protestant Britain flourished, individual freedom and entrepreneurship were on the rise: religious preference was tolerated as discriminatory laws declined, farming discovered science, common lands were fenced, banks were organized, canals dug, turnpikes built, and local governance strengthened as the urban population exploded. Between 1730 and 1780 England began its transformation from an agricultural nation into a "modernized" emerging industrial force. In step with the growing wealth, domestic goods—amenities such as curtains, cutlery, carpets, and clocks that we now take for granted—were suddenly in great demand. To service the need for greater literacy in the evolving economy, educational opportunities broadened with the opening of charity schools and local grammar schools. The demand for books, newspapers, and pamphlets increased as a new reading public emerged, largely with middle-class roots and a Protestant commitment to thrift and hard work. In their goals and ideals the Lunar men, despite their links to the Royal Society, the Society of Arts, and other clubs of the London establishment, were members of this new educated elite, individuals with the freedom, the opportunity, and the money to pursue their passions and ideas.

Beyond political and commercial ambition these freethinkers thought deeply about human behavior and the meaning of life. In what was still an agrarian culture despite growing urbanization, and with technology yet to emerge as the force that it is today, one lived close to the natural world. Thinkers were philosophers as well as scientists. Erasmus Darwin, for example, spent the last decade of his life focused upon his extraordinary compendium *Zoonomia*, subtitled *The Laws of Organic Life*. In it he proposed not only a comprehensive theory of disease—that all diseases were "nervous" and "of the sensorium"—but also that all warm-blooded animals were derived from a single ancestor. From this "one living filament," creatures were differentiated by the action of a "living force" that developed adaptive functions to meet the struggle for food, shelter, and protection, with these advantages then being inherited to the betterment of the species. Thus did the sorting of the ideas found in *Zoonomia* first frame the scientific inquiry into evolution that was to preoccupy Erasmus's grandson, Charles Darwin, half a century later.

In parallel with this search for the fundamental principles governing the natural world, there flourished a curiosity about how to organize society. With the declining influence of the church what was it that would maintain the moral and social order? Is mankind a naturally social animal? If so, is that behavior learned or born within us? What of the freedoms of the individual self? In a shifting culture how is balance between the individual and society achieved and sustained? And in seeking such harmony what role can the market play?

THIS WAS THE AGE OF REASON. The scientific method provided the intellectual engine for Enlightenment discussion. The gathering and dissection of facts through experiment, the detection of common patterns and principles, all contributed to an increase in human understanding. The mantra essentially went as follows: in the pursuit of knowledge reason is paramount, for it is through reason that human progress, no longer tangled in the web of the natural world, will accelerate. As science and individual freedom flourished, the thinkers of the time, such as the Lunar Men, felt they held the future in their own hands: advancing knowledge offered the prospect of infinite social progress—in medicine, in technology, in education, and in the trades. And central to all such progress was an understanding of the reasoning self.

It is to John Locke (1632–1704) that we owe the modern concept of the self—"that conscious thinking thing," as he described it—and of the importance of experience in shaping individual identity. A physician, who in his thirties had worked with the great clinician Thomas Sydenham, Locke brought to the nascent study of mind the rigorous skills of observation, analysis, and comparison that he had honed in his medical practice. For Locke, a man unfettered by the concepts of modern-day genetics, the mind began as a blank slate, a tabula rasa. Through the choices we make we create our identity and in doing so we draw upon the world around us: every step we take is connected to the past *and* to the future—ideas that Lawrence Sterne explored and satirized in his nine-volume novel *The Life and Opinions of Tristram Shandy, Gentleman*, which first began appearing in 1759. Through choice and experience, Locke argued, we are each unique in personality, skill, and social contribution. The civil right to express such individual distinction was to become the foundation for Locke's reasoning on liberty, property, and religious freedom, thinking that later was to profoundly influence the architects of the American Revolution.

While today Locke's ideas may seem utterly mundane, it is well to remember that self-scrutiny was a rare activity until the sixteenth century. In this respect Michel de Montaigne (1533–92), with his introspective essays, may have been the first modern man. Salvation was a collective enterprise in the early Christian church, and even in Locke's time the Puritan doctrine of predestination meant that salvation or damnation was already fixed at birth—not a great stimulus to self-reflection. Also Locke's ideas flew in the face of ready evidence that the behavior of the human animal is far from rational. The turmoil of England's civil strife in the seventeenth century had left few illusions regarding the foibles of man. It was recognized—as Thomas Hobbes had asserted in his magnum opus *Leviathan*, first published in 1651—that human judgment is unreliable. When left to our own devices, we are predisposed to perverse passions, to greed, and to aggression driven by the pleasures and pains of the moment. In championing the virtue of reason in economic and political affairs, therefore, the for-midable challenge was to explain how rational thinking could consis-tently override the passions or the predestiny of one's birthright.

Bernard de Mandeville, on the other side of the fence, saw little value in further debate upon what he considered to be the peren-nial struggle between reason and passion. A man of rascally humor, Mandeville had a practical, if puckish, interpretation of the human condition, particularly when it came to markets. Born in 1670, Man-deville was a Dutch physician who had moved to England at the age of twenty-nine, ostensibly to learn the language. The mores and the people were to his liking, and he stayed, quickly acquiring a taste for British satire. In 1705 he published a doggerel poem, "The Grumbling Hive," that later became the preamble to his book-length essay, *The Fable of the Bees*, in which he proposed that greed and a love of luxury were the engines of economic growth and thus to the public benefit. This did not make Mandeville popular with the churchmen of the day, who preached virtue rather than vice as a mechanism of social con-trol. They publicly dismissed *The Fable* as a nuisance. But that missed the point. Mandeville's essay was a powerful social metaphor: the bee in its industry transforms the pollen that it acquires, just as Watt's beam engine later would transform steam into energy, with profit for both the individual and society. The seed of an idea had been planted, and after much debate it would grow, famously through the writings of

Adam Smith, into an elegant defense of self-interest as the bedrock of a free market economy.

Another at the center of the philosophical debate exploring the dynamic interrelationship between self and society was David Hume. Born in 1711, Hume drew heavily on Locke's ideas of a conscious self and developed them further. In my opinion, perhaps more than any other of his contemporaries, Hume led the thinking of the time away from superstition and idolatry toward the natural sciences. Although the philosophical tools of introspection and astute observation may seem primitive compared to the wizardry of today's investigative neuroscience, Hume's thinking was profound and prescient. He was also precocious, publishing *A Treatise of Human Nature*, considered by many scholars to be his finest work, at the age of twenty-six. Of particular concern to me here is Hume's interest in the "psychology of action"—why we behave as we do—and *the relative roles of reason and the passions.* For Hume *passion* was what motivated action in life. *Reason,* he argued, while quintessentially human, is rarely what moves us, as any modern advertising executive knows full well. In Hume's analysis, to feel passion was to experience a change in self-awareness—be it hunger for food or sex or the more complex strivings of curiosity and social ambition—and it was this shifting balance between the awareness of personal need and perceived social circumstances that prompted each of us to act. Reason was thus "the slave of the passions," largely relegated to the role of strategist in helping us achieve emotional satisfaction.

So here lies the paradox. If Hume was correct and indeed reason is enslaved by passion, then how do avarice and self-interest—as Bernard de Mandeville argued—emerge as a public good? To ask the question another way, what constrains and shapes individual greed and excess, which the eighteenth-century churchmen feared would damage the moral fabric? If we follow the creed of Mandeville, then precious little is the answer: in a market society of individual freedoms we would have to say that avarice is the price of progress. As his colorful doggerel asserts: "Luxury Employ'd a Million of the Poor and Odious Pride a Million more. Envy itself, and Vanity were Ministers of Industry." In the England of the time, where the majority scratched out an agrarian subsistence, constraint of personal initiative—save for the transgressions of the thief and the smuggler—was the accepted norm. Despite the Enlightenment and the growing freedoms enjoyed by the few, for the great mass of humanity the eighteenth century offered little to be enjoyed and much to be endured. It need not be, argued Mandeville. In highlighting man's lust for self-improvement he sought to turn Thomas Hobbes's dim view of human nature into something to celebrate. Mandeville was arguing against mercantilism and the entrenched social controls of the elite to promote instead "laissez-faire" economics and individual free choice. In the face of deprivation, passionate self-interest not only drove us forward; it was also *the engine* of human progress.

The "passions," as the term was used in the early eighteenth century, are today equivalent to those "primary" emotions that are readily apparent in the infant, specifically the capacity to express fear, disgust, anger, and joy. These are the universal emotions driven by the fundamental instincts of self-preservation—by the drives for safety, sustenance, and sex—and as I have described in Chapter 2, they are hardwired into the most ancient part of the brain. The more complex secondary emotions expressed in adult life, such as pity, pride, shame, and guilt, were in eighteenth-century parlance described as the "moral sentiments." Hume considered these emotional states to be learned, calmer than the primary passions, and dependent for their expression upon judgments made against a moral standard. The sentiments were therefore "susceptible to social cultivation," and in Hume's theory of mind this acquired capacity for sympathetic social understanding played a vital role in balancing the drive of the passions in all elements of everyday life, including the marketplace.

Thus for Hume the self—Locke's "conscious thinking thing"—is not a single thing at all but, as he describes it, *"a kind of theatre* [my emphasis] where several perceptions successively make their appearance, re-pass, glide away, and mingle in an infinite variety of postures and situations." Hume's dynamic image of the process of mind as theater is not only evocative—Matt Lieberman might describe it as a delicate dance of the mind's reflexive and reflective processes—but also a metaphor of extraordinary prescience. Essentially Hume is explaining the continuous appraisal that behavioral neuroscience recognizes as characteristic of integrated cortical function—the dynamic give-and-take of information and the formulation of ideas that is the prerequisite to human choice. As I shall elaborate in Chapter 4, the major stage setting for this drama is the orbital-frontal cortex, the most recently evolved and distinctive region of the human brain that is wedged in above the eye sockets. It is here, to use Hume's words, that the brain's adaptive strategy is forged—frequently beyond immediate conscious awareness—as "perceptions" of passion and reason "glide and mingle" to test an "infinite variety" of alternatives. Hume is describing the dynamic mental processes that, in those moments before we take action, serve to inform our thinking, not only through reflective, conscious self-knowledge but also by drawing on the experience of the reflexive, preconscious self.

DAVID HUME'S CONCEPT of mind as a dynamic interplay among competing forces had a powerful effect on his younger colleague and intimate friend Adam Smith. Smith, the Scotsman whose image is on the British twenty-pound note, is now celebrated as the patron saint of capitalism for the economic principles he expounded in *The Wealth of Nations*. Born in 1723 in Kirkcaldy, just across the Firth of Forth from Edinburgh, Smith grew up to be a solitary fellow who spent a considerable amount of time exploring the ideas inside his own head. As a student in Glasgow between 1737 and 1740, he studied moral philosophy and was greatly influenced by Francis Hutcheson, a theologian and freethinker of Scots-Irish descent. Hutcheson had little time for the narrow musings of Bernard de Mandeville, arguing instead that in a free market income that was not spent on luxury would soon find its way to the prudent purchase of something else. Hutcheson believed the self to be a collection of the senses—those consciously registered and otherwise—of which benevolence and morality were particularly important, reflecting an interactive mental process "by which we perceive virtue or vice, in ourselves or others." The interactive principles that lay behind these ideas impressed Smith and in later years were to profoundly influence his own thinking, teaching, and writing. After Glasgow came an unhappy period of private study while Smith was on a scholarship at Balliol College, Oxford—made palatable only by reading Hume's *Treatise of Human Nature*—after which he returned to Scotland and to the intellectual excitement of Edinburgh, then the crucible of the Scottish Enlightenment. There in 1750 he met David Hume, who soon befriended him.

Adam Smith was not a doctrinaire free trader, as he is frequently caricatured, but a careful student of human behavior who thought deeply about social issues. From the influence of his two great teachers, Hutcheson and Hume, he came to recognize that any study of society must begin with an understanding of human interaction as it is expressed in everyday living. Hume had laid the foundations for a social theory of human nature based on *sentiment as a civilizing process*, and Smith soon took up the task with enthusiasm, seeking to align it with his growing interest in moral behavior, commerce, and theories of political economy.

In Edinburgh in 1748 Smith began a series of lectures that were to form the basis of his first great work *The Theory of Moral Sentiments*, published in 1759. Smith, in step with Hume, believed that progress in human affairs was grounded in the passions and the pursuit of life's necessities, but he was repelled by Mandeville's assertion that in the marketplace public benefits arose primarily from private vices. He felt that human nature was expressed not only in an instinct for survival and in the display of the basic passions but also in diverse capacities—

creativity, aestheticism, industry, invention, spirituality, and compassion being among them. Didn't these qualities and an interest in the lives of others, Smith asked, also engage the mind, satisfy the natural appetites, and foster prosperity? Within this framework—as Nicholas Phillipson, a leading scholar of the Scottish Enlightenment and author of *Adam Smith: An Enlightened Life*, has described it—*The Theory of Moral Sentiments* "was Smith's extraordinary attempt to develop a coherent and plausible account of the processes by which we learn the principles of morality from common experience, without descending into Mandevillian cynicism." At its core *Moral Sentiments* is a book about human interaction and the nature of sympathy, "on which all forms of human communication ultimately depend."

In Smith's analysis sympathy—or what he called "social sentiment"—went beyond the ability to communicate one's compassion to others, as Hume essentially had characterized it, to the capacity to imagine what others feel, to what today we call empathy. Consider that you are in a torture chamber, suggested Smith, witness to your brother on the rack. "Though our brother is upon the rack, as long as we ourselves are at our ease, our senses will never inform us of what he suffers. They never did, and never can, carry us beyond our own person, and it is by the imagination only that we can form any conception of what are his sensations. . . . By the imagination we place ourselves in his situation, we conceive ourselves enduring all the same torments, we enter as it were into his body . . . and thence form some idea of his sensations. . . . And we tremble and shudder at the thought of what he feels."

This capacity for fellow feeling through *imagination* Smith considered to be the basis of individual moral judgment and the essential glue that holds a free society together. The moral teaching of the time—an extension of the Christian virtues—was that we must first examine our own actions and use the results of this self-examination to judge the actions of others. Smith turned this idea upside down, arguing that in practice, as social creatures, we first observe the (moral) behaviors of others in infancy, and during maturation, as we become aware that we too are under scrutiny, we learn to judge ourselves. This iterative process of social exchange, beginning in childhood, achieves the self-benefit of an objective self-awareness—an "impartial spectator" or conscience—through which we develop the ability to judge our own behavior and the capacity for self-command in expressing ourselves to others. Sympathy alone is insufficient in holding society together: it is a deeper empathy—*the social sentiment of imagining oneself in the other's shoes*—that fosters moral development and underpins social order.

In these musings on moral sentiment we find conceptual links with Smith's later writings in *The Wealth of Nations*. The intellectual thread running through his examination of moral life in *The Theory of Moral Sentiments* is that a spontaneous and unintended social order emerges through the continuous and dynamic exchange of information among individuals. This concept of dynamic exchange is also the key principle Smith employs in analyzing the system of human relationships that is a market economy. Thus as James Otteson, professor of philosophy at Wake Forest University, has asserted in *Adam Smith's Marketplace of Life*, Smith's writings on human behavior follow a consistent theme, specifically that in the pursuit of mutual sympathy the exchange leads to an ordering of morality in society, while the individual search for better economic conditions spawns the barter and exchange of the market.

Smith's insights are profound. Living in society, we are interdependent and continuously in need of the assistance of others. We seek such assistance in our own self-interest, but we must also appeal to the self-interest of others to achieve what we need, both in seeking affection and in serving our material needs. As Smith famously noted in *The Wealth of Nations*: "It is not from the benevolence of the butcher, the brewer, or the baker that we expect our dinner, but from their regard to their own interest. We address ourselves, not to their humanity, but to their self-love." In the market as in the free society, we seek to establish bargains of mutual benefit through a sympathetic understanding of the mindset of others. While the market may not be the most elegant instance of the exercise of human motivation, in the words of Adam Gopnik—the essayist and *New Yorker* staff writer—"it is the most insistent: everybody has skin in the game." Thus, as in sustaining the moral code, the give-and-take of the market efficiently serves everyday necessity, finding its own natural order not by some preconceived plan but through a multiplicity of peaceable, mutually agreed-upon transactions.

Within this dynamic social framework, Smith asserted, the survival instinct of self-love—what today we call self-interest—was God's "incomprehensible remedy" (or as Mandeville preferred, mankind's "lust for self-improvement") through which a self-regulating economic order could be achieved. When appropriately shaped through barter— through mutually beneficial market exchange—self-interested action made possible a society where the products of individual labor are fairly traded, guided as if by an "invisible hand," thus placing a decent life within the reach of all. In a free-market economy we all become both actors and spectators upon the social stage: we pursue our desires but hold greed consciously in check to win the "sympathetic" acceptance of others and to enhance our personal reputation within the social group. In summary, Smith's argument went, it is the passion of self-love, together with the instinctual drives of curiosity and ambition, that fuel the engine of the market society while social sentiment and the individual conscience of the impartial spectator function as the regulators of our behavior, placing brakes upon deviance and greedy excess.

Smith's formulation of a self-regulating market society is an idealized conception. Under certain social conditions—such as those that still prevailed in the predominantly agrarian economy of Smith's own time—it does have considerable integrity. Given the adoption of a few moral rules—a respect for private property, standard monetary agreements, and honesty in exchange—locally capitalized markets do sustain their own rational order, precisely because they are built upon an interlocking system of personal relationships bound by an accepted morality. But as the eighteenth-century moved toward its close—even as the Lunar men met in Birmingham and Smith labored in Edinburgh over what was to become his *Wealth of Nations*—society was changing, and Smith's delicate balance was changing with it. Today behavioral neurobiology helps us understand why that was so.

Economic markets are complex, homeostatic systems, and like all such systems they trend toward spontaneous order and equilibrium. As shown in Figure 3.1, I find it useful to imagine Smith's conception of market dynamics as an apothecary's balance. Using Smith's language to describe the functional elements, on the left of the diagram are found the drivers of market activity—self-interest, curiosity, love of novelty, and social ambition. From the standpoint of neurobiology these are instinctual survival behaviors rooted in the ancient lizard core of our brain. These behaviors are stable and robust, need little reinforcement, and are the primary passions that motivate us to get out of bed each morning.

On the right-hand side of Figure 3.1, providing constraint and modulation, are the behaviors that Smith labeled collectively as "social sentiment"—the moral self-awareness and self-command embodied in Smith's metaphor of the impartial spectator. These patterns of behavior are intuitive and more complex than the market's instinctual drivers. In neurobehavioral terms these are *culturally determined and learned habits of mind that are predominantly reflexive—that is, preconscious—in operation.* In other words, it is the socially acquired, intuitive behaviors, which Smith proposed as the moral braking system for self-interest, that are the *wobbly* variable in his model. And I mean *wobbly* because the capacity of these social sentiments to constrain greed changes with changing cultural conditions. As the moral sentiment of a society erodes, the market's inherent capacity for self-regulation will shift, with unintended consequences. To pursue

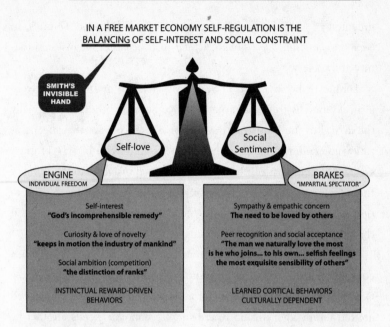

Figure 3.1: Adam Smith's concept of a free market economy is best understood as a dynamic open system that self-regulates. In this ideal conception the engines of market activity—self-interest, curiosity, and social ambition—are tempered by the desire to be loved and socially accepted. These latter sentiments, in Smith's model, are the brakes that curb greed and excess.

my metaphor of *The Well-Tempered Clavier*, with the shifting cultural climate harmony is lost as we find ourselves out of tune.

AND INDEED IN THE late eighteenth century a profound shift was on the horizon. Adam Smith and the Lunar men lived on the cusp of the wave of cultural change that was to deliver the Industrial Revolution. In a few short decades Britain moved from the traditional organization and mindset of an agricultural economy to one dominated by industrialized, capital-intensive production. The behavioral impact of this shift, which we now characterize as "modernization," was documented in 1887 by the German sociologist Ferdinand Tönnies, in *Gemeinschaft und Gesellschaft*, which in translation means "community and society."

Tönnies, who was born in Schleswig-Holstein in 1855, came from a rural family with peasant roots. Hence he had witnessed personally the arrival of the Industrial Revolution and the impact that mechanization and commercialization had upon his native culture. His brother, engaged in trade with Britain, gave him added insight into the mind of the merchant and the emphasis on profit, which was in sharp distinction to the traditional community focus where agriculture, barter, and the skills of the artisan were dominant.

For Tönnies, the transition from community to society lay on a continuum driven by this changing economic order. Sociologically *Gemeinschaft* is the descriptor for a tightly knit community organized around family and kinship where simple economic needs are met by home production and barter. This traditional community is small and stable. No change in behavior among the participants goes unnoticed, and the outlook on life is conservative. Moral sentiment is powerful as a means of social control and is reinforced through folklore, hierarchy, and an organic solidarity forged by the necessities of survival. In short, the individual is subservient to the social group.

Gesellschaft, in contrast, is the modern market society, where Smith's concept of self-interest and the division of labor drives efficiency of production such that consumption and continuous economic growth become essential to its survival. The free movement of capital and the profitable use of money are at the core of the enterprise, with market forces being the sole determinant of price. While the nuclear family still provides a social anchor, it does not dominate individual behavior, and many transient relationships exist that are driven by self-serving motives. Material production is greatly enhanced through this competition among individuals, but Smith's idealized conception of market practice being regulated by social sympathy and moral concern no longer pertains. As the equilibrium of the self-regulating market shifts and disparities in wealth accelerate, the moral regulation of individual behavior declines, and social control falls increasingly to municipal and state agencies.

Today in the developed economies of the United States and Europe the cultural narrative that defines us is *Gesellschaft*. Ubiquitous merchant enterprises, owned and controlled remotely by commercial ventures with a global reach, have replaced the local tethers of parochial self-interest that once bound communities into closely knit economic and social units. This shift in economic organization—transforming as it has energy supply, transportation, and information flow—would have been impossible without the harnessing of fossil fuels. The energy-rich affluence we enjoy today is built upon human ingenuity and the coal seams of yesterday, a history to which the likes of the Combe Mill steam engine stand in simple reminder.

In the meantime the drivers of human behavior have changed little since the Enlightenment. Bernard de Mandeville, it seems, was right after all. Under the rapidly evolving cultural circumstances of a modern, supercharged consumer society, as in my model of Smith's self-regulating economy as an apothecary scale, the balance has shifted dramatically toward the left. Reason, as Hume observed, remains the servant of the passions. Instinct—self-interest that spills all too frequently into greed—is now dominant in motivating market action. In a misreading of Adam Smith's contributions, we have cleaved his philosophy in two and lost its integrity. We focus upon *The Wealth of Nations* as a book apart from the warnings inherent in *The Theory of Moral Sentiments*; classical economics clings to a model asserting that market interference is to blame for all economic crises.

Driving this division is the conviction that in economic affairs human behavior is inherently conscious and rational, a delusion that flies in the face of common sense and the scientific evidence. *Rationality*, to follow the definition of Tony Wrigley, the preeminent Cambridge economic historian, connotes behaviors that "maximize economic return . . . when choosing between different possible courses of action." Similarly, *self-interest* is considered the adoption of behaviors designed to achieve economic advantage for the individual or nuclear family. In both instances *reflective*, conscious deliberation and rational choice are held up as the norm, despite long-standing evidence that we are not consistently rational. Meanwhile *reflexive*, preconscious decision making and the social institutions that shape our intuitive behavior are largely ignored.

It is true that on occasion, in the middle of striking a bargain around some opportunity that we are particularly eager to secure in the marketplace, we may consciously *reflect* upon the motivations of the merchant and how we can achieve the desired goal. But most of the time the choices we make are *reflexive and intuitive*, tuned through the imitation of the behavior of others and the memory-driven templates that have been fashioned from many years of marketplace experience. Here we observe the power of habits of mind—for particular brands of merchandise, for a particular merchant, or for the nostalgia of childhood experience. Thus in the consumer society does the reflective self become the puppet of reflexive choice.

ADAM SMITH'S *An Inquiry into the Nature and Causes of the Wealth of Nations* was published in 1776, the year the American colonists declared their independence from Great Britain. Smith was sympathetic toward their drive for economic freedom, just as many of the members of the Lunar Society were proponents of an American republic. Indeed, the United States of America was conceived of as the Great Experiment—the practical expression of Enlightenment thinking—a democracy to be validated by individual freedom, initiative, and hard work rather than by arbitrary authority or religion. Garry Wills, the distinguished American historian, has suggested in his book *Inventing America* that the construction of the Declaration of Independence reflects the eighteenth-century preoccupations with Newtonian science and moral philosophy. In it Thomas Jefferson—who was well versed in the writings of Locke, Hume, Hutcheson, and Smith, among others—spoke eloquently for what the leaders of the American colonists thought they were or could be.

Thus the Declaration is both a political and a moral document. The body of "self-evident truths"—the pursuit of life, liberty, and happiness that Jefferson deemed worthy of citation—were those forged from individual experience and the collective suffrage of mankind. The philosophical ideal of the Enlightenment presumed responsibility and an inner strength on the part of those individuals living in community, reflecting Smith's understanding of the moral sentiments. Liberty was viewed as the freedom to nurture one's own assets and moral virtues in the pursuit of happiness, and to develop one's own abilities in the workplace. The notion of happiness itself was a dynamic one, reflecting the well-tuned balance of desire and reason as expressed in personal accomplishment and social contribution. In this construct, rather than a fixed state of mind, the emotion of happiness is similar to the concept of price as established through market-based transaction: an ongoing index of the subjective worth that is found in social exchange.

Hence, to the enlightened mind, when the desire for gain outran the ability to satisfy it, the commonsense approach was to bridle one's desire or increase one's productive engagement—or preferably to do both. Failing such a response, the transactional adjustment is lost and misery could be expected. Today we seem to have forgotten that particular lesson. But life in colonial America was challenging—demanding physical stamina and mental ingenuity—and for the privileged Founding Few it fit such a philosophical framework. Indeed, such cultural sentiment is reflected in Benjamin Franklin's autobiography and in his thirteen virtues to be pursued in the development of inner character— perhaps establishing the roots of the self-improvement model still so attractive to the migrant mind of the American.

As is now evident, however, America's Great Enlightenment Experiment has not worked out entirely as planned. This has less to do with the erudition of Thomas Jefferson and the framers of the Declaration than with the nature of the human beast. Fundamentally motivated by self-reward, in the face of affluence we find ourselves prone to patterns of addiction, greed, and corruption. These too are "self-evident truths," although they are more painful to accept than those of Jefferson. Such truths Adam Smith clearly acknowledged—in his rejection of Mandeville, in his understanding of the development of moral sentiment, and in his optimistic striving to justify the rational market mind. Smith appreciated that his vision of a balanced, self-regulating social system based on market exchange was critically dependent upon an intuitive social understanding, but he made the mistake of presuming that such moral affinity would endure regardless of changing circumstances. For Smith in the eighteenth century, wrapped in Panglossian optimism, the conscious mind was king in market exchange, as economists of the classical persuasion still believe. Smith could not foresee a future that within a century would be fired into astonishing economic and social change by the discovery and employment of fossil fuel; nor did the Lunar men or the Founding Fathers.

Even now at the beginning of the twenty-first century we still don't quite understand what we have wrought. Despite a naïve longing to return to what is perceived as the moral simplicity of the eighteenth century and the principles of the Declaration of Independence, as exemplified by the Tea Party movement of the U.S. Republican Party, the world has changed, and the contingencies that mold our behavior have changed with it. In the face of affluence and rampant consumerism our market society is no longer in balance. We have neglected the social institutions that shape the moral autopilots of intuitive understanding—the essential long-term investments that ultimately sustain the equilibrium of the marketplace—and chosen to favor short-term competition and celebrity. Why we tend toward such myopic behavior in our approach to future challenges and where such critical choices are made in the brain is the focus of my next chapter.

Chapter 4

Choice:
The Brain's
Internal Market

> Give me the liberty to know, to utter, and to argue freely
> according to conscience, above all liberties.
>
> John Milton, *Areopagitica* (1644)

IT'S A WARM SUMMER EVENING. The train breaks from the darkness of the tunnel with a whooping whistle. Hugging the craggy hillside, it makes its stately progress toward a small Alpine village. Immaculate in their distinctive blue, cream, and gold livery, the coaches of the Orient Express glisten in the fading light. Knots of people, gathered around the bandstand in the square, turn and wave: outside a church a young couple, just married, are smiling before the cameras. In the train's dining car passengers can be seen sitting down to dinner amid art deco splendor. Then, with another whistle, the legendary express rounds a curve and is out of sight, as quickly as it came.

So what is this—perhaps a paragraph from some article in the *Condé Nast Traveller*; a fragment of nostalgia plucked from a personal diary; or the beginning of a whodunit, Agatha Christie style? Wrong on all counts, I'm afraid: it's a description of what happens on many evenings in an upstairs room of the Los Angeles home of Joaquín Fuster, a distinguished neuroscientist and one of the world's leading experts on memory, choice, and the frontal lobes of the human brain. Dr. Fuster, who has many passions, has long been a model train enthusiast.

"I've loved trains ever since I was a small boy growing up in Barcelona," Joaquín told me when I visited him and his wife, Elisabeth, for dinner one evening. The couple had met as children. "When we were small, we went to the same village for the summer vacation," she explained. But those were difficult years in Spain. Joaquín's father, a physician, had been on the losing side in the Civil War, and after World War II began, Barcelona became a fractious place to call home. For Joaquín, a young boy amid the turmoil, trains and train spotting offered tranquillity.

In Austria in the 1950s Joaquín had developed his special attachment to the Orient Express. After graduating from medical school in Barcelona, he moved to Innsbruck to continue the training in psychiatry that he had initiated in Spain. "I was intrigued by brain anatomy," he explained, "and the clinic where I was studying had an amazing collection of specimens." This fascination plus patient responsibilities frequently kept him working late, sometimes to the neglect of his sleep. But there was a fringe benefit to this nightly diligence. In the clinic, his room overlooked Innsbruck's main railway line, and every evening the Orient Express passed by on its way to Venice, exactly at midnight. The train was a romantic legend in Europe, catering to the famous and the wealthy. Adding fantasy and excitement were the popular mystery tales of Graham Greene and Agatha Christie, set aboard the Orient Express and written in the 1930s. "I never tired of that late-night spectacle and the noise and whistle of the great train," Joaquín confessed. "I found myself imagining the lives of the passengers. It became my late evening's recreation. That was long ago." He paused as his miniature express flashed before us once again. "But as you can see," he added with a smile, "the Orient Express is still speeding past my bedroom, and I'm still thinking about anatomy, memory, and how the brain works."

THE BRAIN'S SPECIALTY is managing information—its acquisition, storage, and retrieval—and choosing among alternatives to craft the actions that are necessary to sustain life. The wiring diagram of the brain is infinitely more complicated, of course, than any railway network. But what the two systems do have in common is that the function of the whole cannot be understood merely through a cataloging of individual parts. Essential to any dynamic understanding of the brain is why and how individual centers are connected and communicate. We are learning, for example, from the recently established Human "Connectome" Project—employing modern imaging technology and computer science to map the brain's pathways—that there are many nodes of local activity that are linked together by high-speed, long-distance connections. This is crudely analogous, in my train metaphor, to how London's extensive Underground rail system is connected by express surface trains to cities in the north and west of England. In both instances the critical factor is that the parts of the system function together as a dynamic whole.

The Connectome project has taken an important step forward in refining our knowledge of the brain's wiring. But that advance will just open a new chapter in our self-searching. Contrary to popular notion, the brain is not programmed like a computer to work in a serial fashion, but rather functions in parallel with information from many different senses being analyzed to achieve optimum benefit—a process not dissimilar to the bartering process that establishes price in the marketplace. What we know of the principles by which the brain achieves this wizardry, the role that memory plays in that achievement, how choices are made, how under ideal circumstance the passions and reason are integrated in that choosing, and why at times our best intentions are thwarted by habit and a preference for short-term reward are the theme of this chapter.

I start with memory in exploring these questions. Memory has been a fascination for Joaquín Fuster throughout his career—he was the first to describe the presence of active memory cells in the primate cortex—for it holds the key to understanding how the brain learns and chooses. Indeed, as an illustration of how memory works, let's take Joaquín's memory of the Orient Express, which from its inception is now decades old. To explain the retention and retrieval of an established memory, we must understand both the brain structures that enable its creation and also the neuronal mechanisms that sustain it.

Thanks to advances in neuroscience, we now know something about the anatomy and physiology of how memory is acquired: we know, for example, that the hippocampus—you will recall that there are two, one buried deep in each temporal lobe—is essential to the acquisition and imprinting of short-term memory. But what about the retention of memories over decades and their retrieval at will: where and how does that take place? Here the prime candidate for memory storage is the cortex, while active retrieval of memory especially involves the frontal lobes, which have long been the focus of Joaquín Fuster's scientific studies.

The brain, like the rest of the body organs, is pliable and renews itself. Thus cortical neurons and their communication networks are constantly being built, destroyed, and reconstituted. In Joaquín's brain, since his first youthful encounter with the legendary express, tens of thousands, probably millions, of nerve cells have been continuously restructuring their *connections* with neighboring cells in response to experience; in addition some have died and some have been damaged; others have been regenerated. And yet over decades all this activity has taken place without deterioration of the good doctor's cherished memory of the Orient Express. Thus on the evidence it is reasonable to conclude that there is no one specific area in Joaquín Fuster's brain where memories of trains are kept: that no individual nerve cell has that responsibility.

An alternative is that memories pertinent to trains, to train travel, to model railways, and so on *persist within a network*—that for neurons remembering and thinking is a collaborative activity. Memories pertinent to the Orient Express are thus sustained through the working relationships—Joaquín calls them *cognits*—that have been developed among groups of neurons. Repeated interaction among these cells has enhanced the richness of the remembrance—the colors, the smells, the sounds, and the emotions—that surrounded the original encounter. This Gestalt—this full grouping—which was first conjured in memory by the grand locomotive passing near the window of the Innsbruck clinic, is now continuously reinforced and refined by each new relevant experience—from the bustle of the Lilliputian village in the upstairs room of Joaquín's house to the real-life pleasures of the train journeys he and Elisabeth take together. Over the years information passing among brain networks has woven a tapestry of personal knowledge that has been further enriched through the power of imagination, that function of mind whereby past memories continuously shape our hopes for the future.

Memory is essential to the fundamental activities of mind, to imagination, and to self-understanding. "There is no such thing as a totally new memory," Joaquín explained to me during our evening together. "What we consider self-knowledge is the memory of facts, the relationship among those facts, and the meaning we attribute to them—gleaned both from past experience and also from what we imagine for the future." And indeed, personal experience confirms such an understanding. Reflect for a moment: close your eyes and listen to the stillness or to the sounds that surround you. Quickly you'll find your mind drifting off either to some remembrance associated with what you are hearing, or perhaps into a daydream about the future. But that image of the future will be closely tied to your personal memories, which include the culture in which you live. Memory has the power to capture not only language and pictures but also smells, sounds, emotions, meanings, and all those essentials that we associate with the subjective experience of the self.

When we recall a specific personal experience, we are not summoning to mind a literal reproduction of past events but pulling together information from different sources, from which we then "reconstruct" the past experience. While the two hippocampi, located in the temporal lobes of the brain, are responsible for the acquisition of memories, long-term memory storage is networked throughout the cortex: the neuronal traces that constitute memory are anatomically distributed in overlapping and far-flung regions of the occipital, temporal, and parietal lobes. Thus the retrieval and association of those trace elements, such as those that you have just conjured in your mind, and their assembly into meaningful memories demands the collaboration of many brain pathways. This is economical in that it avoids the need for us to remember every detail of what has happened over a lifetime, but it also means that we can make errors when remembering the past. Conversely, however, such flexibility in memory is also the key to future planning. By clustering fragments of previous experience to imagine various scenarios that might flow from a particular set of circumstances—life with a particular partner, let's say, or designing a new house—we anticipate what the future may hold. Think of it as akin to a seasoned player strategically planning future moves in a game of chess, only under real-life conditions: it is the capacity to remember the past that enables us to imagine the future.

It is Joaquín Fuster's conviction from long years of study that the aggregation of information that recreates memories of things past and that facilitates imagination of the future is physically represented in the brain's collaborative networks. The Nobel Prize–winning work of Eric Kandel, demonstrating that long-term memory in the aplysia—a large sea slug—is physiologically determined by changes in the signaling strength of the synaptic connections between nerve cells, supports Fuster's assertion and demonstrates how the fundamentals of neuronal action have been conserved across evolution. Similarly the pioneering studies of Itzhak Fried at UCLA, a neurosurgeon who has recorded directly from nerve cells in the brains of patients undergoing evaluation for epilepsy surgery, has shown that clusters of neurons can be specifically and consistently excited by familiar images. Given such evidence, it is reasonable to conclude that the activity and growth of the mind—both the *reflexive, intuitive* mind that I described in Chapter 2, and the *reflective, conscious* thinking that we each identify as the self—has its physical foundation in the connectivity and interdependence of the brain's cortical networks. Any single neuron may be part of many of these active cortical webs—Joaquín's *cognits*—and therefore may be a participant in many memories, learned behaviors, or categorized banks of knowledge. In short, who we are as unique, sentient, and free-thinking individuals is a reflection of the brain's capacity through its networked communication to distill, remember, order, and make choices using the scattered information of accumulated experience.

SO HOW DO BRAIN NETWORKS—these *cognits* of thought and memory—come into being? What drives the evolution of their organization? In simple terms the answer lies in the brain's capacity to learn, from birth and even before, through interchange with the world in which we find ourselves. It's a further simplification but a useful one that the back portion of the brain (the posterior cortex) receives input from the senses, while the anterior region (the frontal cortex) is responsible for decision making and taking action. Joaquín Fuster refers to this process of continuous exchange with the environment as the "perception-action cycle." Perception in this context does not mean just an awareness of the world as it enters the mind through the senses but includes the active sorting of new information and the interpretation of its meaning based on prior experience. Essentially, therefore, as Joaquín remarked during our discussion, perception is a tautology—"we perceive what we remember as we remember what we perceive."

This cycle of perception, learning, and action is the fundamental engine of the mind—both in development and maturity—continuously processing information from the five senses such that the action taken, be that intuitive or by conscious choice, will best meet the challenge or opportunity at hand.

The brain's learning-memory networks of the perception-action cycle, which sustain the gathering of information and inform decision making, are hierarchically organized, and their complexity evolves as the brain matures. Early in brain development those cycles fundamental to survival—the infant's ability to root out the breast and to suck, for example—have been selectively evolved through the experience of the species. Joaquín Fuster has termed these essential networks "phyletic," from *phylogeny*, the study of evolutionary relationships. These reflexive behavioral imprints are genetically preprogrammed but nonetheless operate across a perception-action cycle (see Figure 4.1). For the feeding infant, to elaborate on my example, the sensory *perception* of the mother's *smell*, the *touch* of the breast, the *taste* of milk, and the *sound* of her breathing trigger the motor program that induces the *action* of sucking. As I shall detail in Part II, refinement of this instinctual *cognit* begins immediately after birth when through experience mother and child learn from each other and quickly develop the mutual, loving attachment that ultimately is the origin of trust. The sensory inputs meld to create in the infant's mind the perception of a unique memory network of "mother." And should that rapidly developing memory circuit not be validated when being cared for by an alien "caregiver," a different motor program, one of distress and crying, is swiftly triggered.

Development occurs rapidly in those first months, and soon the infant is working daily on integrating the information perceived through the senses in the service of acquiring new motor skills. So if we return now to my illustration in Chapter 2 of the baby in the crib

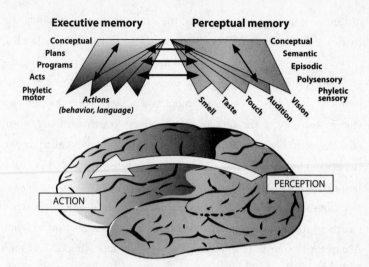

Figure 4.1: The perception-action cycle: Perceiving and sorting information that is incoming from the senses is the fundamental activity of the brain. Following assessment, based on the demands and opportunities of the immediate situation, and tempered by the memory of past experience, action is then taken. Initially these processes are driven by inherited, instinctual (phyletic) templates. These templates are rapidly enhanced by interactive experience during the years of brain maturation and the development of imagination. Ultimately it is the perception-action cycle that enables conceptual and abstract thought, the capacity that exemplifies human behavior. (Illustration based on the work of Joaquín Fuster and presented here with permission)

grasping for a colored ball, we see that *the perception-action cycle is fundamental to the development of habit and the intuitive mind.* Here the infant is already his or her own teacher, fine-tuning the cycle of perception and action through trial and error until the closing of the hand, at just the right moment, is finally mastered and the ability becomes automated.

In contrast to the phyletic preprogrammed memory of the neonate learning to suck, the networks that support many acquired and habitual behaviors—face recognition, feeding, walking, social interaction—develop with less direct genetic supervision. Specific learning in such instances is driven essentially by the strength of the stimulus that carries the information. Thus it is the close proximity of stimuli in time, their repetition and emotional meaning—as we see in language acquisition and grammar construction—that are the most important promoters of a network's development and activity. Here the immense storage capacity of the human cortex offers an extraordinary advantage. At birth this "association" cortex, as it is sometimes called, houses the computer equivalent of many gigabytes of disk space that are yet to be programmed. With maturation, however, improved insulation surrounding the neuronal axons, which are the brain's superhighways of electrical transmission, enhances the efficient transfer of information. A bare axon transmits information slowly, at approximately 20 mph, while those sheathed in the fatty insulation called myelin can conduct electricity up to 270 mph—as fast as the wind in a tornado.

In computerspeak, myelin offers "bandwidth," speeding the brain's ability to transmit information from one local network to another. However, this enhancement takes time. In the ontogeny—a fancy term for the process of development and maturation—of the individual brain, imaging studies indicate that myelination follows a genetically driven chronology. Thus the areas of the cortex responsible for limb movement, essential in learning to walk, and those domains that receive input from the vital body senses, such as sight and hearing, acquire their myelin insulation much earlier than the large association cortex, which continues to mature through adolescence and young adulthood to serve the refinement of abstract thought and complex social behavior. In the full-grown human brain myelin insulation—also called "white matter" because of its pale appearance when the brain is freshly sliced, in contrast to the pink-gray color of the areas where the nerve cells aggregate—constitutes some 42 percent of the brain's volume. Again lapsing into computer language, the mature brain thus combines megahertz processing with gigabyte storage.

This gain in efficiency has great consequence. As the frontal regions of the cortex develop and the neuronal pathways of the brain's associ-

ation areas become myelinated and efficient, the growing infant is liberated from mere physical response to immediate stimuli. Increasingly
the child moves toward conceptual thought and intellectual independence. Language, through which inner thoughts and emotions can be
communicated to others, is the key to this liberation from the sensory
world. Vocabulary expands exponentially, with symbols and imagination commanding an important place alongside the information
flowing from the senses. This leads progressively from behavior that
is principally driven by emotional attachment to others, to the use of
creative intelligence—an autonomous form of information processing,
focused on the future, through which goals and projects are conceived
and choices are made among potential action plans. Such activity, now
codified in language, develops from the broad base of knowledge that
has been acquired—both consciously and intuitively—through continuous engagement with the larger world.

Not surprisingly—although only recently confirmed—this evolving competence in managing worldly challenge is reflected in shifting
alliances among the brain's functional networks. As I explored in the
discussion about habit formation in Chapter 2, we have known for a
hundred years that the brain is in continuous conversation with itself,
even when at rest. MRI technology, however, now makes it possible to
explore, even in infants, the physiological patterns associated with this
internal communication and how they change during development.

That our brain networks are continuously and actively engaged
without our conscious awareness was brought to scientific attention
in the early 1990s, when Marcus Raichle, of the Washington School
of Medicine in St. Louis, reported that the level of brain blood-flow
activity—as measured by PET and fMRI—diminished when subjects
were *consciously* focused upon a visual task. These results came as a
surprise to the investigators, suggesting that "there was likely much
more to brain function than that revealed by experiments manipulating [conscious] demands [of the subject]." In the "resting" state it
appeared that the brain was far from idle. Raichle and his colleagues

labeled this robust "resting" neuronal activity the brain's "default mode" and proposed that it was evidence of ongoing, "stimulus independent" activity among the brain's neuronal centers.

Subsequent studies of individuals at rest—when the subjects lie quietly in the scanner thinking their own thoughts—have confirmed these initial findings of intrinsic, well-organized brain activity. Also, as was suspected, the alliances among the brain's functional networks change with age. In the infant cross talk seems to be determined largely by the anatomical proximity of the neuronal networks. However, in adolescence and early adulthood—when the neuronal superhighways have become myelinated—communication among the major network hubs appears to be driven by common functional purpose. This is also the age range within which underutilized neuronal pathways are "pruned"—destroyed—to favor networks that are being tempered to meet the needs of late adolescence. In other words, those networks particularly active survive at the expense of those less engaged with the world. Thus the networked map of the brain is tuned and adjusted in response to age and experience.

What is clear from the results of these studies—crude though they may be in drawing inference from regional blood flow and electrical activity measures—is that the brain is a busy place, even when we are daydreaming. In these "resting" states of mental activity some 60 to 80 percent of the brain's total energy requirements are consumed. Furthermore, mental tasks that demand conscious engagement add little to this resting energy burden. But what is the purpose of this intrinsic activity? Could it be that the energy consumed by the brain's networks at rest is indicative of the continuous activity of the "perception-action cycle" as we reflexively process, test, and choose among the particulars of the ongoing flood of information that we receive? In our daydreaming—I'm reminded, as I write, of Pooh Bear and his dreams of honey pots—do we catch a glimpse of the intuitive mind at work, reflexively adjusting to the chores and challenges of the everyday world and creatively imagining the opportunities that lie ahead?

Toward the end of my discussion with Joaquín Fuster I asked him what he thought of such an idea. He considered the proposition plausible. "The cortex is always active," he observed. "Through the perception-action cycle the brain is continuously at work adjusting behavior—self-organizing, if you will—to seek the best environmental fit whether we are consciously aware of it or not." To Joaquín consciousness is not a specific function of the brain but a state of heightened activity—especially in the cortex—that *evokes* subjective awareness. "To learn only consciously," he continued, "would clutter our ability to reflect on what we already know. Through memory we have a vast collection of information: hence the brain is acutely attuned to novelty. We continuously assess new opportunities and track any deviation from the expected—whether the repositioning of furniture in a room or a change in the emotional expression of a lover. This information may be brought to conscious attention only later. Indeed a huge proportion of daily life is conducted beyond conscious awareness," he added, "with action triggered by cues in the environment that intuitively resonate with established habits."

Joaquín followed with an amusing story. He had recently returned from a visit to San Francisco, where he had been giving some lectures at a professional meeting. One afternoon, free from his responsibilities, he had gone walking in the Nob Hill district and found himself irresistibly drawn to visit the Cable Car Museum. This seemed rather odd as he had visited on several previous occasions, but he followed his whim anyway and had an enjoyable afternoon. "My initial decision was certainly not a conscious one," he reflected, "but clearly a decision had been made. No doubt my fascination that afternoon with San Francisco's cable cars was nested in memories of my last trip to the city, which in turn is nested within a broader set of preconscious *cognits* tied to trams, trains, and public transportation." Joaquín laughed. "So here we are back to Innsbruck and the Orient Express. That's the perception-action cycle at work. As Freud was fond of emphasizing—although for different reasons—much of the time the brain makes choices without our conscious awareness, and then we rationalize them."

WHETHER CONSCIOUS OR INTUITIVE, *it is choosing among alternatives that determines action.* At times an instinctual drive— intense hunger, for example—will command the decision-making process. But outside such circumstances most of the choices that we make, and the actions that follow, are informed by knowledge gleaned from past experience and incoming sensory information pertinent to the immediate situation. As I have been describing in this chapter, the brain networks that evaluate our perceptions of the world operate largely outside consciousness. Memory helps guide the analysis, which is further shaped by novelty and change—these being fundamental percepts to which the brain is tuned by evolutionary adaptation. Ulti- mately, the process through which we make choices and take edu- cated action is based upon all these streams of information.

Fundamentally the brain chooses in one of two ways. The first is through acquired habit, about which we learned in Chapter 2. *This method of decision making is quick, reflexive, and stimulus-driven, with the brain architecture involved being principally that of the basal ganglia.* This mechanism underpins the brain's autopilots—tuned preconscious responses—that initially may have been acquired with conscious awareness but that have become intuitive. This decision making operates efficiently in a stable environment where actions taken have predictable and consistent outcomes.

The second method the brain has for performing decision making, which is my focus here, is fundamentally through a process of internal competition, where the relationship between an action taken—actual or imagined—and its consequence is analyzed and the information retained and coded for future reference. *This process of goal-directed action and decision making is primarily conscious and reflective and depends upon the integrity of the orbital-frontal cortex.*

The reader will remember that the orbital-frontal cortex, also known simply as the prefrontal or "executive" cortex, is the most forward portion of the brain tucked in above the eye sockets of the skull. Little was known about the function of this densely packed labyrinth when I was in medical school in the 1960s. In fact the frontal lobes were a student's nightmare. *Gray's Anatomy* offered the usual elegant drawings with a Latin name for each of the hills and valleys of the crinkled surface—names that we were forced to commit to memory in the absence of any facts to bind our understanding—but that was about it.

Classical stories in the medical archives, such as the tragedy of Phineas Gage, did offer intriguing clues, however, and suggested that the frontal cortices play an important role in planning, emotional control, and social behavior. In 1848 Gage, working as the foreman of a railroad construction gang in Vermont, suffered severe brain damage when a tamping bar he was using was driven by an accidental explosion to pierce his upper jaw, exiting through the left side of his forehead. Amazingly Gage survived the ordeal, but from that time on his calm, responsible behavior was replaced by impulsivity, emotional outbursts, and social indiscretion. Subsequently, neuropsychological assessment in persons suffering comparable frontal lobe damage, combined with brain imaging, has confirmed similar patterns of behavior and verified the executive role of the prefrontal region in regulating choice and planning.

But what of the choice that leads to action? What enables that critical step? Morten Kringelbach, senior research fellow at Queen's College, Oxford, and professor of neuroscience at Aarhus University in Denmark, believes that the key to unlocking these mysteries is acknowledging the central role of pleasure in driving human behavior. "Pleasure as a motivating force goes beyond the evolutionary imperative of physical survival," Morten explained to me one afternoon during a visit to his laboratory at the Warneford Hospital in Oxford. "Think about it. For most of us, sensory pleasures and social interaction are equally as important as eating, perhaps even more so. Those who no longer experience pleasure—those who suffer anhedonia—society considers sick, and many die by their own hand. Pleasure is central to life." As director of Hedonia: TrygFonden Research Group, and an acknowledged leader in pleasure research, Morten Kringelbach speaks with authority.

As Morten explained to me, the process of choice within the brain is dynamic and interactive. The picture that is coming together from human imaging and animal experiments confirms that the orbital-frontal cortices—there are two of them, left and right, side by side—provide the integrative forum for decision making, but that the responsibilities for processing the information upon which any choice depends are shared among several complementary domains. Unfortunately some of the old anatomical terms, derived from Latin—ventral, dorsal, medial, and lateral—remain important in orienting us to this new geography and need to be repeated here to help with my explanation. A simple aid to memory and to keeping things straight, as Morten suggested, is to think of each lobe as a room. Then, standing in the middle of the right lobe, in front of you is the ventral surface of the cortex, behind you is the dorsal pole, to the right is the lateral boundary and to the left is the inner medial wall, which then abuts the complementary medial wall of the left cortical lobe. In processing the incoming information, each area has its own set of responsibilities. In broad terms it is the medial area of the frontal cortex that continuously monitors incoming information to evaluate its potential value for pleasure and reward, whereas the lateral cortex is preoccupied with control, particularly inhibition of potentially pain-inducing actions and the modification of established behavior patterns.

From a meta-analysis of many studies, both his own and those of other investigators, Morten has constructed an anatomical map—which I reproduce in Figure 4.2—that is useful in understanding how information flows into this complex region of the frontal cortex, and the analytic functions that are performed there. In complement to Joaquín Fuster's perception-action cycle Morten's studies confirm that it is in the posterior part of the brain that perception first becomes organized. The thalamus, which is the brain's sensory collection center, aggregates information flowing from the five principal senses of taste, smell, touch, hearing, and vision together with stimuli arising from the body organs and continuously relays it forward to the posterior (dorsal) region of the orbital-frontal cortices. As it advances, this rich influx is integrated with information flowing from the vital emotional centers of the ancient limbic brain. These centers include the hypothalamus, which is responsible for hormone release and the homeostatic balance of many essential body functions; the hippocampus, where memories are created; the amygdala serving as the brain's emotional sentinel and social early warning system; and the insula, which is tuned to receive information from the body's inner world.

Thus, essentially, there are two parallel interactive cycles of perception and action: a "thinking" cycle, or cycle of reason, which courses through new cortical structures and the *lateral* prefrontal cortex, and an "emotional" cycle that integrates information from the limbic structures and the *ventral* prefrontal cortex—two cycles that in their cross talk create a dynamic and balanced whole.

This continuous inflow of primary information then continues its forward passage to initiate the action phase of the perception-action cycle. As the gathering of facts continues, knowledge from networks honed by the memory of previous experience is added to the mix, and this multisensory assemblage of information is assigned value regarding potential for reward or punishment. As is evident in Figure 4.2, the brain area responsible for this evaluative process receives its name—the ventromedial orbital-frontal cortex—from its anatomical location. When a potentially rewarding opportunity is encountered, the executive cortex figures out the value of the opportunity from its

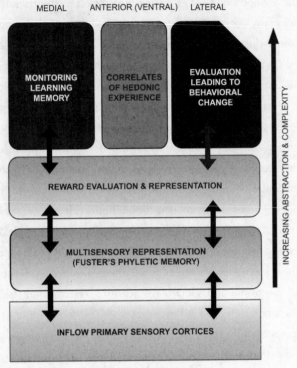

MEDIAL   ANTERIOR (VENTRAL)   LATERAL

MONITORING
LEARNING
MEMORY

CORRELATES
OF HEDONIC
EXPERIENCE

EVALUATION
LEADING TO
BEHAVIORAL
CHANGE

REWARD EVALUATION & REPRESENTATION

MULTISENSORY REPRESENTATION
(FUSTER'S PHYLETIC MEMORY)

INFLOW PRIMARY SENSORY CORTICES

INCREASING ABSTRACTION & COMPLEXITY

POSTERIOR (DORSAL)

Figure 4.2: Choice and the executive brain: The diagram represents the functions of the frontal cortices (the right half is illustrated) as information moves forward and choices are made. Decoded sensory information continuously flows into the frontal lobes from the primary sensors of the brain and body—from the organs of touch, smell, taste, hearing, and vision. As it advances, the information is integrated through the activity of the posterior parts of the prefrontal lobes and assigned a reward value as it moves forward. From there the new information can shape behavioral choice (through the ventrolateral prefrontal region), be compared with past experience, and then be stored in memory (in the ventromedial cortex) or be assessed regarding its potential hedonic (pleasurable) experience. The subjective reward value of the incoming experience also is modified by the prevailing internal state of the body (e.g., hunger). Continuous communication among the prefrontal cortices and other brain regions, such as the amygdala and the nucleus accumbens, further assesses risk and refines the choices that are made. (Illustration based on the work of Morten Kringelbach and presented here with permission)

potential for pleasure when compared to previous experience: it is only then that the optimal behavioral action is chosen. When we choose something to eat, for example, studies suggest that the orbital-frontal cortex anticipates the subjective pleasure and nutritional value of the food available based on past experience and current information and then decides the potential reward value of eating it.

As Morten suggested during the afternoon of my visit, if this all seems a little complicated, then try thinking of the process as a virtual market operating within the brain—a place where information is collected, value is established, and choices are made. Imagine that you are in the market to buy something significant, let's say a new car. What are the assessments—the checks and balances that you would go through—to ensure that the vehicle you buy is the one that will best serve your needs, that you can afford, and that you will enjoy driving? To make such a choice, most of us first gather as much information as is possible about the product, its availability, the company that makes it, our past experience with similar vehicles, its relative price, and so on.

This process, familiar to each of us, is one comparable in many ways to that which goes on in the orbital-frontal cortex at the culmination of the perception-action cycle. Different pathways within the brain—different functional networks—bring information to the orbital-frontal cortex where they compete for distinction, just as in a marketplace. In the brain, however, the index of "support" for the choice ultimately adopted—or "purchased," if you will—is based not on competitive price but on the number of neurons firing in unit time and/or the signal strength of the synaptic connections between participating nerve cells, until a level of critical discharge is reached and action is initiated.

In the brain, making choices is not a sporadic activity but a process designed to produce continuous, adaptive improvement with pleasurable experience as the goal. To follow the market analogy, the orbital-frontal cortex maintains a sophisticated online evaluation of all the business transactions, including associated opportunities and disappointments, in which you have been previously engaged—a comprehensive catalogue that enables rapid response to changing circumstances. This together with the brain's network plasticity offers great flexibility in choice and action.

The reward value—the subjective pleasure—associated with any prior experience is stored in memory and recorded by the ventromedial region of the executive brain, a brain area found to be particularly active in Marcus Raichle's "resting" blood flow studies. Thus, as Morten Kringelbach describes it, *the ventromedial area of the frontal cortex is the guardian of preference based upon memories of previous pleasures.* I think of it as that part of the cortex that establishes hedonistic value and fuels the engines of self-interest— the "animal spirits"—that drive Adam Smith's model of the self-regulating market.

The ventro*lateral* prefrontal cortex, on the other hand, is the braking system of Smith's model, focused primarily on planning and making choices that will keep us safe for the future: *the ventrolateral cortex is thus the brain's agent of "self-control."* Should curiosity or the pleasures of self-indulgence compromise safety or sensible adaptation, it is the ventrolateral prefrontal cortex, especially on the right side of the brain, that springs into restraining action. Think of it, therefore, as analogous to a voice of conscience, or to Adam Smith's impartial spectator.

IN THE MARKETPLACE barter is all about balancing the risk of loss and pain against the reward of pleasure and profit. And that is exactly what the orbital-frontal cortex has evolved to do. In simplistic terms, the ventrolateral prefrontal cortex is concerned about risk while the ventromedial prefrontal region is resolutely committed to hedonistic pursuit. Ideally the two brain regions are tuned through experience to collaborate when it comes to choice of action. To paraphrase what

David Hume emphasized two centuries ago, while it is passion (the ventromedial cortex) that drives us, any call to action is played out within the theater of reason (the ventrolateral cortex) where "perceptions . . . glide and mingle" to test an "infinite variety" of alternatives. *In reality, however, the two brain regions are inherently in competition.* This becomes particularly evident when the timing of a reward is entered into the equation. Why, for example, do we procrastinate in making long-term plans, both as individuals and as a society? Why do New Year resolutions last only for a week or two? A personal anecdote will help illustrate my point.

In Los Angeles, in the neighborhood where I live, there is a small French-Canadian bistro named Soleil. It's along Westwood Boulevard, on a corner close to the bookstore and just down from a string of Iranian shops. The people who go there seem to like each other. It's good value, lively, and unpretentious. Pictures of Vincent Van Gogh's famous sunflowers are on the wall, and there's something suggestive—intended, I'm sure—of the artist's little house in Arles, except I know the cooking is better, much better.

Luc Alarie, the owner-chef, is from Montreal. He's a big man with an impish grin: he might be imagined playing hockey for the Montreal Canadiens, if he weren't so generous and funny. The menu is everything you ever hoped for in a French bistro; escargots, boeuf bourguignon, grilled steaks with peppercorn sauce, and of course french fries. Once you've dug into a basket of those thin, crispy fries at Soleil, you're hooked. As a confirmed addict, I try to be circumspect, going only with friends and insisting that we share.

On the particular January evening I have in mind there were three of us. We were celebrating something, I can't recall exactly what, but we were in a good mood, and so was Luc. There was plenty of banter. We had eaten well too, despite the New Year resolve to cut back on the calories: escargots, a tasty coq au vin, wine, and the essential basket of fries. We agreed we were stuffed and content: no dessert tonight, thank you, we told Luc when he made his rounds, just the bill. *"Mon dieu, c'est impossible,*" cried our host, hands in the air. "Tonight I have prepared the special Montreal caramel cheesecake, just for you!" No, no we protested; we're full. "For this, *mes amis, mais non!*" retorted Luc. We protested again, not a bite more, until finally Luc withdrew, looking crestfallen. We gave a sigh of relief. The bill arrived. Then suddenly Luc was back, grinning broadly and bearing a plate with a slice of his latest triumph—the caramel cheesecake—together with three forks. "Just a little taste," he explained, placing the dish proudly before us. We exchanged glances. "Go. Try it," added Luc, still smiling. We looked at each other again. Two minutes later the plate was empty.

There is nothing unique about this little pantomime, of course, for it is repeated every evening in millions of restaurants across America. George Ainslie, who is professor of psychiatry at Temple University in Philadelphia and one of the first to study this phenomenon, calls it "inter-temporal or delayed discounting"—when in the face of imme- diate reward future outcomes are undervalued. Ainslie's studies con- firm my experience at the Soleil restaurant: essentially what happened was that the short-term anticipated pleasure of the tasty cheesecake momentarily outweighed the long-term value of avoiding rich foods. For the brain in the short term it is not the logic of a decision but internal barter that establishes value.

A cornerstone of classical economic theory is that human beings exercise rational self-interest when bartering and choosing—that over time we are dependable in decision making, consistently seek- ing maximum utility. If this were so, then our preferences could be described by an *exponential* curve, where a larger reward would always have greater value than one that is smaller, regardless of its timing. Unfortunately such an orderly pursuit of goals is far from the norm. Laboratory studies confirm Ainslie's concept of intertemporal bargain- ing, with the timing of a potential reward significantly influencing the final decision. Thus human decision making is best described as being *hyperbolic*. As the possibility of receiving a small reward draws closer in time, it becomes more attractive until, briefly, it is preferred over a larger opportunity that is delayed.

The study of intertemporal discounting offers a special window through which to observe the brain's internal market in operation. Research using fMRI technology confirms that separate brain systems are responsible for evaluating immediate and delayed rewards. In general these studies suggest that short-term impulsiveness, as we would predict, is driven by the ancient limbic structures and the nucleus accumbens, which is home to the dopamine reward pathways. These ancient systems are in league with the ventromedial orbital-frontal region of the cortex—which is deeply involved, as you will recall, in tracking the subjective pleasure associated with prior experience. The assessment of the potential payoff from investment in long-term reward, on the other hand, is the responsibility of the ventrolateral regions (the brain's braking system) and the dorsal regions of the prefrontal cortex especially on the right side of the brain—all of which fits well with the analysis provided by Morten Kringelbach, which I reviewed earlier.

Of particular interest is that both the long-term *constraining* and *liberating* roles exerted on behavior by the ventrolateral orbital-frontal cortex appears to be *independent* of reward timing: it's simply that the brain's capacity for constraint loses out to the lure of potential reward when the short-term bartering becomes intense. The orbital-frontal network, which we know to be involved in long-range planning, delayed gratification, and abstract thinking, is dominant in activity when the potential reward is in the distant future, but as the reward moves closer in time, its comparative influence diminishes, and the short-term pleasure seeking of the ventromedial cortex, the limbic system, and the dopamine-reward system rapidly prevails in determining choice. This is the same brain architecture that research has found to be consistently associated with impulsive behavior and addiction, which helps explain why other sensory triggers associated with desire—including touch, smell, and sight—are closely tied to craving and impulsive behavior. Also, on the mundane level, it aids in understanding why food tastes that we rarely encountered in our evolutionary history—such as sweetness reflected in caramel cheesecake—can easily override good intentions and a well-satisfied appetite, simply because of the powerful promise of hedonic gratification that such food evokes, especially when you can see and smell it.

SO WHAT HAVE we learned? One lesson is certain: in our choices, we human beings are short-term opportunists; we are wired that way. In the language of neuroscience, without conscious effort to achieve the contrary, delayed discounting will trump responsibility. Over the centuries, when we were small in numbers and coping with dangerous and depriving environments, this propensity to grasp immediate opportunity served us well in the fight for survival. But the world is changing: now there are many of us—many billions—and why, how, and what we choose will make a critical difference over the long term. Sustaining a focus on the future is particularly challenging in the consumer-driven society, regardless of political persuasion, when immediate gratification becomes the coin of the realm. With the complicity of the conscious self, in our intuitive habits we find ourselves drawn into a Faustian bargain, one that limits our capacity for long-term planning. In exchange for an abundance of immediate choice, delayed discounting becomes the brain's default mode; inadvertently we are retuning and rewiring our neural architecture, further reinforcing our propensity for short-term opportunism.

On the surface the brain's two systems of choosing—that of the *reflexive*, stimulus-driven decision making of habit and the goal-directed *reflective* choice, where the action taken is sensitive to consequence—appear to be distinct entities. In reality, however, they overlap in their function and responsibilities, and each can reinforce the behavior of the other. Both can help determine what we do next. In a feedback loop of learning and memory, how habits are tuned either reinforces or inhibits reflective choice.

Habit, as I have noted before, *is potentially an intuitive force for good*, both in fostering efficiency of mind and in sustaining the cultural web that knits together human society. So in Los Angeles, even on a Sunday morning when there are few cars on the road, I intuitively drive down the right side of Wilshire Boulevard despite it being an eight-lane highway with plenty of space for creative maneuvering. This is habit—reflexive tuning—actively at work supporting public safety. I do not think about my behavior. When visiting England, however, even though I was born there, my retuned, reflexive American mindset is dangerous, and I must consciously pay attention when driving on the left.

In the social context habit is conformity. Such social norms are evident in all cultures—in dress codes, in diet, in mannerisms, in beliefs, and so on—and they can be extraordinarily powerful in shaping behavior. In our home culture how much time we spend consciously thinking about any social norm—driving on the right; whether global warming exists; that self-interest, economic growth, and the consumer society are good for America—is an inverse measure of its influence. Once a cultural mindset is pervasive, however, the orthodoxy becomes self-reinforcing, and we conform without thinking. We "rewire" the brain's tuning, or as the psychologist Joshua Epstein has described it, writing in *Computational Economics*, "we *learn* to be thoughtless."

In doing so we compromise choice. In "thoughtlessly" becoming economically and emotionally dependent upon habitual consumption, we distort the brain's internal market. The habit centers of the basal ganglia, now in cahoots with the pleasure-loving ventromedial prefrontal region and its limbic allies, do battle against the scolding constraint of its neighbor the ventrolateral prefrontal cortex. It's not much of a competition, as I discovered when faced with Luc's caramel cheesecake. When immediate opportunity reinforces our hedonistic preferences, the capacity for personal restraint loses most of the time. Today, in our headlong, turbocharged commercial pursuit, we have inadvertently overtaxed the brain's internal braking system. As individuals and as a society, we find ourselves off balance.

Chapter 5

Market Mayhem:
Of Museums and Money

> This division of labour, from which so many advantages
> are derived, is not originally the effect of any human wis-
> dom. It is the necessary, though very slow and gradual
> consequence of a certain propensity in human nature
> which has in view no such extensive utility; the propen-
> sity to truck, barter, and exchange one thing for another.
>
> Adam Smith, *The Wealth of Nations* (1776)

I SPENT THANKSGIVING 2008 in New York City and over that
weekend visited an exhibition, *Beyond Babylon*, that had just opened
at the Metropolitan Museum of Art. In retrospect its focus—the
trading practices among Mediterranean city-states in the late Bronze
Age—seems ironic, even satiric. Only ten weeks earlier trading on
Wall Street had taken a dramatic and dangerous downturn, just as the
Bronze Age economy, some four millennia earlier, had staggered and
suddenly buckled.

Over four catastrophic days in mid-September the Dow Jones average had plunged a thousand points, only to whipsaw back on talk of
possible broad government intervention. By the end of the week the
world had lost Lehman Brothers, a 158-year-old investment bank,

and AIG—the insurance giant American International Group—had declared that to avoid bankruptcy it needed a $70 billion bailout from the Federal Reserve. It was a week, as *The Wall Street Journal* observed with uncharacteristic lament, that was destined to change American capitalism. Shocks of this magnitude had not been felt since the Great Depression, and soon the world's financial markets were frozen in fear. By early October virtually every traded asset seemed to be collapsing: in just one week the S&P 500 index would lose over 20 percent of its value, affecting investors worldwide. The Great Recession, the first of the new millennium, was under way. Much as the interwoven fortunes of the Bronze Age dynasties had suffered, similarly the whole financial fabric of the global economy appeared ready to rip apart.

Using what I learned from my museum visit and the financial meltdown of 2008, in these next pages I draw out the common neurobehavioral threads that have characterized our market behavior over millennia. But more particularly, using the finance industry as my case study, I will highlight how the ancient instinctual driver of myopic self-interest, together with shifting cultural habits and changing social regulations, eroded self-restraint to trigger market mayhem. I conclude, as Mark Twain is purported to have observed, that while human history may not repeat itself, it surely does rhyme, offering valuable lessons for the future.

MARKETS EMERGE WHEREVER people congregate: along a riverbank, in a courtyard, and on a village street. The ideal marketplace reflects human need and desire, a distillate of our labors, hopes and fears. In contemporary Western culture we accept that fundamental to market exchange is the freedom to choose. It is the seller and the buyer together that determine the value of the goods, based on personal preference. Without the freedom of individual choice and the protection of property, there is no market. Thus today we defend markets, as Adam Smith described them, to be "the simple and obvious system of natural liberty." This is our contemporary understanding, but it is one that has been in evolution for thousands of years.

Barter and exchange are older than the practice of agriculture. The mutual interchange of favors—the reciprocal grooming seen in nonhuman primates, or the exchange of gossip in our own species—plays an essential role in sustaining group cohesion in social animals. Long ago we learned that such reciprocation was a fine alternative to fighting: "if you scratch my back, then I'll scratch yours," as the saying goes. Once we outgrew the social economy of the nomadic hunting band and began to live in larger, relatively stable groups with tasks divided among individuals, it was a natural evolution to build upon such reciprocity—be it for affection or to satisfy physical need—offering to others what we did not require for ourselves. Similarly as communities grew in complexity, trade among them became essential to survival. Rarely could a single cluster of individuals, however skilled and talented, provide everything that was needed, often even at a subsistence level. Thus as human settlements evolved—long before money was invented to facilitate market exchange, and an eternity before Adam Smith published his influential tome—the division of labor and the trading of surplus goods was a social imperative.

In the late Bronze Age the Mediterranean was a trading hub. This was pressed home at the Metropolitan exhibition by a brilliantly colored satellite image of the eastern Mediterranean, rimmed to the north by the mountains of Anatolia. It was a reminder that four thousand years ago this punch bowl of blue water was central to commerce, supporting a vigorous sea trade that complemented overland caravan routes and was vital to the transport of grains, oils, and precious metals among the hinterland empires and their ruling families.

At the core of the exhibition were artifacts salvaged from a Bronze Age trading vessel, which had been discovered off the Turkish coast. Carbon dating of wood found aboard the ship suggests that it sank around 1300 B.C., making it the world's oldest known shipwreck. Cape Uluburun, after which the wreck was named, is a spit of land on the southwestern coast of Anatolia situated just before the peninsula crumbles into the Aegean Sea, creating the scattering of islands that on the map appear as stepping-stones to Greece. It is an area of stunning beauty, as I can attest from having sailed there. On many days a turquoise sea complements a sun-drenched sky of azure blue with scudding white clouds hanging over red sandstone cliffs. But it is dangerous too: the currents close to shore are treacherous and the rocks jagged, and with the weather patterns given to violent storms, even in the summer months, it can be a deadly place—as it had been for the Uluburun merchants.

The wonderful thing about ancient shipwrecks is that they provide a unique slice of history, where the mundane details of life—in peace and in war—are frozen in time. So it is with the Uluburun wreck: in addition to some ten tons of Cyprus copper plus tin from Central Asia—potentially enough bronze to equip a small army—it was carrying amphorae filled with oils, olives, and grains, as well as a rich cargo of finished goods. This was a vessel of considerable wealth making its way west to the Aegean Sea.

The late Bronze Age is a particularly colorful period in Mediterranean history, one remembered and embellished in the epic poems of Homer. Presuming the carbon dating to be accurate, the Uluburun vessel would have met its fate approximately a century before the violent siege of Troy by the Mycenaean Greeks and the collapse of the other hitherto vibrant trading empires in the eastern Mediterranean. For the previous several centuries sophisticated feudal societies had thrived in the region, including the Hittite empire of Anatolia, a superpower of the era.

Trade had been essential to the growth of the great empires and cultural centers of the aristocracy, which when not allied with one another were frequently at war. Money was unknown. Commerce flourished among these ruling elites as a sophisticated barter system, the oldest form of human exchange. This practice was ritualized as reciprocal "gifting"—essentially a prenegotiated contract—where ambassadors and merchants representing the powerful feudal families delivered cargoes of dowry or tribute, favors that later would be repaid through further gifting. Overland caravans connecting the great cities of Egypt, Mesopotamia, and the Hittite empires of the Anatolian peninsula were complemented by the seafaring Syrians and Canaanites—and the powerful Mycenaean Greeks—who traded between North Africa, Cyprus, Crete, and the Aegean. Driven in large part by the need to acquire essential raw materials and staple goods, this economic interdependence also promoted fine craftsmanship and an expanded cultural understanding.

Bronze was a commodity particularly prized and traded. The dull brown metal that we now associate with church bells, plumbing fixtures, and statues commemorating the Great War is one of the most versatile of alloys. Its discovery—through trial and error in the smelting of metal ore—had marked a significant technical advance. Created primarily from copper, strengthened by combining it with tin, bronze was the essential metal in the manufacture of tools, weapons, and body armor and was something to fight over, much as we fight over oil today. With the island of Cyprus being a principal source of copper ore, sea trade was not only attractive but also fostered the transport of other cargo: pottery jugs being carried from Greece were filled with oil or with wine from Egypt, to be exchanged for grain from Babylonia or ebony from Africa.

Sea voyages during this period of Mediterranean history were risky and dangerous. Navigation was primitive, and vessels were square-rigged, which means they sailed best with a following wind, essentially limiting sea travel to the summer months, when northwesterly winds prevail in the eastern Mediterranean. Thus a ship setting sail from Greece had a fair chance of finding Africa. But the return voyage had to be made counterclockwise, keeping the coast of the Levant and Anatolia in sight. That helps explain why the Uluburun wreck was found so close to shore: caught in an unexpected squall, a heavily laden squared-rigged vessel frequently ended up on the rocks, with little chance of survival.

And indeed the Uluburun vessel was heavily laden. Personal artifacts recovered suggest that the merchants had set sail from Tell Abu Hawam, a Canaanite port in what is now northern Israel. Also, judging by the number of copper ingots and the dozens of mint-condition Cypriot bowls and tableware packed in large ceramic jars, the ship had made call in Cyprus before continuing its journey west, hugging the shoreline of Anatolia. It must have been just days later, failing to navigate the rocky promontory of Cape Uluburun, perhaps in a storm, perhaps through error, that it foundered. Skittering down a rocky escarpment, the broad-beamed vessel came to rest in deep water, complete with crew and cargo, there to remain for more than three thousand years.

Archaeological detective work indicates that three or four Syrian-Canaanite merchants were aboard the ship. There's also good evidence that two Mycenaean Greeks of elite status were traveling homeward. Two bronze swords and elegant personal effects including tableware, razors, and beads—all of Mycenaean manufacture—plus drinking sets and knives from that region support this conclusion. A third, rather shadowy figure, armed with sword, spearheads, and a mace, appears to have been from northern Greece or even the Balkans, implying that he may have been a mercenary employed for protection of the ship's company and its cargo against piracy.

Certainly the Uluburun's cargo contained much that would please a pirate. The extraordinary workmanship reflected in the gleaming objects beckoning from behind their safety glass that afternoon at the museum was a reminder that the powerful dynasties of the age not only competed for bronze to maintain their military might but also sought to outdo one another artistically. I found the artifacts on display compelling: their beauty dispelled any notion that a nimble mind, a dexterous hand, and an instinct for design might be recently acquired human attributes. In this era before money, prestige items of high quality were a mark of social status, just as now, and indispensable as gifts. But they were also essential in the payment of bribes and tolls for those seeking access to goods and raw materials not available at home.

Since Adam Smith we have come to think of a market economy as driven by personal choice. You like something, and you have the money—or the credit—and you simply buy it. Not so in the Bronze Age. The economy of the time was shaped not by individual consumption but by the exercise of power among ruling families. These so-called palace economies were hierarchically organized and rigidly controlled, with all goods and services being the property of the ruling monarch. Such communities, sometimes thirty or forty thousand strong, emerged initially in fertile valleys and were built upon an agricultural surplus: this was then mobilized to administer a tithe economy, to sustain an army, to indulge the whim of a priestly-warrior class, and eventually to support a social elite living in luxury. A successful agricultural village, where the inhabitants worked side by side, was thus slowly transformed into a hierarchical society.

Maintaining order in such centrally controlled economies and protecting the wealth accumulated was not easy for the ruling elite. Natural hazards were always lurking, but ever present too, given the cunning of men, was the fear of fraud and deceit. To guard against such risks, the powerful families assembled not only large chariot-based armies—hence the voracious appetite for bronze—but also employed their own overseers. These loyal traders and "ambassadors," such as the Mycenaean Greeks thought to have sailed with the Uluburun, were responsible for determining the value of the goods traded and for ensuring the security of their exchange.

The value of most commodities was determined by weight. Thus some 139 weights were salvaged from the Uluburun wreck, most well used. Some were cast in the shape of animals—a frog, a duck, a reclining bull, the head of a lion, and even a fly—presumably for rapid identification.

Accuracy mattered: hence seasoned merchants had to hand a set of weights for the precise measure of valuable metals such as gold and silver and another for assessing the value of heavier goods. In the bulk bartering of oils and grains, volume was widely accepted as a rough measure of weight and thus value. Two handled amphorae—the tall elegant earthenware jars, miniature painted versions of which can be found in every tourist town in Turkey and Greece—were the shipping containers of the day. When crafted with a conical base they were easily and securely stowed by pressing them into the sand of the ship's ballast. Hence amphorae were used for the sea transport of just about everything, including wine, olive oil, grains, fish, and even pottery.

By the late Bronze Age goods were traded over vast distances and across lands where diverse peoples spoke many languages and merchants regularly spent months, even years, away from home and family. Thus the *securing* of transactions against the risk of fraud was an ongoing problem. Although the cuneiform inscription of clay tablets was widely used for accounting and for sending messages among the elites, most people could neither read nor write. It was the widespread adoption of "seal" stones, employing the universal language of pictures, that first sidestepped this problem and helped reduce the risk in international trading. A "seal" was a carved cylinder of rock crystal or some other semiprecious stone that served to identify the bearer: think of it as the forerunner of the personalized credit card. The seal was carved with symbolic figures and pictures that were specific to its owner and to his place of business, such that when the seal was rolled over wet clay or wax, the resulting set of images created a unique signature. When it became time to "seal" a business deal—a phrase that remains with us—this simple tool provided a tangible record of ownership, receipt, or purchase.

Bronze Age trade was "profitable" when it sustained a political alliance. Hence the distribution of goods was driven principally by relationships among families and palaces, not by individuals and prices. Profit seeking and haggling were reserved for fringe markets operating in neutral territory, where powerful but hostile empires could trade through emissaries. These markets also gave an opportunity for local producers to trade beyond their immediate social circle. A fringe benefit of this cultural mix of mogul and market was the flowering of creativity among many professionals and artisans. The major dynasties competed for the best warriors but also for the finest builders, physicians, poets and musicians; and for the most exotic works of art. The result was a far-reaching web of international trade fostering extraordinary human enterprise.

AND THEN, MOST SUDDENLY, it all came tumbling down. Within a few short decades, between approximately 1200 and 1150 B.C., the economies of the eastern Mediterranean feudal states collapsed, bringing to an end the Hittite, Trojan, and Greek-Mycenaean empires and severely challenging the stability of Egypt. Exactly what happened is still a matter of intense debate among scholars. The ultimate impact, however, is clear: as Robert Drews suggests in his authoritative study, *The End of the Bronze Age*, politically and culturally the collapse was a catastrophe greater than the fall of the Roman Empire. At the core of the mystery are descriptions of well-armed attackers who came in from the western Mediterranean, from the Aegean and beyond, to decimate vital port cities and commercial centers. In the nineteenth century archaeologists called them the "Sea People," and the name has stuck. It is unclear, however, whether these marauders were the root cause of the collapse or itinerant pirates plundering the already internally crippled but still rich feudal empires.

One controversial but intriguing proposal put forward by Eberhard Zangger, a geologist educated at Stanford University and now working in Switzerland, suggests that the events leading up to the Greek-Trojan war and the siege of Troy in approximately 1195 B.C. hold the key to the riddle. Drawing inspiration from archaeological evidence and the historical narratives of Homer and Plato—admittedly stories of literary license that were several hundred years in genesis—Zangger argues that the equilibrium of political and military power in the western Mediterranean was shifting in the late Bronze Age.

The growing strength of these dueling Aegean peoples—the Mycenaean Greeks and the Trojans—was straining the long-established and previously dominant Hittite empire of Anatolia, which was also being challenged from the east by Assyria. Under this pressure and seeking to control their vital source of copper and the supply routes of grain from Egypt, the Hittites had invaded Cyprus, further angering their seafaring western neighbors. Troy and its allies, for their part, had slowly achieved control of the many islands in the eastern Aegean from which, some suspect, the "Sea People" may have come. The Trojans also controlled the important maritime trade route through the Dardanelles to the Black Sea, thus exacerbating their long-standing conflict with the Mycenaean Greeks and ultimately leading to the siege of Troy to which Homer gave poetic immortality.

While, as some believe, changing weather patterns with periodic drought and the disruption of local crop production may have worsened the mounting pressures faced by the rulers of these great trading dynasties—it is well documented that the Hittites had such problems—in all probability at the root of their sudden collapse was a commercial interdependency that had outgrown its asset base, triggering rivalry, mutual suspicion, and increasing dysfunction. The wealth of the feudal Mediterranean states was built upon the exploitation of natural resources that were not evenly distributed—they never are—and it was this disparity that for hundreds of years had served to drive a thriving trade. At the center of commerce was the barter of grain to feed the workforce, copper to equip the armies, and timber to provide energy for smelting and wood for construction. As these assets dwindled, the struggle to control resources essential to economic strength and the defense of established empires promoted protracted hostilities, as exemplified by the Mycenaean-Trojan wars.

Just as today fossil fuels are central to our conflicts and struggles—and to our affluence—so was timber essential to the Bronze Age economy. In the smelting of ore, charcoal makes a hotter fire than wood, but under average conditions it takes one ton of timber to produce about four hundred pounds of charcoal. And that was just the beginning. The working of metal, clay firing for pottery manufacture, and the construction of ships, dwellings, and palaces all demanded timber. By the late Bronze Age the appetite for wood was straining the natural cycle of organic renewal. Egypt had practically no trees, and the famed cedars of Lebanon had long been depleted. Thus in all probability, in the decades prior to their systemic collapse, the great trading nations of the Bronze Age already were running out of their energy source, having expanded beyond its natural supply. A complex, interdependent economy founded upon intense competition among ruling elites had overreached and become unsustainable.

The final collapse of these early eastern Mediterranean dynasties came swiftly. As trade and supply lines became disorganized, critical shortages of food and fuel began to emerge that made it politically impossible for the rigidly controlled palace economies to adapt. With commercial opportunity and military resources declining, the feudal leadership weakened, along with the capability for defense, opening opportunities for insurrection by those previously suppressed. Thus among the bands of hungry seagoing predators were those who in the aftermath of protracted war plundered to secure their own survival. The economy of the Mediterranean world stumbled out of balance. Trade disappeared as vital port cities and palaces of fabled riches were razed and burned: those who survived retreated to the countryside in an attempt to secure their future amid a simpler, agriculture-based economy. As Zangger describes it "civilizations that had been shaped by aristocrats became societies of herdsmen and shepherds. When the fighting was over, entire languages and scripts had vanished." Indeed it would be several centuries before the Greek city-states, now revered as the cradle of Western civilization, grew to prominence and regenerated the familiar cycle of trade, competition, and conflict.

THE LIGHT WAS FAILING and the air distinctly colder as I left the exhibition and made my way down the steps of the museum and into Central Park that November afternoon. With the gray warmth of the day trapped by the growing chill, a mist was forming over the lake and spreading among the trees. All seemed curiously in order; but with the Wall Street mayhem still fresh in my mind, I was in a reflective mood.

Great museums are part of humankind's collective memory, places where a multitude of enduring objects conspire in myriad ways to tell the story of who we are, of how through curiosity, craft, and conflict we have sought to shape our world. Amid today's helter-skelter existence museums offer up thin slices from the great slab of memory that is human history. For me an appreciation of what has passed is the prerequisite to understanding the realities of the present.

Alone with such thoughts, I turned and made my way back through the park to Fifth Avenue. The pace of the strollers had quickened. The vendors too were hurrying, eager to pack their stalls away before evening fell upon them. Here was the modern-day vestige of the nomadic Bronze Age merchant—those who, with a set of weights and a seal of identity in hand, had conducted a vibrant international trade with little more than a precise memory, craftsmanship skills, and a good supply of intuitive sense: no laptop, no cell phone, no barcode, not even an abacus. It was a reminder that for millennia the fabric of commerce has been stitched together by a human thread: by our abiding passion for barter and exchange.

So how may we better understand the cycles of expansion, explosion, and collapse that over centuries have dogged that passion? What explains the giddy boom and bust of modern finance? For me, as a behavioral scientist, such oscillations in behavior reflect the gyrations of a dynamic, open system. In 1969 Ludwig von Bertalanffy, a father of systems theory, was one of the first to propose the idea that vital systems—of which the human mind and market economies are prime examples—avoid disorganization and collapse by maintaining an interactive equilibration with their surroundings through the consumption of energy. The fundamental feature of such self-regulating living systems is the capacity to explore and adapt to prevailing circumstance by choosing among alternatives.

Friedrich August von Hayek, the eminent Austrian economist who won a Nobel Prize in 1974 and was influenced in his thinking by Bertalanffy, was fascinated by the concept of a common thread linking market and mind. In midcareer Hayek published *The Sensory Order*, an exploration of the brain as a self-organizing and goal-directed system that seeks homeostatic equilibrium through the prioritizing of competitive information. In his later writings, by extrapolation, Hayek saw the free market as a similar self-correcting open system. Markets, he believed, are not a political construct but a natural product of human social interaction.

In any society the central economic problem is how best to organize production and employ available resources in order to satisfy the needs and desires of many different people. Allowing those individual decision makers to respond competitively to freely determined prices, Hayek argued, was the best way to order widely scattered information about the wealth of the material world and its application to need. The resources of labor, capital, and human ingenuity would thus be appropriately allocated in a manner that could not be mimicked by a central planner, however brilliant. Hence while the market is a result of self-interested human action, Hayek asserted, its self-correction does not result from human intention. Rather through the actions of numerous individuals who have the freedom to choose—equivalent in a biological system to, let's say, the individual neurons of the brain—a spontaneous order emerges that has a well-structured, dynamic, and self-correcting social pattern.

Such thinking is resonant with Adam Smith's much-quoted market metaphor from two centuries earlier describing homeostatic balance: the market in an open society behaves as if guided by an "invisible hand." In behavior the human mind and free markets are both natural, extended orders—open, dynamic systems—created by the interaction of billions of neurons or millions of individuals. Through the choosing among alternatives to exert individual preference, the system as a whole moves toward equilibrium: so do the economist and the neuroscientist find common ground.

The common operating principle of these dynamic systems, biological and social, is that they are regulated at all levels of organization by mechanisms—comparable to the brain's perception-action cycle described in Chapter 4—that provide continuous behavioral correction. These control mechanisms are information-driven feedback loops operating around set points tuned to survival. Collectively they integrate knowledge about the supply chain of raw material and its rate of consumption into a life-sustaining dynamic whole. Simple examples of such feedback loops are setting product prices in a market system and, in the living brain, sustaining a stable supply of glucose energy derived from a wide variety of ecological sources.

The set points around which such systems operate can adapt to a changing environment—can tune to prevailing circumstances—but ultimately the system's vital equilibrium will be compromised if driven to extreme. Thus privation of available resources (as illustrated by dwindling timber supplies in the Late Bronze Age) or maximization (as reflected today in an abundance of high-calorie foods) can distort or disable essential regulatory mechanisms. This disturbs the system's capacity to sustain its balance. It is an illusion therefore to think of dynamic systems—markets or brains—as infinitely adaptive. Consistent and objective feedback of information is essential not only to growth and resilience but also to exercising healthy constraint. Without such regulatory feedback instability of function emerges that if not corrected will lead to collapse.

The economic system of Bronze Age society, viewed within this dynamic context, was clearly brittle in its capacity to adapt to change. While opportunity and risk, as in today's world, were the equation around which the economic system operated and sought balance, natural resources were limited and the fear of conflict ever present. These were the variables *constraining* economic development. The *drivers* of commercial growth were the instinctual behaviors of greed, self-interest, and fascination for novelty (as I described in the earlier chapters), but each was distilled now through the acquisitive appetites of a handful of powerful, intensely competitive ruling families. Merchants benefited from the security of the regional monopolies granted to them by the elites, and in return they were expected to secure the sources of raw materials and exclusive markets essential to prestige and maintaining dominance. But these feudal city-states, which were rarely self-sustaining, rigidly controlled the production and distribution of all staples and luxury crafts. When resources were abundant, the elites overseeing these palace economies achieved a precarious social balance with other powerful families through gifting and barter. During uncertain economic times without the benefit of accurate, timely communication, the essential element of trust quickly decayed, to be replaced by fear and paranoia, spurring aggression, conflict, and ultimately system-wide collapse.

In biology a disturbance of regulatory feedback is similarly a prescription for self-destruction, as is confirmed by the uncontrolled growth of cancer or the self-destructive chaos of mania or anorexia nervosa. This also pertains to the modern-day "self-regulating free market," which is not free in the generally accepted sense of the word. As Adam Smith postulated, an idealized small market does produce its own rational order, founded as it is on feedback loops of self-interested exchange. Extended capital markets too must operate within established regulatory safeguards if they are to remain in dynamic equilibrium. What is evident from the study of the cell turned cancerous is equally true for the market system that falters through fear or is overwhelmed by greed: regulation matters.

* * * *

SO WHAT EXPLAINS the Great Financial Crash of 2008, given that American business long ago embraced the theory and dynamic principles of Adam Smith's self-regulating free-market ideology? What went wrong? From the sociological perspective, the answer is a simple one; as John Komlos, professor emeritus of economics at the University of Munich, has observed, "we are no longer living in Adam Smith's village economy." The cultural and physical contingencies, he argues, that regulate modern-day markets—despite being tempered by central banks and antimonopoly legislation—are dramatically different from those of Smith's time, which "presumed a dominant (self-regulatory) morality that no longer is valid."

The modern banking industry offers an example of this loss of "moral tuning" and self-correction. Today's financial markets are principally controlled by an oligarch of powerful international institutions that have become profoundly influenced in their behavior by the myopic pursuit of short-term profit. This pursuit has been aided further by a willful disruption of the social mechanisms designed to provide regulatory feedback and the increasingly abstract nature of money.

In today's world, money and finance have replaced the Bronze Age "gifting" of tangible assets as the principal regulators of economic activity. Operating a market economy on the basis of barter is cumbersome: essentially you must first find the person who has what you want and hope that they will want what you have. Beyond the village such effort becomes tedious, as the Bronze Age merchant knew only too well. Some agreed-upon and regulated system of exchange therefore becomes essential. Thus the ancient trader's insignia sealed on clay may be considered the forerunner of both "money" and credit—a promissory token to be exchanged later for the goods received or delivered. Over subsequent centuries gold and silver evolved as an intermediary method of exchange, simplifying accounting and later functioning as a reserve of value, to greatly increase the efficiency of markets.

For any market to find equilibrium and operate efficiently, however, *trust among individuals* must remain at the core of the exchange, as in the village economy. Money extends that trust, inferring that as in a "gentleman's agreement," its face value will be honored. In the modern economy banks in their simple form are designed to mediate that trust; those depositing their savings in the bank make it possible for credit to be extended to others. Savers receive a financial return on their investment while, within certain limits, still being able to draw upon their funds when needed. Once upon a time—indeed, within my own living memory—such local banking was conducted on a handshake. If, as a trusted community member, you needed a loan for a car, the first step was to consult the bank manager. In concept the social purpose of today's financial industry is comparable: to allocate the savings of American families to their reliable and most productive use.

But that ethos has changed, and banking has changed with it. Now the major international banks are increasingly focused, as their primary mission, upon speculative investment as a source of increased profit for managers and shareholders rather than upon customer service. Furthermore, for the average American in the electronic age, money as a tangible asset is fast becoming invisible, reduced now to a string of numbers that provide a record of the pay we receive, the expenses we incur, and the money we owe. In everyday experience the exchange of silver and gold is no longer associated with money. Even paper money is disappearing, replaced increasingly by plastic cards of credit and perhaps, in the near future, by virtual "bit" money. And yet this abstract concept of "money" has become ever more central to our lives and tightly equated with "the market." The gyrations of abstract-seeming financial markets and the banking industry are now the world's metric of economic health. It is the oscillation of a set of numbers on a computer screen that makes us rich or poor.

Hayek, in *The Fatal Conceit*, warned against such abstraction: "The moment that barter is replaced by indirect exchange mediated by money, ready intelligibility ceases." The Greek city-states at the beginning of the sixth century B.C., arising as a phoenix from the dark centuries that followed the Bronze Age collapse, were the first to use money in our contemporary, abstract sense. Most important, as the Greeks discovered, with money comes a new form of power. Reciprocity; the sharing of possessions; kinship; ritual; complex negotiation— with sufficient money such concerns are no longer primary. It is not trustworthy interpersonal relationships but the possession of money that determines social dominance, making possible a predatory power where money alone can satisfy needs and slake all desires. While it is possible to have too much to eat, too much to drink, and even too much sex, in the abstract one can never have enough money. The old instinctual regulatory feedback loops no longer pertain. Although in mythology the fable of King Midas decries the appetite for gold and riches as moral travesty, in reality few individuals in today's abstract, credit-driven world seek to limit their acquisition of "money" and its promise of material pleasure.

IN RETROSPECT THERE is a consensus that easy credit, excessive borrowing, and the complex bundling of home loans helped spur the U.S. housing bubble and fuel the subprime mortgage crisis that led to the global fiscal seizure of 2008. Economists give the quaint name *moral hazard* to such jeopardy, and yet the story began innocently enough a decade earlier when a group of young entrepreneurs at JP Morgan Chase dreamed up a new way to increase their trading profit. Faced with a global savings glut and low interest rates in the closing decade of the twentieth century, pension funds and other endowments were demanding safe, higher-yield investments. Similarly the big international banks were exploring innovative ways of managing risk by bundling loans into portfolios that were then credit-financed and sold on as individual units, thus reducing the amount of bank capital needed to cover potential defaults.

By the late 1990s, as the excitement of the dot.com boom declined and with the ongoing liberalization of banking laws, federal regulators accepted the concept of creating such "credit derivatives." The finance industry, including insurance giants such as AIG, responded with enthusiasm. At first all was well since the portfolios were constructed largely from the assets of companies with proven track records. As the opportunities for short-term profit were recognized, however, there was a hunger for more. Soon home mortgages, which were in plentiful supply, were being added to the pot. A herd mentality quickly took hold, and within a decade the derivatives market had exploded to $12 trillion. But problems were emerging. The securities were complex and difficult to understand, even for those selling them, and risk was virtually impossible to accurately assess. Because the income of the hustlers was tied to the units sold, however, this detail was largely ignored: credit derivatives, mortgage-backed securities, swaps, and other mysterious financial instruments were packaged and repackaged and were soon being offered across a growing global market, creating unknown trillions in imaginary wealth.

The poor investment quality of these mortgage-backed securities was apparently of little concern to the banks selling them, focused as they were on short-term profit. Research from the University of Chicago business school, using data collected by government agencies from three thousand zip-code districts, suggested that the explosion of mortgage growth was tied to easy credit being offered, particularly to those individuals least able to afford it. Districts where households frequently had been rejected for home mortgages prior to 1996 had the highest rate of approval in the boom years between 2001 and 2005. These districts, which were identified as "high latent demand" zip codes, were also regions of declining income and poor employment growth during those same years. In other words, the standard of risk being applied to loan evaluation was so far reduced that it became probable that with a downturn in the economy many individuals would default on their loans.

Fundamentally, for the capitalist enterprise to grow, it must partner with individuals and harness their desire to invest, buy, or borrow as a source of new finance. Traditionally, even before the Industrial Revolution, economic growth was driven by capital accumulation and investment. With the invention of the modern consumer society, however, indebtedness through easy credit has become an accepted vehicle for financial partnership, especially in the United States. In fact, the "debt economy," based on an assumption of continuous growth, is an American invention. After the Second World War, through the Bretton Woods International Monetary Agreement of 1944, the U.S. dollar assumed a unique position in international trade, with the major world currencies being tied to its value, which in turn was linked to gold. When Richard Nixon severed this link between gold and the dollar in 1971, the world's circulating money supply grew rapidly, fostering easier credit and an exponential increase in borrowing. In many rich countries and particularly in the United States, in addition to government spending private debt was encouraged. The government gave tax breaks on home mortgages and on corporate borrowing, making debt acceptable both as a means of driving market growth and as something desirable, creating in tandem a new economic paradigm.

The explosion of credit in the American economy—by 2007 debt had exceeded $50 trillion—not only fostered the housing bubble but also changed our habits. It distorted self-regulation, diminishing prudent behavior at all levels of the market, to create a destabilizing positive feedback loop, as diagrammed in Figure 5.1. The ancient chain of survival behaviors—the perception of opportunity, risk assessment, and chosen action followed by the feedback cycle of reward or punishment—had been compromised by the promotion of an illusion of continuous economic growth and the cultural encouragement of myopic, short-term profit taking.

Perhaps for the first time in human history, it was the possibility of reward rather than of punishment that dominated in the calculus of risk. In distorting the objective evaluation of risk, easy credit provides a false sense of security about the future. It retunes the brain. In

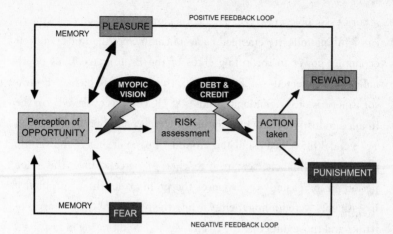

Figure 5.1: Risk, debt, and the perception-action cycle: Easy credit, tolerance of debt, and a focus on short-term financial gain distort the natural balance of risk and reward that is integral to the brain's perception-action cycle. In the language of dynamic systems, it fosters a positive feedback loop that is unsustainable, leading ultimately to implosion and systemic collapse. The 2008 fiscal crisis is an example of such implosion.

addition it feeds our preference for immediate reward—just as the caramel cheesecake served my short-term pleasure and made me ignore my long-term goal of maintaining a healthy body weight. Through using credit we can receive today what we otherwise would have to postpone until tomorrow, if even then. The debt incurred, however, also mortgages our future. Easy credit systems, therefore, can lead to spendthrift behaviors as when we avoid the fine print on the credit card agreement and fail to notice that debt incurs a 30 percent interest rate. In neurobehavioral terms, easy credit builds intuitive habits that hijack the brain's perception-action cycle.

In rational moments most of us agree that mortgaging the future to excessive debt is not prudent behavior. In the run-up to the 2008 fiscal crisis, however, homeowners, investors, the banks, and the government were essentially doing just that, all accumulating debt until as a nation the United States was awash in a tsunami of credit. Greed became rampant as speculative investments and the mortgage-backed securities bubble grew ever larger. In parallel the leaders of America's banking industry emerged as an oligarchy, not dissimilar in their economic power to the ruling elites of the Bronze Age. This dominance was reflected—as Deepak Lal, the James S. Coleman Professor Emeritus of International Studies at UCLA, has observed—in the finance industry's changing share of U.S. corporate profits. Between 1973 and 1985 it had oscillated around 16 percent, but in the run-up to the global financial seizure it reached 41 percent. Over this same period an increasing proportion of the profits from these speculative investments were finding their way into the pockets of the managers of banks and those directing the insurance and credit-rating industries.

With a focus on maximizing immediate return, compensation in America's finance industry exploded until in 2007 the average banker's paycheck was 181 percent of the average executive pay in comparable private corporations. In a typical scenario, when the annual profits of a bank were divided, half of that profit was paid out to the bankers themselves. With everything to gain and little downside to risk, both intuitive and rational self-monitoring was in retreat, and Adam Smith's impartial spectator became an anecdote of history. Greed and unbridled ambition had co-opted reason.

Justification of the extravagant compensation packages followed a familiar refrain: driven by the market, substantial bonuses were needed to retain the best minds. But such profligacy had public consequences. In Britain in December 2009 the Bank of England pronounced that "if discretionary distributions [for which read bonuses] had been 20 percent lower per year between 2000 and 2008, the major British banks would have generated around 75 billion pounds of additional capital—more than what was required from the public sector during the crisis."

With hindsight the facts are simple. Beginning in the 1980s, America as a nation largely abandoned any social constraint of its banking industry, and many other rich countries followed. The traditional divisions between commercial and investment banks were removed, and high-risk "casino" banking became commonplace in both the United States and Europe. Beyond the obvious appeal of such speculation to our ancient instinctual cravings, in the run-up to the subprime housing debacle other perverse incentives were also operating. Derivative financing by the banks, for example, was highly leveraged, being derived principally from public offerings. With little of their institutional assets at risk, this further diminished any sense of personal jeopardy, both for individual bankers and for insurance agencies such as AIG. In consequence, as the tide of speculative investments rose, the value of the derivatives sold was no longer grounded in marketable assets.

Indeed, in the wake of the debacle the debts of the major private banks involved were moved swiftly to the public ledger out of fear that their collapse might bring the world's financial systems down with them. Not only were the banks "too big to fail," but their leaders were "too big to jail." Therefore, apart from Lehman, most of the senior managers of the "megabanks" escaped virtually unscathed from the crisis, thanks to government rescue. This lack of negative feedback—specifically the fear of potential punishment for the choices made—violates a fundamental premise of the corrective action necessary to promote behavioral adjustment in any dynamic system. Despite greed and unparalleled risk-taking the oligarchy involved in the financial crash came away essentially unharmed.

IN CONTRAST, FOR THE MAJORITY of Americans the financial crisis was of great impact. It is clear in retrospect that growing social inequality, which only worsened following the 2008 collapse, was also driving the instability of America's financial system. In the post–World War II years between 1952 and the 1980s the richest 1 percent of American households earned approximately 10 percent of the national income. By 2007, in contrast, 23.5 percent of America's earnings were flowing to the top 1 percent. Such disparities had not been seen since the 1920s, just prior to the Great Depression.

Patterns of spending across America suggest that this social disparity was playing a significant role in the ballooning of debt. For those living at the economic margin, freeing up credit eases many difficulties—for the short term—and acts as a temporary means to promote economic growth. Debt-fueled spending on luxury goods and services by poorer households—what *The Economist* has labeled "trickle-down" consumption—in the years prior to the 2008 crisis had been driven, in part, by efforts to match the profligate habits of the celebrity rich. Raghuram Rajan, of the University of Chicago Booth School of Business, proposes in his book *Fault Lines* that it was hence a *combination* of social inequality and the easing of credit restrictions that helped prime the financial crisis.

Although the average citizen may find it hard to identify the social deficiencies that enabled the banking oligarchs to run away with millions of dollars, many of the perverse incentives that drove the bankers' actions have been similarly shaping the behavior of all of us. While it gives satisfaction to pillory Wall Street and the international financiers as the villains of the 2008 madness, they are minor actors when it comes to the larger narrative—a drama of imprudent habit, debt, and self-deception in which we each played our part. In the famous words of Walt Kelly's *Pogo* cartoon strip, "We have met the enemy and he is us." The conflict is within our own heads; projecting it onto others is an effort at self-solace. Reflecting upon our own behavior, it is we—in our myopic quest for more—who collectively drove the credit bubbles and helped make possible the bankers' acquisition of their millions. As active agents in promoting the growth and ultimate overreach of the consumer society, we must assume our share of the responsibility for its financial stumbling.

We may argue, of course, that there were extenuating circumstances. During the last twenty-five years of the twentieth century the American economy was in recession only 5 percent of the time, compared to 22 percent of the previous quarter-century. Reflexively such long periods of uninterrupted expansion foster a mood of complacency. In our intuitive habits, especially those who grew up in that era, we began to assume that the good times would never end. We learned to be thoughtless, falling into the sin of extrapolation—that the future will be like the immediate past. But what we failed to acknowledge was that in America's case a substantial proportion of that economic growth had been built on debt that eventually would have to be repaid. Before 1985 American consumers saved on average about 9 percent of their disposable income, but by 2005 the comparable savings rate was zero as mortgage, credit card, and other consumer debt rose to 127 percent of disposable income. With Uncle Sam similarly awash in red ink, in our desire for more we have transformed America from the world's bank to a debtor nation.

Ours was a Faustian bargain. In the last three decades, aided and abetted by the enticements of consumerism, *we have been busily retuning our neural architecture.* From the perspective of behavioral neurobiology, in cahoots with the pleasures of consumption *we have disrupted the brain's perception-action cycle, resetting the intuitive balance between the hedonistic ventromedial cortex and the constraining ventrolateral cortex*, thus disrupting the autopilots of the brain's internal market. Passion has prevailed over reason: we have created a bubble-promoting positive feedback loop, favoring short-term self-interest over the longer-term advantages of prudent self-constraint.

ADAM SMITH BELIEVED that it is the influence of society that transforms people into independent, moral beings. In Smith's mind the process was far from passive, as I explained in Chapter 3; rather it emerges from lifelong social interaction. Thus, ask who is responsible for moral development, and there is no single answer because it is a collective liability. Nor is the shaping of moral sensitivity haphazard; rather it is founded in objective self-awareness, a quality of mind that we accrue through the careful study of others—by first imagining ourselves to be in another's shoes and then learning from that experience by comparing the subjective sentiments evoked with the actions that we observe.

In this way moral concern develops through social exchange. The process is an iterative one. Ideally, over time one becomes one's own best critic, creating in the mind an intuitive capacity to monitor personal thoughts and actions and to learn from that monitoring, essentially viewing one's own behavior from the perspective of an outsider. You will recall that Smith personified this intuitive facility as the "impartial spectator," an entity that helps moderate the perennial struggle between passion and reason. Think of the "spectator" as a friendly moderator, working to achieve harmony or, in Smith's words, to establish the foundational virtues "of self-denial, of self-government, of that command which subjects all the movements of our nature to what our own dignity, honour, and the propriety of our own conduct, require."

The collective noun for these basic virtues is *character*—a sense of self-direction, an acceptance of personal responsibility, and the ability to regulate one's own emotions, especially to defer immediate gratification in favor of future goals. Character is built, not born. Ironically, however, just when we need it most—given the character-draining temptations of the consumer society—discussion of how "good" character is built is an unfashionable subject, largely ignored in today's public debate.

This is regrettable, for the prosocial virtues of individual character, consistently expressed, underpin the culture of mutual trust that is essential to civil society. Trust is the sentiment that arises in a community when honest and cooperative behavior is the regular and shared norm. The human drive for attachment—Smith's social sympathy—and the competitive social behaviors exercised in market exchange are two sides of the same coin. When individuals habitually work together in a free society, the integration of these two fundamental social behaviors—the pursuit of meaningful fellowship and the search for improved economic circumstance—become the coinage of success. It is through such interaction that a stable social order is ensured, together with a market society that serves both individual initiative and the common good. The lesson is that markets cannot be divorced from the culture that sustains them: societies enjoying high trust develop strong social capital and prosperous economies.

But the reverse is also true. As trust declines, the social glue erodes. And in the aftermath of the 2008 global debacle, trust was at low ebb. When for several weeks the international financial system was frozen in fear, it was a crisis driven by a loss of basic trust among investors, bankers, governments, and the average citizen. Subsequently the trust barometer continued its fall as a seemingly endless list of improprieties emerged: the British members of Parliament were fiddling their expenses; some elected leaders in the United States were driving their municipalities toward bankruptcy with the promise of overly generous pensions; federal agencies were seeking hundreds of millions of dollars in penalties from major financial institutions, both in the United States and abroad, for their part in the subprime scandal; and then in the summer of 2012 came definitive evidence of attempts by major banks to manipulate LIBOR, the London Interbank Offered Rate, which sets the short-term costs of bank borrowing.

This unfolding story not only calls into question the integrity of the financial and government institutions involved but also the moral and ethical character of those in leadership positions. Even more relevant is that it emphasizes, as I have highlighted in these first chapters, the value of understanding how the human brain works. From the perspective of behavioral neuroscience, the 2008 financial collapse was predictable: fostering individualistic, short-term, reward-driven, and debt-fueled consumption breeds risk-taking and addictive behavior. An ethos of unbridled self-interest, gambling, and casual dishonesty had given birth to greed and fraud in high places, calling into question whether the market model we now pursue is in itself destructive of trust, character development, and cultural balance.

Calls to regulate international finance came thick and fast after the meltdown, and certainly they are needed. But one doubts whether, alone, such externally imposed regulations will be enough: regulators cannot oversee the millions of transactions that go on in the world, let alone monitor the ethics of those who promote and oversee them. No, unfashionable though it may be, it is time—in these days of technical abstraction, time starvation, personal stress, and family fragmentation—to return to an investigation of how "good character" may be built and to the social institutions that best foster that vital construction.

This is my focus in Part II.

Part II
PROLOGUE

How to Live?

THE GREEKS CALLED IT *ataraxia*, the state of being unperturbed, of tranquillity and peace of mind. For Epicurus it was the foundation of *eudaimonia*, the joy of human flourishing. Two thousand years on, Adam Smith was in agreement. Smith considered happiness to be born of tranquillity and enjoyment—the fruit of a well-tuned brain.

But human beings are not given to serenity. Tranquillity does not come naturally to the human mind: *ataraxia* is a highly cultivated state achieved through hard work and the self-discipline that we call character. Such tuning arises from awareness of the true nature of the world and an understanding of the limitations of our being. To achieve such self-command, we must first accept ourselves for who we are: instinctually driven, curious, self-interested, focused on the short-term, and ruled by habit. These core human attributes are tempered by extraordinary powers of reason—of perception, analysis, imagination, and choice. But we are also deeply social beings with a need for fellowship. The challenge of a life well lived is to meld these selves together in harmony, blending reason and passion to promote individual wellbeing and a sustainable human future.

Ours are privileged but confusing times. Nothing is more antithetical to the cultivation of *ataraxia* than the narrative of a debt-fueled consumer society, which in its promotion of material gluttony and creeping inequality flirts with self-destruction. But how do we dig out from under this seductive avalanche? Adam Smith considered three cardinal human values—fairness, benevolence, and prudence—to underpin a stable social order. These elements of character are grounded in the bonds of infancy and crafted over a lifetime. It is through their nurturance and promotion that social fellowship is exercised. Future thriving, as an individual and in the social realm, is a matter of conscious choice and shared responsibility. Healthy children flourish in healthy families, healthy schools, and healthy communities. Collectively we prosper in habitats that are designed with humans in mind, and through markets that foster opportunity and choice. The mix for a vibrant human future has not changed, as I explain in these next chapters.

Chapter 6

Love:
Weaving the
Web of Trust

Mary had a little lamb,
Whose fleece was white as snow.
And everywhere that Mary went,
The lamb was sure to go.

Sarah Josepha Hale (1830)

How selfish soever man may be supposed, there are evi-
dently some principles in his nature, which interest him
in the fortunes of others, and render their happiness
necessary to him, though he derives nothing from it,
except the pleasure of seeing it.

Adam Smith, *The Theory of Moral Sentiments* (1759)

FOR THE VERMONT SHEEP FARMER the final weeks of winter
blend hope and insecurity. The sun is stronger and higher, but the
nights remain intensely frigid. Despite sunny days the northwest wind
can still knife its way into the bone, even through the warmest parka.
The Easter moon, cresting in late March, promises the coming of

spring but casts its silvered light across frozen pastures. And it's there on a clear night that you can see them, in ghostly silhouette. Out of the woods, and dancing to a mating chorus of howls, yelps, and falsetto yips, they circle ever closer. It's lambing season, and after lean winter months the coyotes are hungry.

During those waning, chilly weeks before springtime the potential of a coyote raid is just one of the concerns that keeps my daughter among her sheep on many nights during lambing. Helen started her flock of sixty or so purebred Icelandic sheep a few years before her own daughter was born. Indeed Wren, whose birthday is in February, spent her first lambing season peeking out from a pouch worn underneath her mother's down parka, getting a close-up view of the births and feedings. Every spring since then—Wren is now five—she has followed Helen around the barn, tending to the newborns, absorbing the social habits of their mothers, and occasionally being knocked sideways by a head butt from a ewe who thinks she's someone else's lamb.

The sheep and their ways fascinate Wren. In the warmth of the house, after barn chores are complete and supper is over, her regular bedtime request is "more stories about the sheep." Wren's favorite is about Russett, the old ewe with craggy horns and a tarnished copper fleece. Russett is a baby snatcher; her maternal instinct is so strong that each year, before she has delivered her own, she tries to steal lambs from the other mothers. Initially after Russett joined the herd, Helen was unaware of her tricks. So one morning when she found Russett with a white ram and Shy, another young mother, with one white ewe, she presumed that both sheep had delivered single lambs overnight.

Icelandic sheep are vigorous creatures. After fourteen hundred years of evolution in the Spartan hills of Iceland, the newborn will begin nursing within a few minutes of taking breath. In response ewes "nicker" constantly to their offspring and rapidly know the infant by its smell and voice. Thus, mother and lamb are bonded within moments of birth. So seemed to be the case of Russett and Shy, with both babies nursing well and sticking close to their mothers. Clearly, thought Helen, the lambs were bonding normally.

So, as Wren's favorite story goes, all was well until four days later, when Russett gave birth to her own twins. It was a particularly cold night, and the new lambs would have needed milk rapidly after arrival. But Russett's adopted white ram was already much bigger and stronger than the newly born twins and was drinking a lot of her milk. So by the time Helen got to the barn on her routine visit, an hour or so after the birth, the newborns were chilled and weak, with tongues so cold that they were unable to suckle. Taking the lambs back to the farmhouse, Helen bundled them in a box next to the woodstove and fed them with a stomach tube every hour for the remainder of the night; one lived and the other died. The one that survived was Ruby, the farm's first bottle baby. She lived in the kitchen for a week and tottered around with Wren, who had just turned one at the time and was learning to walk.

"Tell me more," Wren always asks eagerly at this part of the story, adding sternly after a pause, "you shouldn't steal someone else's babies." And so her mother proceeds: Helen was now wise to Russett's game, and for the next couple of years all was well. Then just as it seemed that Russett had given up her old habit, the baby snatching was back. A young yearling named Juno gave birth to twins, and before Juno knew what was up, Russett had convinced one of them that she was its mother. Helen, no longer fooled, separated Russett, but returning the baby to Juno was no easy task.

With the lamb removed, Russett became totally distraught, throwing herself repeatedly against the wall of her pen, while Juno, a flighty and confused first-time mother, wasn't comfortable nursing a rescued offspring that smelled like another's child. And so, as it must be in farming practice, Helen explains to Wren how she returned the little rejected soul to Russett, hoping that when Russett's own lambs arrived, she would manage to nurse them all, which fortunately she did.

Wren sighs with satisfaction. "But that Russett is bad," she comments, offering some moral closure to the tale. "Babies need their real mummies if the bad wolf comes." For Wren the sheep stories are reality-based precautionary tales—much as were the stories of the Brothers Grimm for children two centuries earlier—for vulnerable lambs indeed do fall victim to coyote raids. Perhaps that is why Wren—as an expression of nascent maternal instinct, or out of her own anxieties—will take my hand when walking among the sheep in springtime so that together we may ensure that all the lambs know their mothers and that no one is crying or lost. As the little shepherd to her flock, Wren already understands the importance of emotional attachment and social order.

So it was that when Wren was aged three, Ruby, the lamb she had helped rescue and raise, had her own baby lamb. Much to her parents' surprise, Wren was beside herself. Helen couldn't figure out what was troubling her daughter until Wren explained through her sobs that Ruby was her "little sister," and now with her own baby to feed things could never be the same. It was a poignant moment in a young girl's evolving sense of love and loss. But so too does Wren's distress illustrate how attuned we are, even at a tender age, to the complexities of a social world that is unique to our species.

THE RAPID ATTACHMENT of a lamb to its mother in the late days of a cold Vermont winter is driven by mammalian instinct, behavior essential to the lamb's survival while waiting for the sun-filled, playful days of spring. The bond is formed immediately, triggered by the smell and warmth of the mother, for without it the newborn's death is certain within hours. Carried within the phyletic memory of our species, human beings share this mammalian instinct for parental-infant bonding. From a broad range of studies we now recognize that the attachments that Wren witnessed and nurtured in the sheep herd are driven by the same neuronal chemistry as in ourselves. That which bonds ewe to lamb similarly bonds Helen to Wren. The chemistry of this bonding is the chemistry of love.

As I shall explore, this same elixir primes the development of trust and the social bonds essential to building character and community. Contrary to the competitive images conjured by Madison Avenue, in a healthy society personal fulfillment is founded not simply on shopping and self-interest but also on cooperation and caring. Indeed, *a unique capacity for caring and mutual trust is the hallmark of the evolution of our social behavior as a species and of our development as individuals.* It is in our own self-interest, through better understanding of others, to promote the flourishing of such affiliation. How we navigate our early experiences with love and loss shapes the intuitive self-knowledge that drives much of our social interaction as adults. In turn, it is the collective expression of such social sentiment that provides stability to our cultural institution—infusing meaning into the stories we tell through literature, art, music, and theater—and sustaining the social webs that provide many of life's most valuable rewards.

How, in infancy and early childhood, these interactive social webs are woven is the focus of this chapter; and why and how, in the school years, they form the essential lattice upon which learning and character are built, is my subject in the next. That we understand and foster a healthy maturational process is vital to our well-being, and thus the discussion across the two chapters is intimately entwined. But also there arises a fundamental question as we look ahead: do we have the collective and political will to nurture and promote the self-command essential to a sustainable human future?

Let me begin with sexual bonding. What does science tell us about this elixir of love? Interestingly human beings are among the 3 to 5 percent of mammals that ever practice monogamy, be that through serial attachment or by selectively mating with a single life partner. Of those species that have been studied, which team up in stable pairs and share the responsibility of raising their offspring, it is the prairie vole—a small rodent that inhabits the grasslands of North America—that is most celebrated. Like humans these little creatures have a complicated social organization, and we have learned much from them about the genetics and chemistry of the attachment bond. This is because in mating behavior prairie voles are truly steadfast, usually taking only one partner in a lifetime. Their mountain cousins, on the other hand, are promiscuous.

What explains such dramatic differences in attachment behavior? you may ask. It is a question that has long fascinated Larry Young, a neuroscientist and professor of psychiatry at Emory University. As a graduate student in Texas, Young studied the molecular mechanisms underpinning variation in the sexual behavior of lizards, before moving on to Emory where he worked with Thomas Insel, now the director of the National Institute of Mental Health in Washington, D.C. Building on Insel's pioneering work, Young has discovered some intriguing differences between the mountain and prairie voles. To put it simply, summarizing many years of research, in contrast to its Casanova cousin the faithful prairie vole has many more receptors for oxytocin and vasopressin—the hormones of attachment and affiliation—in the brain regions that are most critical to reward and reinforcement.

These "love" hormones of oxytocin and vasopressin are released when prairie voles have sex. Simultaneously there is a comparable rise of dopamine in the nucleus accumbens, the reward center of the brain and an integral part of the basal ganglia where habits are constructed. In other words, in the prairie vole's brain the reward centers of sex and attachment are interwoven. After the first intense sexual encounter, which can last for several hours, monogamy becomes driven by conditioned habit that in its repetition continues to make the prairie couple feel good. In human terms, the little creatures "fall in love." However, when the prairie vole's "love" receptors are chemically blocked, as Young has done in his experiments, and oxytocin and vasopressin hormones are unable to attach to their respective binding sites, the bond between the prairie partners fails to develop. In its behavior the prairie vole then becomes a mountain vole.

So was Russett's thievery, which so disturbed my granddaughter, driven by a mutant combination of "love" receptor chemistry and reward? It's a possibility. We know that in sheep oxytocin has a major role in mother infant-bonding and that smell, as any sheep farmer will tell you, also plays an integral part in the process. It was for this reason, of course, that Juno did not accept her own lamb after Helen returned it to her. After being suckled by Russett, the infant just did not smell "right." And smell is pertinent not only to prairie voles and sheep but also to us. There's plenty of evidence that smell and close attachment are intimately intertwined in human bonding, including between father and child. There is also considerable variation in the human vasopressin gene among individuals, which may help explain why some of us are more consistent and content in our relationships than are others. Nor, reciprocally, is Wren's attachment to the lamb she had nurtured unusual: human infants as young as eighteen months will show concern for others and will provide comfort to those who are crying and in distress.

IT IS FROM THIS FUSION of evolved biology and propensity for mutual caring—phyletic memory forged initially in the crucible of survival and tempered later by the experience of reward and reprimand—that human beings crafted the most complex social order of any creature on this planet. In achieving this evolution it has helped that the human infant is a magnet for the attention of others, just as is the frisking lamb in spring. Even Charles Darwin, who seems to have been a rather shy and retiring man, was fascinated by the smiles and babbling of young children. Indeed in 1872 he wrote *The Expression of Emotion in Man and Animals*, which is not as famous as *On the Origin of Species* but equally important for any reader interested in social communication. We have all seen it: grown men bending over a baby carriage, grimacing, and speaking in high-pitched coos and musical syllables. While babies may seem utterly helpless, they have an enormous ability to change the behavior of those around them.

Sarah Hrdy, a professor of anthropology at the University of California, Davis, suggests in *Mothers and Others: The Evolutionary Origins of Mutual Understanding* that it is precisely this ability of human infants to engage persons other than their biological mother that sets us apart from the great apes and that builds the platform for our extraordinary gift of social interaction. She points out—based on the studies of still-existing foraging tribes in central Africa—that before the invention of towns and cities, babies spent over half their time with individuals other than their natural parents. Hrdy believes that it is precisely because the human infant is so vulnerable, and for so long, that humankind is uniquely collaborative. Our social success has its origin in the strategy of "cooperative breeding," where the responsibility for nurturing the young was a collective one, simply because it was necessary.

In all likelihood our forebears lived largely in isolated bands of extended kinship. In tough times survival depended more upon collaboration and a healthy web of social relationships than on any one individual's heroic success in combat or the hunt. Peaceful interaction with others enhanced self-preservation and supported the successful rearing of children, to common advantage. Starvation was the stark alternative to this reciprocal caring. Thus the working mother is not a recent invention: indeed, the evidence is that under demanding circumstances fathers too became caregivers.

The early challenges to human survival were the deprivations of habitat and an uncertain food supply. Hrdy suggests that intergroup aggression was probably rare in hunter-gatherers, both in our own hominid species, *Homo sapiens*, and in *Homo erectus* before us. In part this was because until recently there were relatively few of us on the face of the Earth. *Homo erectus* marched out of Africa many hundreds of thousands of years ago—these particular progenitors were around for about 1.6 million years before becoming extinct—and yet the archeological evidence of their presence is sparse. So why, asks Hrdy, since we were so few in number, would any tribe fight with a potentially competitive group when moving a few kilometers could secure an alternative hunting ground?

Support for this live-and-let-live proposition comes from the extensive studies of Polly Wiessner, a distinguished cultural anthropologist who has worked among the !Kung and other Kalahari Bushmen for over three decades. The Bushmen, sometimes called the San, are the indigenous peoples of southern Africa, having lived in the same semiarid desert region for some eighty thousand years. Weissner reports that among the Bushmen people the cultural norm in sustaining extended kinships is a system of gift giving, storytelling, and visiting—a social technology similar in function to the "gifting" economy among the wealthy dynasties of the Bronze Age that I described in Chapter 5. Fighting *among* kinships to secure survival is less common than fighting for a preferred sexual partner. In many groups the social convention of arranged marriage discourages even this behavior, recognizing that such self-seeking competition siphons off energy better spent on the foraging and hunting that sustains the viability of the group as a whole.

The necessity of maintaining a stable social order, therefore, appears to be rooted in the extended vulnerability of the human infant. Gift giving creates long-standing ties and a network of socially interdependent partnerships that are supportive of children. From these bonds the capacity for mutual trust emerges, with the mother as the first trustee. Such caring, expressed generation after generation, becomes embedded in the cultural intelligence—commonsense knowledge— that the best hedge against privation and crisis is to pool risk by networking. As Weissner has described in her studies of the !Kung, when "the wellbeing of any individual rests heavily in the hands of others," the security of the whole group is enhanced.

BUT WHAT SUSTAINS our sociability in our affluent society? In the self-absorption of modern times—when we no longer live together in small economic groups and everyday challenges are refracted through a commercial lens—is social sentiment eroding? Affluence certainly taps into our instinctual strivings and fosters myopic self-indulgence, as I described in Chapter 1. And yet in moments of disaster like earthquakes and great storms, or following aggressive tragedies like mindless mass murders, strangers leap to the assistance of those who suffer. When in 2004 India was hit by a massive tsunami, those who fared best were not individuals of material wealth but those most socially connected within their community. Mutual caring, it appears, remains a collective human attribute.

One expression of this ingrained disposition is the human sense of fairness, which you will recall Adam Smith considered among the cardinal virtues of character. Such evenhandedness can be demonstrated in clever laboratory experiments, such as the Ultimatum Game first developed by the German economist Werner Güth. In this game two players are asked to divide a sum of money between them, or perhaps share some goody such as a slice of cake. One of the players—the proposer—puts a proposition to the responder, seated in another room, who then may accept the offered division or reject it. Under the rules of the game, however, the responder is not passive: should he or she reject the proposed sharing, then both players receive nothing. Universally, and this experiment now has been performed across many cultures, individuals rarely accept a share lower than 20 percent. But interestingly this fraction is well below the portion of 40 to 50 percent that the proposer usually offers.

Many researchers believe that beyond the blood ties of immediate family it is this unique human sense of fairness—together with the brain capacity to keep track of the many complicated interactions involved—that enables large groups of individuals to live together in harmony and trust. Essentially what holds a trusting society together and marks our humanity is the sentiment that others should be treated as we wish to be treated. Personal rejection, and the subjective sense of others being poorly treated, are both experienced as painful. Thus in context Wren's worried response to Russett "stealing" another ewe's lamb reflects the childhood emergence of such caring virtues.

From the perspective of behavioral neuroscience, these mirrored sentiments registering fair and unfair social practice are behaviors comparable to those I have discussed before, intuitive habits built from experience upon a phyletic template. As my UCLA colleagues Naomi Eisenberger and Matt Lieberman have shown—you will recall meeting Matt in Chapter 2—such habits help shape how we interpret and react to the complexities of the social world. Furthermore, from their work and that of others, it is becoming clear that in monitoring the emotional ups and downs of social interaction the brain uses the same neurochemistry that encodes physical pain and pleasure.

This explains, as Adam Smith observed in *The Theory of Moral Sentiments*, why we *feel* the pain of a brother on the rack. And a moment of introspection will produce examples from your own experience. From a mundane episode of modern times, a friend recently recounted to me how her husband—who has an artificial hip and suffers chronic debilitating illness—had been subjected to an unnecessary and intrusive body search at the hands of airport security guards after his metallic joint triggered the alarms. "I was enraged at the unfairness of it all: his pain was my pain," she recounted.

Our physical and emotional experiences are intertwined. The reward networks through which the *physical pleasures* of food and sex are recorded—the medial orbital-frontal cortex, the amygdala, and the dopamine-rich nucleus accumbens of the basal ganglia—also record the *emotional pleasures* of social engagement and acceptance by others. Conversely *physical pain* is registered in the posterior portion of the cingulate cortex, in the insula, and in structures set deep in the ancient midbrain. Similarly the *emotional distress* of social rejection— measured in the laboratory through the subtle exclusion of a participant's avatar in a computerized game of catch—is not only registered through the same brain structures but the stress that is induced also triggers an inflammatory immune response. Thus the brain circuits involved in gauging the social and physical experience of pain and pleasure are closely linked.

The love hormones of affiliation and emotional regulation, which as we have seen are so critical to survival in the neonate, also play their role in adult life through modulation of these social brain networks. In the Ultimatum Game oxytocin, administered as a nasal spray to the proposer, increases generous offers by a massive 80 percent, while feeding the responder a diet low in tryptophan, thus depleting brain serotonin levels, decreases the acceptance rate of unfair proposals. Habitually programmed brain networks thus are modulated by emotional chemistry to tune our behavior under changing social and physical conditions. Each is a pillar of our survival equipment: mind and body are indeed one. However, while the avoidance of physical pain is largely instinctual—no second lesson is needed for a child to avoid a hot stove—the capacity to understand another's situation and to modulate one's emotion accordingly are mental abilities learned as the brain matures and as we interact with others. In broad terms this capacity is called empathy, and it plays a critical role in the development of the well-tuned brain.

THE MENTAL FACILITIES for *empathic understanding* that are central to trust and social cohesion develop slowly, founded on the attachments of infancy. The empathic virtues of fairness, patience, and compassion for others do not spring fully formed into existence: rather they are built incrementally and fixed in mind by memory, meaning, and habit. Let me return to the youthful experiences of Wren by way of illustration. In what has become a rarity in modern times, family life and the economic center of Wren's experience are one and the same. Knoll Farm in Fayston, Vermont, where she lives with her parents and older sister, is not only a working farm but also the home of the Center for Whole Communities, a foundation devoted to developing just what its name implies.

In the summer when the center's workshops and seminars are in full swing, the place is buzzing with people with distinct opinions and ideas, many from different cultures and from places far and wide. Wren's experience during these summer months is one of varied and intense interaction. As a result, in her social development she is constantly struggling to find personal meaning in the intricacies of her experience—to integrate emotional engagement with a reasoned analysis of what she is learning. This integration of emotion and reason is a central task of the web-weaving and tuning essential to growing up, and it's not easy.

Wren is small-boned, almost pixielike, with bobbed brown hair and twinkling hazel eyes. But like all healthy young children, that little package contains astonishing energy and a curiosity that is insatiable. Living with animals, adults, and a sister five years her senior, Wren's curiosity is well served. In particular she is a fountain of knowledge about the goings-on at Knoll Farm and the responsibilities that come with being a farmer. I remember one evening in the late summer when together we were given the responsibility of doing the evening chores—feeding the chickens and collecting the eggs; making sure the sheep were secure in their pen; and selecting some vegetables from the garden for supper. Wren made it clear from the beginning that I was her helper. I was given precise instructions not only on how to conduct myself around the animals but also on the priorities that we should follow. Central to the whole was a continuous stream of animated conversation: her mobile face, expressive hands, and well-modulated voice left no ambiguity regarding her intentions and my part in our exercise. Thus when my performance fell short of expectations, I was gently reminded as to the nature of my duties.

By now you may be inclined to dismiss Wren as a little girl too big for her britches. But in fact, understanding her behavior within the context of normal childhood development helps illustrate how reason and empathic awareness begin to spin the web of habit. Acts of sharing and working constructively together—behaviors complementary to empathic concern—are heavily dependent upon an intuitive conformity to common goals, especially in difficult times. It is during such times that outliers and nonconformists make things complicated: better by far to shape behavior ahead of any crisis by encouraging collaborative habits. Among the Kalahari Bushmen, for example, children are taught to divide the food they receive and offer half of it to another: the gifting of their personal beads to a playmate is another tradition. But in addition to leading by example, another way of shaping social behavior is by mild and consistent rebuke.

Wren, no doubt having been the object of this technique of gentle shaping, now intuitively encoded, was interested in practicing her skills as we worked together around the farm. I was the new kid on the block and needed to be schooled. Wren had learned the nuts and bolts of caring for chickens and for sheep not only through instruction but also from her own observation and the preconscious assimilation of habit—routines of behavior that she was eager to pass on to me. At a practical level she saw it as her job to make her wishes clear and to teach me the important farm routines, but in doing so she was also exercising her own emerging sense of mastery. In regard to her own behavior, Wren was beginning to exercise the habit of *self-command*, a function of the maturing lateral prefrontal cortex.

TO CONSISTENTLY SHAPE the capacity for self-command, childhood learning must be built upon those stable emotional attachments that are forged in infancy. As every attentive parent knows, young children are able early to make their wishes clear. An innate capacity to express fundamental emotion through the facial musculature—signals of fear, joy, pain, and distaste—is apparent within the first few weeks of life. Similarly babies can read the emotions of others. Substantial portions of the human brain, particularly the frontal cortex and the parietal-temporal region, are given over to recognizing faces and to interpreting the emotions they convey, as new parents quickly discover when amusing their offspring by pulling funny faces or sticking out the tongue.

Charles Darwin, experimenting with his infant son, noted that when the maid pretended to weep, the child appeared sad, despite being too young to have learned the association. Such emotional behavior, Darwin concluded, must be built into the pith of the person—an inherited instinct of survival that engaged the world instantly. It is in the newborn that the tuning of communication begins. The young mother interprets a preprogrammed grimace as a smile, and in the process of caring for her baby she smiles back. The phyletic neuronal program thus activated in the baby's brain perceives the pleasures of that caring as reward, and the pattern repeats itself. This interactive loop of positive reinforcement within the security of the developing love bond between parent and child nurtures the later development of complex social behavior.

Faces fascinate not only babies but also adults. The ability to read facial expression is essential to our social understanding throughout life. It is through the face that we perceive the comforting concern of a lover, or that we relax amid the smiles of friends. Reading facial expressions is a preverbal, universal mode of human communication. This capacity is deeply wired, as has recently been confirmed in a unique study from Israel, which compared the facial emotions in blind persons with those of sighted members of their families. In joy and sadness family members who are blind from birth exhibit similar facial expressions as their siblings. Emotion, expressed instinctually through the facial musculature, is the primary human language.

Building upon this emotional signaling, the human brain is also tuned to engage with the social world through astute observation and mimicry. Implicitly we study and copy the behavior of others, coming to understand their intent by imagining ourselves in their place and, by association, the emotion they must be feeling, as Adam Smith astutely described two centuries ago. We now know that these fundamentals of imitative behavior are enabled in the brain by what have aptly been described as *mirror neurons*. This research has begun to offer a richer understanding of the brain mechanisms whereby motor habits develop, and even of how young children build upon their fascination with faces to master the art of social communication.

Mirror neurons were discovered accidentally in 1996 by a team of Italian scientists led by Giacomo Rizzolatti, when studying how the brain initiates movement. As the story goes, the brain cells being monitored in one of the monkeys began to fire as the animal observed a graduate student about to eat an ice cream cone. The monkey had not moved. Similar observations had been made earlier involving peanuts and raisins and other kinds of food; when the monkey heard or saw others eating, even though the animal was not actively participating in the feast, cells close to the motor area of the cortex fired in unison.

It was soon discovered using a variety of imaging techniques that similar mirror neuron systems are peppered throughout the human cortex and potentially are involved in everything from the silent imitation of the physical actions of others to intuitive understanding. In addition to clustering in brain regions responsible for perception and movement, mirror neurons are found in brain areas associated with the ability to understand the emotion and intentions of others—areas such as the temporal lobe, the posterior parietal lobe of the cortex, and the insula, which plays an important role in our subjective awareness of inner bodily states and the perception of pain.

Marcus Iacoboni, a neurology professor at the Semel Institute for Neuroscience at UCLA, believes that the insula cortex helps modulate the instinctual drives of the old lizard brain, thus promoting empathic understanding. So how does empathy go beyond sympathy? you may ask. Broken into its elements, *empathy is the ability to "feel" the emotional state of another and to "project" oneself into the situation they face*—and in so doing to create a virtual understanding of their subjective experience in one's own mind—while continuing to "discriminate" oneself apart, as an autonomous individual.

Thus in an fMRI brain-imaging study, conducted by Iacoboni and his colleagues, where the subjects were asked to either imitate or to observe emotional facial expressions, the *insula blood flow was greater during imitation* than during observation. This suggests that the insula is indeed an active player in understanding the emotions of others. Conversely, and in support of this possibility, the researchers also found that when the insula region was neurologically damaged, the sufferer was impaired in recognizing emotional signals, with empathic understanding compromised.

Beyond the laboratory, however, a fundamental question is what behaviors do the brain's mirror mechanisms facilitate in everyday life? One intriguing possibility, put forward by Rizzolatti, is that they "provide a direct understanding of the actions and emotions of others, without [the need for] higher order cognitive mediation." In other words—cast your mind back to my conversation with Joaquín Fuster in Chapter 4—*the mirror systems of the brain, acting in concert with the perception-action cycle, enhance the capacity to make swift, reflexive choices based upon intuitive habit.* This frame of understanding helps explain, among other things, the extraordinary efficiency of acquired habits. The brain's mirror neuron systems not only tune the physical skills required to improve our tennis game; they also help us navigate the social world intuitively and efficiently.

The social ability, through these mental gymnastics, to perceive the intentions of others has acquired in psychology the eloquent title *theory of mind.* It is argued that the mental capacity to operate within a social web of great complexity is an important evolutionary step, distinguishing our own social behavior from that of other primates. By observing the behavior of others and going through the subjective exercise of reproducing what we observe, we gain a better understanding of the other individual's thoughts and feelings. By so doing, we implicitly presume that they too have a mind—hence the title *theory of mind*—accepting that the mind observed is unique and distinct from our own. Indeed, at its zenith, such empathic ability is often construed as wisdom. But most intriguing of all—and most tragic—is that in some children this fundamental capacity for social understanding does not develop normally.

I am referring, of course, to the syndrome of autism. Autism is a developmental disability where, among other symptoms, the understanding of the emotional expression of others is impaired. Indeed, some autistic children are frequently so distressed by the complexity of social relationships that, if left to their own devices, they will become preoccupied with inanimate objects and ritual behaviors. A study conducted by the developmental psychologist Mirella Dapretto—in which mildly autistic children were asked to imitate emotional expressions from photographs—revealed that the brain's mirror neurons were relatively inactive in autistic children compared to those whose social behavior was developing normally.

The difficulties experienced by autistic people in the school and work settings emphasize the extraordinary importance of the social world in defining who we are. While we each begin forging a personal self as early as sucking milk, the developmental process unfolds over time and is far from linear. As Leslie Brothers, a psychiatrist, has emphasized in her book *Friday's Footprint; How Society Shapes the Human Mind*, while we might like to think of the brain as a neutral scribe of what we experience—as a good newspaper reporter might strive for objective assessment—such a simple metaphor is far from accurate when it comes to the development and tuning of the self. Rather, it is through continuous social interaction that a child comes to acquire the cultural habits of mind that shape the brain's organization—ultimately honing through reason the skills of speech and written language—to complement emotional awareness and build the amalgam of biology, experience, and imagination that creates personal meaning and a unique self.

WREN, AT THE AGE OF FIVE and in the quest to understand herself and her world, is on the cusp of creating her own theory of mind. At this age the interplay between early childhood attachments and a growing fascination with cultural experience is actively shaping self-awareness. Thus Wren is slowly moving from the concrete to the abstract through fantasy. She has begun the development of the psychological tools and habits she will require to know why and how the world presents itself as it does. In her imaginative play she tests her perceptual understanding through action—*becoming* the farmer, the cook, and the mother—by drawing her sister, parents, and those willing into her games. A box becomes a table, the corner of the barn a house, the broomstick a horse; and with the family dog as trusted companion, the garden shed is transformed into a fort from which to explore the somewhat scary far reaches of the blueberry patch, yet to be pruned of its spring growth. It is through interactive play that Wren develops, as do all children, an abstraction of her experience that is uniquely meaningful to her and separate from the real objects in her world.

Play is an iterative process. Just as when we learned to ride a bicycle or to catch a ball—when the task was to coordinate the brain's hand and eye motor systems—so do we seek through imaginative play to integrate the brain's networks in the perception-action cycle of emotion and reason. Each generation learns these truths anew until they become infused with personal meaning and ingrained as habits of character—those shared canons of ethical behavior that bind us together in common cause. Wren is at the beginning of that journey, for it takes a decade or two to achieve the balance and social maturity that we associate with adulthood. This is in part because the emotional and reward systems of the ancient brain come "online" at a much earlier stage in development than do the frontal cortices, which are heavily dependent upon myelin insulation for efficient function and objective decision making.

Adolescence, in this regard, is a particularly challenging time. Frequently forgotten, however, is that much of the behavior that emerges in the turmoil of adolescence is framed by the experience of what has gone before. The attachments and habits of mind developed during the latency years—essentially those between ages six and twelve—and the peer relationships that are built during that same timeframe play a significant role in how the "terrible teens" unfold. Along with budding sexuality emerges a heightened sensitivity to peer group interaction and social standing, which when harnessed appropriately is an asset in building character. With the frontal cortices yet to reach maturity, however, the newly awakened passions of the ancient limbic brain can also outrun young people's nascent capacity for reason and self-control, especially when they are stressed. Under such circumstances, and commonly when they are in the company of peers, risk-taking behaviors can rapidly escalate, sometimes with tragic consequences.

This is where consistent parental and cultural guidance becomes important. Strong and well-established family ties mitigate such behaviors. My colleague Andrew Fuligni and co-workers, using fMRI technology to better understand the brain regions involved, have shown in a series of studies that meaningful family relationships can buffer adolescent risk-taking. Employing a measure of self-control together with the Balloon Analogue Risk Task (BART), which is an engaging game that correlates well with real-life adolescent risk behaviors such as sexual promiscuity and smoking, the investigators studied forty-eight young subjects. In the BART game the participant has a series of opportunities to inflate a virtual balloon: the greater in size that the balloon becomes, the more money there is to be made. But should the balloon become overinflated and explode, then money is lost. Those youngsters with strong family ties, especially those who reported contributing to the chores and the other necessities of living as a family unit—an informal measure of empathic concern—showed greater restraint in balloon pumping. Associated with such restraint was reduced fMRI activity in the brain's reward centers, and greater activation of the dorso-lateral prefrontal cortex, which as you will recall is part of the brain's braking system and regulator in chief when it comes to emotional behavior. Such studies suggest that sociability and responsible self-command are closely aligned in their development with empathic understanding within the family.

Mary Gordon, the Canadian educator and social entrepreneur, recognizing the importance of strengthening sociability, believes that empathic skills can be usefully taught in the school setting. Indeed, Gordon has demonstrated such in an innovative classroom-based parenting program that includes children as young as three. Each class "adopts" a baby, preferably one about six months old at the outset, and the parent—usually the mother—together with a trained instructor visits the classroom once a month for a school year. During a typical visit the students gather around the baby, who is lying on a blanket, to observe his or her behavior, to ask the mother questions, and to imagine the child's temperament, what is being communicated, the meaning of sounds being made, and so on. The young students, watching the engagement of mother and baby as the infant matures over the school year, come to appreciate through their own empathic awareness not only the meaning of the baby's behavior but also implicitly that of their own siblings, family members, and peers.

The Roots of Empathy program, which began in the 1980s at a family center in Toronto, is now taught in English and French across Canada with the endorsement of the Ministry of Education and has reached more than 68,000 children. Founded on "the wisdom of babies," as Gordon describes it, the goal is to strengthen the development of a child's *moral imagination*—the uniquely human capacity to empathize with others and to respond appropriately in society. While in the developed nations we remain committed to the idea that parents and the nuclear family have the most important influence upon a child's development of empathic awareness, the acquisition of those skills is heavily dependent upon being the fortunate *recipient* of them. Sadly, as family structures fragment in the twenty-first century, such consistency in human interaction is harder to find. This is the cultural inconsistency that Gordon seeks to mitigate. And indeed the Roots of Empathy program has been shown to reduce bullying and aggression in school. But Gordon has a larger goal: in fostering "moral imagination" in children, she hopes to strengthen the web of self-awareness and responsibility that is the foundation of sharing and trust.

WE HAVE NOW SEEN that through early bonding, the capacity for moral imagination, and a consistency in character building, the human animal is predisposed to creating strong empathic societies. But in the social webs that we weave, how does the brain keep everything organized? How do we keep track of the myriad relationships that are involved? Beyond the cooperative drive, what is it that distinguishes us from other social animals in sustaining the capacity for large group living?

Human social groups are far greater in size than those of other primates, where collaborative relationships are sustained largely by mutual grooming. But even in the monkey world where affiliation is highly structured within both social and kinship networks, keeping track of friends and enemies can be a challenging intellectual exercise. The ability to do so appears to be associated with brain size. Robin Dunbar, director of the Institute of Cognitive and Evolutionary Anthropology at Oxford University, believes that it is the computational demands of living in social groups that has led to the unusual growth of the primate cortex; and reciprocally that it is the size of the new cortex that ultimately determines troop size. In support of his thesis Dunbar has calculated that the neocortical ratio—the size of the new cortex compared to that of the total brain—is highly correlated with mean group size in thirty-six different varieties of primate.

Dunbar argues that the size of the functional group in human society is similarly correlated, as in the primate world, with cortical volume. Human groups are too large to be sustained by social grooming, of course. Parenthetically Dunbar has calculated, somewhat puckishly, that if searching for lice and burrs *were* the glue holding human society together, then each of us would be spending some 42 percent of our waking hours doing exactly that! But such levity aside, Dunbar's ratio offers some important insights into the natural social order of human interaction.

In *Homo sapiens* the new cortex has a volume of approximately 1,000 cubic centimeters while total brain volume is 1,250 cubic centimeters, a ratio that is 50 percent larger than that found in any other primate species. By extrapolation Dunbar predicts that in human society stable group relationships can be sustained to a maximum of approximately 150 persons. As he suggests, this number—now referred to as "Dunbar's number"—has an uncanny resonance with the size of the many communities recorded early in human history. So the size of a Neolithic village in Mesopotamia eight thousand years ago was approximately 20 to 25 family dwellings, or some 150 persons. Or consider the great eleventh-century survey conducted by William the Conqueror, familiarly known as the Domesday Book, which showed the average village population in England and Wales to be of comparable size at 150 to 180 persons. Similarly throughout history the basic fighting unit in professional armies has remained stable at around the Dunbar number. In the Roman era, a centurion commanded approximately one hundred men, and it varies little in the combat units of modern times.

Such fighting units have incentives to work together, just as did the villagers of ancient settlements, or the Kalahari Bushmen in their collective struggle against a depriving environment. But what of contemporary democratic societies, where many thousands live together in cities that in turn are clustered within nation-states that number millions of souls? How are such vast conurbations sustained? Beyond the immediate acknowledgement that civic law and the means to enforce it become necessities, two important insights help us understand this conundrum. First is knowledge of the microstructure and self-organizing nature of human social networks, and second is the critical role played by language.

Despite Dunbar's calculation of 150 people being the constraining limit for meaningful interaction, he has never asserted, as some have implied, that such groups are uniform in their structure. He merely predicted that beyond that number of friends and acquaintances, we have limited brain-processing power to keep relationships organized, let alone to nurture the extended associations. While modern technologies have facilitated communication, there is no evidence they have increased our ability to sustain a larger number of meaningful relationships.

So what are meaningful relationships? Recent social research validates common sense: most individuals maintain a cluster of close confidants but also enjoy a larger group of friends and acquaintances. Think of your social network, if you will, as a series of concentric circles with yourself sitting in the middle. The innermost layer—perhaps no more than five or six persons—is composed of those, including family, with whom you share personal confidences and to whom you would turn in times of emotional turmoil. Beyond this intimate circle lies a group of fifteen to twenty friends whom you contact frequently—sharing sympathetic understanding and similar perspectives on life—and with whom you are close enough that their illness or death would be deeply distressing. A further network of perhaps fifty individuals—for reasons yet to be explained the numbers within each widening concentric circle seem to increase by a factor of three—are those with whom we stay in touch but see only irregularly. Thus the average social network extends as a series of hierarchically inclusive subgroupings, with intimacy, meaning, and trust declining as the time invested in each friendship diminishes.

It emerges, therefore, that the larger the social network, the weaker are the ties among individuals. The number of intimate connections that any one person can maintain is limited both by the time and the intellectual effort required to sustain them. Of course, some people are better than others at the social network game: Bill Clinton immediately comes to mind as a paragon of communicative competence, as were Winston Churchill and Ben Franklin before him. Individual differences clearly do exist and indeed may be prewired. Emerging evidence from fMRI studies, for example, suggests that the ventral portion of the medial frontal cortex plays a critical role in determining social aptitude, further validating Dunbar's hypothesis that it is the new cortex that has given humans our edge in social communication. But beside social aptitude, the skill that Clinton, Franklin, and Churchill share is that of extraordinary verbal facility. It is language—in complement to intelligence and empathic understanding—that has been critical in our social success.

WE DON'T KNOW WHEN human language emerged, for it left no physical trace in the archeological record comparable to the use of tools or fire. What is obvious, however, is that while people can speak, our closest cousins, the chimpanzees, have only limited verbal communication even though they may have a primitive theory of mind. Yet we share some 98 percent of our genetic material with the chimp. So what has made the difference? Nature is inherently conservative in its evolution. Segments of the genetic code that work well—those templates that code for the building blocks that are well adapted to environmental circumstances—are retained across species. Only when a change in code emerges, through mutation or recombination, and proves itself under the challenge of natural selection to be more adaptive does evolutionary shift occur.

The first hint that the facility for language might have evolved from a fortuitous mutation that is not enjoyed by the chimpanzee came from the burdens carried by a family of individuals living in London. Among three generations of this kinship—known in the scientific literature as the KE family—almost half of the members suffered from difficulties in speaking. Their incapacities were not just in the articulation of words and the construction of sentences but also in controlling the fine movements of the face and mouth that are essential to creating the phonetics that support language expression. In 2001 the neurogeneticist Simon Fisher, then a graduate student at Oxford University, together with fellow researchers in London and Oxford, found that the gene FOXP2 in affected family members, located on chromosome 7, had an architectural fault that impaired its regulatory role in the neuronal and neuromuscular development essential to speech production.

FOXP2 is one of a set of "master" genes, highly conserved during evolution, that play important roles in setting up the basic machinery of life. Thus yeast cells, mice, dogs, and the great apes show little difference in the FOXP2 genes they carry. The human version, however, differs slightly from that of other primates by two base pairs, a slight coding difference that was so beneficial that it spread rapidly through our ancestral population—what scientists call a selective sweep—potentially to facilitate the development of language. Interestingly our close cousins the Neanderthals, from which *Homo sapiens* diverged 300,000 to 400,000 years ago and who became extinct some 30,000 years ago, appear to have carried the same mutation.

The chimpanzee, however, from which we diverged five to seven million years ago, does not. The small instructional changes in the human FOXP2 gene compared to the chimp variant determine the differential activity of a whole cascade of other genes—genes known to be involved in the brain's control of motor function and in the formation of the face, skull, cartilage, and connective tissue. Thus the human FOXP2 gene guides the activity not only of other genes within the brain itself but also those enabling the brain's control of the mouth muscles, vocal cords, and breathing system essential to the phonetics of speech. Hence, although the FOXP2 gene should not be considered, in and of itself, "the language gene," when it swept through the human population some 100 to 400 centuries ago, it does appear to have facilitated the *development* of complex language.

This fortunate shift immeasurably improved our social adaptation by enhancing communication, which facilitated group size and stimulated cortical brain growth to create a positive feedback loop that gave *Homo sapiens* an extraordinary evolutionary advantage. Conversation proved not only efficient and informative but also entertaining and fun. Chattering works well with many different chores and under varied social circumstances.

What we particularly like to talk about is each other. We call this new "grooming" behavior gossip, and it's the bread and butter not only of Facebook, the talk shows, and the tabloid press but of each one of us in sustaining everyday social interaction. Eric Foster, a professor of management at the University of Pennsylvania's Wharton School, who has made an extensive study of gossip, concludes that social topics involving everyone present or third parties are the focus of conversation some two-thirds of the time, with, perhaps surprisingly for some, "little empirical evidence that women gossip more than men."

AS EVERY PARENT KNOWS, along with chatter and language in childhood comes questioning. From an early age children ask many questions—by the fourth year, literally hundreds of them every day. Gossiping in adult life may be understood as an extension of this developmental stage when children begin to imagine events they have not witnessed, and people they've never met. Through this imagining we begin construction of the set of inner maps that sustain our own unique web of sociability. In childhood it's an essential exercise for the nascent mind—akin to the physical play that tunes habitual motor skills—whereby an intuitive order is placed upon the world, with fact distinguished from fantasy, an essential forerunner to the formal task of schooling and literacy.

For a five-year-old such as Wren, the questioning marks the early imaginings of a stable group of attachments that in adulthood become the basis of consistent, real-life social interaction. The development of such imagined, fixed systems of interrelationship, as Maurice Bloch, the Anglo-French cultural anthropologist, has described them, is the foundation of human culture. Although in reality all is fluid in the give-and-take of everyday life, it is through such imaginings, as I shall discuss in Chapter 10, that we craft a cultural system—political, legal, moral, and social—that is of enduring capacity. It is this ability to imagine a future of stable social engagement, with both individuals and institutions, that we call trust. Trust, in all its complexity—a maturational process nurtured first by the mother-infant bond, tuned in meaning through empathic awareness, and honed in efficiency by intuitive understanding—is something uniquely human.

But in that genesis, trust is also something uniquely fragile. Reflect for one more moment, if you will, upon the milestones in the emotional and intellectual development of a five-year-old child such as Wren, as I have described them here. In just a few short years—from the early security of a mother's love through the anxious ambiguities of novel caregivers, shifting attachments, and the beginnings of peer sociability—the infant mind adopts the preconscious efficiencies of habit, slowly forges self-awareness, and begins to embrace imagination and language. In the ideal world, these achievements weave the delicate web that sustains a child's capacity to place their trust in others. This web of trust, in its collective expression, is the foundation of human society.

It is also a web easily broken. A depressed mother, marital discord in the parents, neglect, significant trauma, the privations of poverty, and the excessive indulgence of affluence: for decades it has been known that such challenges can compromise not only the progression of early developmental milestones but also permanently scar individuals, compromising school achievement and predisposing them later in life to anxiety, depression, and self-destructive behaviors. What was not accepted until recently, however, is that such demanding "external" social conditions have the power to profoundly influence the most basic of "internal" biological processes, including the gene expression that shapes our behavior.

The lesson is that the genetic prescription we each carry does not alone determine our destiny: but the interaction of that prescription with family, culture, and experience certainly does, with powerful effects upon how we think and feel and how we will live in adult life. This interactive process, pursuing my analogy to Bach's well-tempered clavier, may be thought of as the first steps that we take in the "self-tuning" of the brain—and the beginning of a lifelong personal journey. For each of us, however, in these helter-skelter times, the challenge is whether it remains possible to achieve such qualities of character development when the consumer culture barely sustains them. And yet how skilled we eventually become in our self-tuning has important implications, not only for personal resilience but also for public and social policy—shaping the choices that we make, the cultural institutions that we promote, the cities that we build, the food we eat, and the respect we have for the natural environment. And perhaps most important of all, as the cycle continues, it shapes how we flexibly educate the next generation of children for what is an uncertain future.

It is to this latter subject that I now turn.

Chapter 7

Character: Education and Self-Command

A very young child has no self-command; whatever are its emotions, whether fear, or grief or anger, it endeavours always by the violence of its outcries, to alarm as much as it can, the attention of its nurse, or of its parents. When it is old enough to go to school, or to mix with its equals, it soon finds that they have no such indulgent partiality. It thus enters into the great school of self-command; it studies to be more and more master of itself: and begins to exercise over its own feelings a discipline.

Adam Smith, *The Theory of Moral Sentiments* (1759)

A Clerk ther was of Oxenford . . .
And gladly wolde he lerne, and gladly teche.

Geoffrey Chaucer, *The Canterbury Tales*
(late fourteenth century)

WE ARE EACH, THROUGHOUT LIFE, both student and teacher. But how to learn and what to teach? Is it just the facts, as Mr. Thomas Gradgrind in Charles Dickens's *Hard Times* insisted? "Now, what

I want is facts. Teach these boys and girls nothing but facts. Facts alone are wanted in life." But of course, as with many of Dickens's characters, Gradgrind repents by the end of the saga, recognizing that facts emerge from curiosity, imagination, and a sense of meaning. The attempted transformation of children into emotionless mechanical robots, dutifully spouting rote formulae and facts, just didn't work. Human beings with all our hopes and fears, argued Dickens through his characters, are not utilitarian machines.

That was in the mid-nineteenth century, but the debate goes on. After all, some facts are valuable—as are the habits needed to acquire them—and learning factual information even can be made fun. So believed my own physics master, Mr. Wesson, whom I can see as clearly now as when he stood before our class at the grammar school, insisting that the date be written "in my way." Mr. Wesson had each of us living in bemused terror: should we be caught looking out the window, there soon would be a hand on the collar directing that we pay attention to the work not the world. And yet we loved the man and his many endearing eccentricities. Probably in his sixties—it's hard to judge the age of one's elders when one is young—Mr. Wesson had the peculiar habit of leaving his cheeks unshaven, twirling and playing with the two wiry clumps of facial adornment as he paced and lectured. That he kept his trousers up with braces, supplemented by a length of Bunsen burner tubing tied around the waist, and that he told extremely funny jokes, many of which were self-deprecating, just added to our fascination. He was an eccentric and a caring one at that, which in addition to his insistence upon a disciplined approach to study—"to secure your future, my boy"—made him an exceptional teacher.

Mr. Wesson, with all his oddities, understood how to craft the habits of self-reliance that are the foundation of character and lifelong learning. We all agreed that he had a unique way of prodding us out of complacency and providing a new perspective on the world. Thus when in the second year of my lessons with him he died suddenly from what was rumored to be a carcinoma, there was a pervasive sadness in the school. Looking back, I remember only fragments of the facts that he taught me: but the capacity for study and a fascination with ideas, the qualities at the core of his instruction, have stayed with me. Beyond the facts, Mr. Wesson was a great teacher.

SO WHAT MAKES a great teacher? What are the elements of excellent instruction, and how do they work together to determine high performance in students? What marks the best performing schools? Thanks to a program that was established in 2000 by the Organization for Economic Cooperation and Development (OECD), which tracks the academic achievement of fifteen-year-old students in reading, math, and science across its thirty-four member countries, we are now able to engage such questions, directly comparing educational philosophy and achievement across varied instructional systems and cultures.

The results have been surprising. That the major reason for student failure in school is lack of financial investment, as many teachers' unions in the United States have argued, turns out not to be the driving issue. As I will further explore in this chapter, disparities in finance are important variables, as are sociocultural factors, but money alone does not determine differences in scholastic achievement. Indeed, the OECD's Program for International Student Assessment (PISA) suggests that a nation's financial investment may account for less than 10 percent of the variance in overall performance. The United States, for example, recognizing that it was falling behind other developed countries, increased public spending per student, after correcting for inflation, by 73 percent between 1980 and 2005. Nonetheless student achievement measured by the PISA survey remained stubbornly entrenched in the lower rankings. While some individual states, most notably Massachusetts and Connecticut, performed well when considered individually in the 2009 survey, as a nation the

United States ranked 17th, 31st, and 23rd in reading, math, and science respectively. Furthermore, although in the 2012 survey a slight trend toward improvement was apparent in the U.S. math and science scores, its international ranking was essentially unchanged. The United Kingdom, with average performance in math and science and above average in reading, similarly did not improve its performance between 2006 and 2012. This is in contrast to other regions studied—Shanghai-China, Singapore, Canada, Saxony, and Poland being among them—that consistently have done so.

Intrigued by such differences, the international consulting firm McKinsey, in a study published in 2007, investigated twenty-five of the best-performing school systems in the world. It concluded that three things mattered most: first, securing the best people to become teachers; second, supporting them in their continuing professional development; and third, ensuring that high-quality instruction was consistently and equitably available to every child, regardless of circumstance.

One country that comes to mind in reading this prescription is Finland, which stands as an exemplar when measured by the academic accomplishments of its students. This little country with a population of some 5.4 million people has consistently achieved an upper ranking in the PISA surveys since their inception in 2000. Described by *The Atlantic* magazine as "the West's reigning education superpower," Finland is also unusual in that it achieves its high rankings with only small variation among student test scores, showing that consistently high academic performance is possible across all socioeconomic groups. And yet on close inspection, by comparison with the prevailing Western obsession of injecting market competition into education, or the pressure cooker system of rote learning and cramming employed in East Asia, Finland's formula for success seems something of an anachronism.

Finland's prevailing philosophy, first and foremost, is to develop an *equitable* system of instruction for students—the third element of McKinsey's triumvirate. Second is to recruit only those with the best minds to become teachers, paying them good wages from early in their career and giving them considerable responsibility and independence thereafter. In Finland, on the average, 10 percent of applicants are admitted into the teaching profession: this intense competition ensures that only outstanding individuals succeed. Over five to seven years at an established university, the would-be-teacher earns both an undergraduate and a master's degree and is expected to develop a strong academic record in addition to demonstrating excellent interpersonal skills in the classroom. Once graduated, teachers have autonomy and freedom in their approach to curricula development, together with the opportunity and encouragement to develop their own educational focus. Thus teaching in Finland is a profession that is desirable, prestigious, and dynamic.

In the Finnish school system exams are infrequent, being replaced by thoughtful assessments of each student by their individual teachers, with personalized plans crafted regularly for refinement and remedial exercise. Rather than a model of intense competition—of spot tests and a race to the top—instruction is collaborative, indeed almost leisurely. Students do not enter elementary school until the age of seven; the day is shorter than in most schools in the United States or Britain, and creative, playful engagement with the natural world is encouraged. The result is an educational environment of low stress with an emphasis on strong personal attachment, promoting both happy students and satisfied teachers. It seems too good to be true, but given Finland's repeated success in the international rankings of academic achievement, something is obviously working. Pasi Sahlberg, director of the Center for International Mobility and Cooperation at the Finnish Ministry of Education and Culture, in his book *Finnish Lessons* emphasizes that it is not competitive school choice that is important in achieving excellence but rather the equitable distribution of opportunity for all students, regardless of their economic background. Finland's educational system thrives not upon stimulating student rivalry but through fostering collaborative learning and strong problem-solving habits.

Constructing educational systems that work is not rocket science, but neither is it simple. The 2007 McKinsey report, linking quantitative results from the PISA study with the qualitative insights of their own investigations, has helped elucidate what distinguishes high-performing school systems. The findings question, for example, whether structural reorganization contributes much to student success. Both Britain and the United States have experimented with school integration, decentralization, choice, and interschool competition. Of themselves, none of these models are associated with consistent improvement in student achievement. Similarly, from a review of more than one hundred studies, lowering student-to-teacher ratios alone, independent of teaching practice, appears to have little impact on student performance except at the lower grade levels.

So how may we make sense of these findings? If we step back for a moment and consider the McKinsey report within the context of what we know about human development, what the Finns have demonstrated in their thirty-year experiment makes good sense. The Finnish experience reminds us that it is the personal bond between trusting students and dedicated, skillful teachers that lays the foundation for academic success. In the Finnish classroom, to quote Pasi Stahlberg, the critical ingredient is "placing [personal] responsibility and trust before [test] accountability." It is a reminder that in the free society, beyond the acquisition of facts, education serves a moral purpose— the development of individual character and the capacity for self-directed growth. I call it the Wesson effect.

The Finnish experiment promotes some important questions. Has the Anglo-American model of secondary education derailed because we have ignored the humanitarian and developmental aspects of learning? Have we forgotten that throughout life, but particularly when we are young, we learn best from the trial and error of personal experimentation, in a secure environment and guided by those we trust? In the face of growing economic competition abroad and declining student performance at home, have we opted for the short-term fix? In choosing corporate-style top-down planning and metric-driven, market competition—rather than tackling the perennial challenges of promoting professional excellence, achieving equal student access, and strengthening the relationships among teacher, pupil, and family—have we inadvertently encouraged bifurcation in educational opportunity and student achievement?

From the perspective of the behavioral neuroscientist, four simple words describe the ecology of educational development: *attachment, meaning, habit*, and *trust*. These words form *a progressive sequence*, and they will be recognized as reflecting the *maturational process* that I described in Chapter 6. A fifth element is *opportunity*, and when that is present, the educational-maturational cycle continues throughout life. For all of us, as social animals, *attachment* is primary; it is within the security of mutual attachment that personal *meaning* develops; and from the confidence that social meaning brings grows empathic understanding and the efficiency of intuitive *habit*. It is through the educational-maturational cycle, as these elements are woven together, that *self-awareness* develops, together with personal well-being and the capacity to *trust* others. Similarly, through this progression, we develop the skills of self-reliance—the capacity for self-tuning and the thoughtful adaptation to circumstance that we call character. Should the sequence be neglected or disrupted in its maturation, however, then we stumble.

In our struggles toward maturity and autonomy we build upon our inherited platform of temperament, but it is what we learn from each other and the habits that we acquire that largely shape character. From the perspective of neuroscience, think of it as the brain's perception-action cycle at work—an extended dance whereby emotional sensitivity melds with growing intellectual awareness of the external world to create the intuitive habits, the guiding beliefs, and the capacity for executive action that characterize mature human behavior. This, for Adam Smith, was "the great school of self-command," an iterative process whereby we become "more and more master" of ourselves, to exercise the melding of passion and reason in collaborative harmony. It is through self-command that the brain is tuned.

THE QUALITIES OF SELF-COMMAND that flow from a broadly based system of education are also essential to sustaining a vibrant market economy. The United States was one of the first nations to recognize the importance of this equation. As Claudia Goldin, the Henry Lee Professor of Economics at Harvard, has detailed in her writings, America's promotion of mass education during the twentieth century played a key role in its economic success and rise to world dominance. The roots of this achievement are to be found in the primary school movement of the nineteenth century, later enhanced by the rapid growth of high school enrollment in the early part of the twentieth century. By the early 1960s the U.S. high school graduation rate was over 70 percent, far higher than in the European nations. This growth went hand in hand with the growing demand for a literate and skilled labor force to sustain America's established leadership in technology, manufacturing, and international trade.

But today, fifty years later, this enviable position has ebbed away. "Education Slowdown Threatens US," proclaimed a *Wall Street Journal* headline in the spring of 2012. And indeed today, despite their aspirations many young Americans are not as well educated as their parents. Remarkably, while 70 percent of high school graduates enroll in college, many never obtain a degree or diploma; 43 percent of the students who entered as freshmen in 2002 had not received a degree six years later. As a result, as a percentage of population, the United States now lags in the proportion of its citizens attaining a top college degree. In 2009 fourteen of the world's developed countries in the world graduated a higher percentage of individuals from college than did America. Yet the United States spends a greater portion of its GDP on higher education than any other nation.

A partial explanation of these demographic shifts, including the failure to graduate, is that the cost of college education in America is soaring, putting it out of reach of many middle-class families. Higher education in America has bubbled into being a growth industry: fees at American universities rose five times faster than inflation between 1980 and 2010. In 2013 for the leading private universities of the Ivy League, the cost of tuition alone was hovering around $40,000 per year. Even for the public-supported colleges and universities, beset by cutbacks in state funds, in the first decade of the new millennium the annual cost of tuition and fees rose 72 percent to just under $9,000. In consequence, student debt now exceeds that of credit card debt in the United States, ballooning from $41 billion in 1999 to $87 billion a decade later.

These numbers reflect the growing bifurcation in the educational opportunities available to young Americans. This is also true for British students. While America's leading universities remain among the best in the world—of the one hundred top ranked institutions, 50 percent are in the United States—and house faculties of extraordinary achievement in both science and the arts, the rising cost of attendance is constraining access. The evidence is growing that America is falling behind in the development of a flexible and broadly educated citizenry. A 2005 study funded by the Pew Charitable Trusts, based on a sample of 1,827 graduating students from 80 randomly selected two- and four-year private and public colleges, found that of those individuals graduating with a four-year degree, only 50 percent had basic quantitative and literacy skills, such as assessing the comparative value of potential purchases or following the logic of a written argument. This does not bode well for the nation's future.

Ideally education helps develop the student's capacity for creative thought and communication, which in a democratic society is an essential social good. Unfortunately, however, in a competitive, market-dominated culture, it is easy to fall into the Mr. Gradgrind trap. Prioritizing the acquisition of facts for their economic value has the inherent danger of stifling a student's innate creativity by reducing the learning process to a test-driven product line. The purpose of attending a "good" school becomes largely to secure a "good" job, one that will generate the economic returns of the "good" life, with little attention paid to what living a "good" life actually entails.

Such an assembly-line approach is in many ways a covert form of central planning that views young people as commodities to be fit into preconceived parameters in hopes of ensuring their future economic contribution. But the relationship between a vibrant economy and facts acquired in college is not fixed. Given the rate of technical innovation in the developed economies and the shift away from direct human labor, it is difficult to predict the labor force America will need in the next decade, let alone the next century. Common sense would suggest that it is better to make the cultural investments necessary to teach students to think for themselves, providing them with the self-discipline required to hone the intellectual skills that will serve them and society, over a lifetime of adaptation and learning.

In a market-driven consumer society such as the United States, however, not to maximize economic gain is considered failure. The inherent danger in educating principally to foster market growth, however, is that while the search for new goods stimulates technological innovation and consumer desire, the democratic society's need for collective wisdom is less well served. Under economic pressure, as James Engell and Anthony Dangerfield note in *Saving Higher Education in the Age of Money*, "parents and students no longer choose the best education that money can buy . . . [but] are faced with choosing which college . . . will buy them more money." In a competitive society it is understandable that families ask how their investment will serve to secure a lucrative position in the volatile job market of globalization.

But if only an economic analysis is offered to justify the value of college, then institutions of higher learning fall short of their broader educational responsibilities. Thus we drift toward the consumer-oriented university.

The fundamental truth is that buying an education is different from buying a refrigerator. Students are more akin to fine craftsmen than to consumers: they are not passive recipients of product but create knowledge within themselves through interaction with mentors, peers, and others who have a significant presence in their lives. The result, a balanced self, is a powerful instrument for economic good. Thus what guarantees employment and happiness in a rapidly changing world is what has always guaranteed it: achieving the ethos—the strength of character and self-command—that ensures lifelong learning and responsible citizenship. I would argue that honing the qualities that make for such character strengths—critical thought, analytical skills, a sense of justice, aesthetic appreciation, and empathic awareness—is the central task of higher education. The outcome of such a delicate process cannot be measured merely in market terms, as when one seeks the "best buy" refrigerator. Higher education needs to embrace responsibility for the development of student self-awareness and for disciplined understanding of the human condition. In short, it is through broad educational opportunity that we ensure leadership tomorrow.

THE BRITISH ECONOMIST John Maynard Keynes, who graduated with a mathematics degree from Cambridge in 1904, believed in such an ethos—that the primary social role of the university is to develop intelligence and character by honing the student's skills of reasoning and communication. Once that foundation is in place, Keynes argued, the details of any chosen profession are easily acquired.

Today, a century on from Keynes, George Bowen, who lectures in management studies at Queen's College and the Saïd Business School at Oxford University, is in staunch agreement. I first met George on a ferryboat that was making a stormy crossing of the Irish Sea—nothing life endangering but uncomfortable enough to get people into conversation—and we soon stumbled upon our mutual interest in education. George, who came to his teaching career after several decades as an executive in the global textile industry, is a passionate supporter of the tutorial, which since the nineteenth century has been the hallmark of undergraduate study at Oxford and was a tradition informally established long before that.

The essay is the core exercise in developing the skills of reasoning and communication, George explained to me one afternoon, as we sat amid portraits of grim-faced kings and long-gone princes in the senior common room at Queen's College. "I know it sounds simplistic," he said, settling into his armchair with a cup of coffee, "but the under-graduate literally comes to Oxford to learn how to write essays. Each week during the academic year the student writes a mini-thesis on a study topic that is chosen with their tutor." The primary objective is to acquire the discipline of making a logical argument that supports their personal conclusions.

"I tell my students," continued George, "that if they want to argue that the moon is green and not yellow, then that is fine. We are not arguing about right and wrong. I just want to see how well they can construct an argument and whether the conclusion reached is logical. I want to see in the first couple of paragraphs what they understand their topic to be before setting out to explain that understanding. We don't want all the answers up front, just an indication that they have given thought to the topic before they started writing. The task is then to review the literature in brief, to develop their argument, and to bring their thesis to an intelligent conclusion.

"The essays are marked thirty percent on structure, thirty percent on content, and the rest on the strength and originality of the argu-ment," he continued. "This means that the student must not only become familiar with the primary authorities on the topic, but also bring their own sources and authors to the party. We do not want the students to tell us what is in books—they are meant to have read that stuff—but to juxtapose and integrate their own ideas in comparative discussion."

In George's experience a weekly one-hour tutorial, in combination with essay writing, enables the mentor to assess the personal skills and knowledge of each student, progressively raising the bar until the discipline of analytic thinking is achieved. "So you're on your own," reflected George. "There's no alternative but to buckle down and work. We teach a key lesson for life, the secret to unearthing reliable information, thinking logically, and making sound judgments."

In fact, as I proposed to George that afternoon, his real business at the college was not in teaching management but in the development of good habits within a supportive and caring relationship. In mastering the discipline of the essay the student was honing the brain's capacity for intuitive learning and releasing the power of the orbital-frontal cortex—the executive brain—to do what it does best, to think and to choose. George nodded. "The essay is merely the vehicle," he agreed, "while the interactive tutorial format strengthens the good feelings between student and teacher." He found this particularly valuable for some of his foreign students, including those from the United States, many of whom were unfamiliar and uncomfortable in offering opinions of their own. "It comes as a bit of a shock," George remarked, "because many of them are used to just assembling facts, to concentrating on content and on regurgitating the book or the notes, rather than pushing them aside and thinking for themselves."

The skill set, I suggested to George, was similar to that of a good psychotherapist, which is to start from where the individual feels comfortable and from there to discover what they find meaningful (that is, to employ the progressive sequence of the maturational process—attachment, meaning, habit, etc.—as I outlined it earlier in this chapter) rather than to dive straight into abstract discussion. "Exactly," George replied. "So in the beginning, I try to have some in-depth, meaningful talk with each student: where they're coming from, where they are in their thinking, and where they would like to be in a few years' time. I build on that conversation and particularly on areas where they've done well. What we're teaching is often highly abstract—the creation of wealth, management failure, and so on—and it's necessary to relate the essay writing and course of study to what they can grasp easily, especially at the outset. So I might connect the abnormal profits in the luxury goods market to a young woman's interest in designer handbags. Or I hitch a boyhood interest in aircraft modeling to the problems of Boeing Aircraft, a company that despite its dominant position in the industry faces the challenge of Airbus, which enjoys government support. In short I try to frame the new with what's familiar."

George paused for a moment. "Oxford is a very peculiar place," he continued, waving his hand at the assembled portraits on the wall. "It is a private charity and has been so for about one thousand years. Students who come here often choose to do so because of the tutorial system. The essay is our heuristic tool. Rooted in the Greek litera-ture of Platonic and Socratic argument, it was dusted off during the Renaissance and reinvented to become a basic educational form. So the lure of Oxford, and places like it, remains this type of intimate education. Basically, when it comes to autonomy and discipline, we practice what we preach: unlike many universities no one sits in on my tutorials. Presumably if I were doing badly I would be told, but in general having come out of business this is a very strange professional world! Productivity and efficiency are not defined the same way as in the marketplace, but nonetheless individuals with fine leadership skills continue to emerge."

But what of today? I asked. Oxford and comparable universities are elite institutions, to which only a minority of students gains access. What of the rest? "Yes, that is the challenge," George agreed. "But let's not lose sight of the forest for the trees. The goal of a liberal edu-cation is to encourage people to use their imagination and to think for themselves—no easy task in today's affluent world of predigested, instant information. We are privileged here: the students are bright with strong educational backgrounds, and on average eager to learn. I accept that privilege, but it distracts from the point that I'm making. The legacy and history of these ancient institutions teaches us that human beings learn by example: it is through the intimate relationship between student and teacher that thought is disciplined and self-command is achieved. This is the key to lifelong learning. And it works. As student confidence grows, so do flexibility and the appetite for facts, which in today's world are ever changing. That is the lesson we must take away from here and from places like it."

WRITING NOW ABOUT MY conversation with George Bowen, I find my thoughts drifting back to the English grammar school where I was a student in the 1950s. George is right. We know that the formula for academic success lies in the student-teacher dyad maximizing the progressive sequence of the educational process, for that is how the human brain, over millennia, has worked its magic. But how in modern times do we serve the needs of a greater number while preserving that intimate progression? Ironically, I believe that it was our zeal to solve this conundrum, while inadvertently forgetting the role of intimacy in the educational process, that has fostered the growing bifurcation of opportunity in the Anglo-American model of secondary education.

Within two decades of my attendance at the grammar school such institutions had essentially disappeared in Britain, having been replaced by the "comprehensive" model. The hope for this change, as George and I discussed during our afternoon together, was to serve the greater good by improving access to higher education. The effort was unabashedly a copy of the American ideal—championed by John Dewey and others early in the twentieth century—that the bedrock of a democratic nation was universal access to secondary education, providing opportunity for all.

The shift in Britain had come in reaction to the adoption in the 1940s of a system where children were tested and academically divided at the age of eleven, sending some 25 percent of them to grammar school and the rest to schools emphasizing vocational training and practical skills. In the baby-boomer postwar years, in a nation seeking to recover its economic vitality, many considered such constraints wasteful of potential talent. Thus, taking lead from the U.S. model, the comprehensive school program, which abandoned the exams at age eleven, was introduced in 1965 with the goal of increasing the number of students achieving university entrance. No longer would social class limit educational opportunity.

Certainly at midcentury the U.S. system of comprehensive schooling was yielding some impressive results. A 1968 study by the National Academy of Sciences provided evidence that America had become "the leading producer of mathematical talent in the world." And yet acrimonious debate regarding America's competitiveness was never far from the surface, especially in the immediate post-Sputnik period, when fear of Soviet domination began to drive educational priorities in science and technology. Also America was growing fast: between 1960 and 2012 the population of the United States grew 74 percent, from approximately 180 million to 315 million. High schools too were growing in size and changing in character as the nation adopted an industrialized, assembly-line approach to producing the skilled workforce necessary for an expanding economy.

Consolidated for economic efficiency and requiring large parcels of land, the secondary school increasingly moved to the edge of town and adopted a sprawling, sometimes modular design not dissimilar from the suburban homes that surrounded it. Beginning in the 1970s, with mandatory busing to promote racial integration in certain communities, many students found themselves far from home in unfamiliar neighborhoods; walking to school became impossible. The physical learning environment also was changing. Following the energy crisis of the 1970s, school buildings were sunk deeper into the ground, with a trend toward grouped windowless classrooms and flat roofs. Gone were the scholastically inspired Gothic and Renaissance styles of earlier decades, when schools reflected local civic pride: the new motive was corporate, with minimal ornamentation.

Soon the majority of the new high schools were enrolling 1,500 students or more, with some having 4,000 or 5,000 adolescents. A supportive educational environment with individual instruction and a relationship of trust between student and teacher were early casualties of this impersonal growth. Predictably, as the progressive sequence of educational maturation was disrupted, a decline in motivation and academic achievement followed—especially for students from disadvantaged and low-income families—together with an escalation of behavioral problems and violence. By 1983 it was recognized that something was seriously amiss. Amid growing concern the Reagan administration released *A Nation at Risk: The Imperative for Educational Reform,* focused principally upon secondary school education. Noting that over the previous two decades, as just one measure of growing mediocrity, there had been a consistent drop in the Scholastic Aptitude Test scores of college-bound seniors, the commission questioned whether America's educational system was up to the task of delivering a workforce that was competitive with those of the other developed nations.

Over the same time period similarly disturbing trends were evident in Britain's effort toward comprehensive schooling. As George Bowen remarked during our discussion, "the vision of opportunity through equal access was to be applauded but the implementation strategy was appalling. We underfunded the new schools, built bad buildings, and had students packed forty to fifty in a class. That is not a recipe for success." Again, in Britain as in the United States, those children particularly disadvantaged were from immigrant and deprived backgrounds, with 20 percent of the students leaving school at sixteen and a substantial number dropping out even earlier, according to an OECD report published in 2012.

For many families, the comprehensive high school system was no longer perceived as an adequate preparation for college. Soon in both Britain and the United States those families who could afford it, and some who could not, were sending their sons and daughters to private or parochial schools, Although only 7 percent of Britons are privately educated—it's about 11 percent in America—they disproportionately hold privileged places in business, the professions, and the nation's political hierarchy. Thus at Oxford and Cambridge approximately half the undergraduates have been privately schooled. A similar pattern of private secondary school education that secures privilege—and one equally entrenched—is to be found in America, where mobility between the social classes is now lower than in most European countries. The industrialization of the secondary school, designed to secure college entrance for a larger number of students, has not only failed miserably in its goal but has also compounded the problems that it first sought to resolve.

THE DISPARITIES AND ongoing failure of America's industrialization of secondary education is readily apparent to Susan Corbin, who juggles each day to remedy its unintended consequences. Since 2000 Susan has taught at El Camino College, a two-year public community college that enrolls 25,000 students in Torrance, California. Torrance is an urban, oil-producing region bordering the Pacific Ocean, southwest of Los Angeles. Not given to despondency, Susan was smiling broadly on the hot afternoon that we met at a coffee shop, close to campus. "You're probably wondering why I'm so happy today?" she volunteered, as we greeted each other. "Well, it's early June, the semester's almost over, and my students are making progress. That's all good news for a community college teacher!"

In her looks, Susan Corbin is as Celtic as her name: brown wavy hair, blue eyes, and an engaging smile. I had first met her at a hospital reception a few months earlier, through her husband who is a physician. That year we were in the midst of California's budget problems, which had included draconian cuts to education, and I had expressed my interest in learning more about how a dedicated frontline teacher coped with such challenges. In subsequent conversations it became apparent that Susan's approach to helping her mostly disadvantaged but college-bound students improve their learning skills drew intuitively upon many principles of behavioral neuroscience, so I became eager to learn more about her method and practice.

"When I first started at the college," Susan began, "I was shocked by the grim reality faced by many of the students. Supposedly I was teaching college-level courses, and yet some 85 percent of those enrolled in my classes had only precollege capability in reading and math. But fascinatingly there was little stigma attached to such inability." She had been a philosophy major in college and had worked as a journalist before going to graduate school, where she had focused on sociolinguistics and literacy studies, making her an excellent candidate to take over remedial reading as her initial assignment. "I was surprised to find in those early weeks," she recalled, "that my colleagues were giving vocabulary worksheets to students whose comprehension was essentially that of early high school—sort of asking the student to memorize the pieces of a jigsaw without benefit of seeing the picture on the box cover. That seemed to me dangerously counterproductive: if you believe as a teacher that acquiring language and writing skills is stringing words together with little attention to their meaning, then your students are unlikely to read with any great skill. I was not immediately popular in the teachers' common room."

Initially being an outsider to the teaching profession—the well-trodden path of the teachers' training college had not been hers—Susan had felt uneasy in taking a rote approach to vocabulary and literacy. Later, recalling her own experience as a youngster heightened her discomfort. "My parents when teaching me to read had invited me to crawl into their laps," she explained. "My father was a graduate student at the time, so for all I knew we were reading a

physics book, but with a singsong voice it potentially sounded interesting to me." Reflecting upon that experience, Susan realized that
she had never consciously memorized vocabulary. "It's the sitting in
the lap—the intimacy and shared attention—that begins the process, not the words on the page. And yet when we're dealing with
disadvantaged kids in high school, or precollege students in remedial
classes, we somehow think that rote memory is the answer. Well, I've
discovered it is not. Remedial students, in particular, need a sense of
belonging. Once that trust is established, then the successful teacher
can focus on gaining the student's interest, something equivalent to
my father's singsong voice. Many students have experienced reading
only as something mechanical, with a college degree a strictly utilitarian step toward a better-paying job. Vocabulary books just don't
shift that preconception." Perhaps, Susan wondered, pondering her
dilemma, the students should be reading rap songs in class or something equivalent. Looking back, she remembers the thought as seeding an important idea.

Susan learned quickly, in befriending her trainees, that the majority
of her disadvantaged, working-class students thought differently about
education than was the experience in her own family. Most had few
books in the their homes growing up. Although they were obviously
determined and smart, having sought out community college despite
many obstacles, reading a book was a contrived activity. Written information was something shared in their families; letters received were
read aloud. It was considered odd to do things by oneself. Thus a student might have acquired the habit of sitting alone at a desk but without tutoring did not have the analytic skills to benefit from the lesson
in front of them. Similarly other family members didn't understand that
studying meant two hours in a quiet corner with the TV turned off.

Furthermore, many of the students in Susan's classes had already
passed the high school equivalency test, which was confusing to the
parents. "So," she told me, "I commonly am asked the question, 'If
my daughter went to high school, why is she now taking ninth-grade

English again?' It's one of the missteps in America's educational system: the children coming from deprived backgrounds are not accultur-
ated to the process of learning, so we slip them through their exams as
a short-term fix." She paused for a moment. "Why study? Good study
habits are tough to build. It's easy for me to teach the language of
responsibility in the abstract, but not so easy for the student to be
intuitively responsible when faced with the demands and materialism
of their everyday existence. Without the meaning that comes from
understanding, it's impossible for them to take the long view."

"So in the last year or two," Susan continued, "in remembering the
idea about rap songs, I've changed my practice. I provide the meaningful social context first and start working on habit building later."
By way of illustration, she described to me how, in a remedial reading class, instead of giving out the assigned text, she and the students
were reading books as a means of developing good study habits. "Yes, I
know," she said, smiling again, "it's mundane, but also revolutionary in
a small way. I start off with *The Pact*. It's real-life biography written by
three doctors who grew up on the streets of Newark, New Jersey, met
in high school, and made it into medical school through friendship and
mutual caring. Students love it. The book speaks to them. Many times
I've had young men who've known the gang scene here in Torrance—
kids who've been to jail—weeping as we read. For these kids the social
context strikes home: the young men weeping in class also had a pact,
but the wrong one. The habits and loyalties of the gang world had not
served them. They too wanted membership and social meaning: they
too wanted to be understood. They just took the wrong turn."

Once the book has the students engaged—once the emotional
investment in the subject matter and the characters is secure—Susan
begins to emphasize those habits of mind required for self-propelled
study in an academic setting. First she introduces the idea of opinion
and choice as the bases of analytic skill, asking "which passages in this
book are real to your own experience, what resonates with you emotionally about the story?" She also encourages her students to speak to

each other about their opinions, something which, as Susan explained, many are afraid to do at first, fearing that they will be made to look foolish. But with practice and classroom interaction trust develops. New perspectives emerge, and individual students begin writing about those ideas that interest them. Susan avoids complex questions about grammar. "My goal at this stage is to strengthen the ability to reason from personal experience," she told me. Similarly, to get the students to read out loud, she sometimes suggests that they pretend to be actors—to deliver the words from the book as if they were their own, thus introducing the skill of speaking to an audience as an important mode of social communication.

"My whole idea is to build confidence starting with a familiar subject, in a secure emotional setting. And it's not lost on the students that it all unfolds just from reading together," Susan explained, smiling again. "I'm an energetic participant, of course. Just as it's motivating to read the pages of a book that is meaningful, so is it motivating if your teacher responds thoughtfully. I try to establish the idea that we each read one hundred pages a week, which at first seems crazy to my students. But because of the trust that has seeded itself in the classroom—not only between me and the class—but also among students themselves, they become willing."

"Then after a few weeks, when we've got into our stride, I move on to *The Seven Habits of Highly Successful People*, by Stephen Covey. That's a very different book, of course, and more complicated than *The Pact* because it's asking you to get inside your own head, to be aware of yourself as a unique individual. It's more difficult to talk about our own habits and feelings. So I tell the students they can use themselves or the characters from *The Pact* if they are more comfortable with that. In fact some colleagues scoff that *Seven Habits* is *too* complex, but I'm comforted by the memories of when I was in school, which I share, that I didn't understand everything I read, especially on the first pass. I got what I could out of my lessons, and I tell my students that's all you can do. That's sufficient as a beginning.

"The important thing is to be honest in stretching yourself: to be learning new ways of doing things, new self-discipline, and to reach beyond your comfort zone. I tell them learning is a bit like boot camp for the mind. The students who have been in the service really get that idea. They're among the best self-directed students—they know how to listen and take advantage of what they are told." She paused again. "In fact they make me realize," she continued, "that valuable life skills should not be confused with going to college. Frankly, I'm not sure we've been straight with the American people. Somewhere along the road we've sold the idea that it's college that ensures the future and gives people value. And yet a skilled plumber makes a good living and is more than valued when needed, as we all know from personal experience."

George Bowen had said the same thing. "In Britain we're always being influenced by this Athenian image of the public school, devaluing the skill of the hand against the skill of the head." Neither Britain nor the United States has good technical schools. There's no tradition of secondary education setting the stage to acquire vocational lifetime skills. In Germany, on the other hand, about half of all high school students choose vocational training after the age of sixteen. More than 40 percent become apprentices: in America the figure is less than 1 percent. Youth unemployment figures in the two countries reflect these cultural differences. In the United States unemployment is about 15 percent for sixteen-to-twenty-four-year-olds; in Germany it's half that. It's a lost opportunity: failing to bring young people into the workforce is a significant drag on the American economy.

It also reflects a mismatch between what the labor market needs and what the educational system is producing. So 15 percent of taxi drivers in the United States have a degree and 25 percent of sales clerks, even 5 percent of janitors. Only at the top end of the educational spectrum, for those with postgraduate degrees, does education and the job market come together with any precision. Young people are beginning to take notice. When Siemens, a German company, opened up fifty apprenticeship positions comparable to those it routinely offers at home—in mechanical engineering and computer science—at its North Carolina operation, it had two thousand applications, but only 10 percent of those applicants passed the aptitude test.

It was Susan's opinion that it would not be difficult to realign the community college system to provide greater support to such public-private partnerships. In Germany it's a cooperative model, created between employers and trade unions, guaranteeing that the apprenticeship-vocational college program supports the qualifications needed by industry. The trainee receives an allowance each month while in training, and about half stay on at that same company after graduation. "I have a number of students who would go for that," Susan said with a smile.

SUSAN CORBIN IS A GIFTED TEACHER, laboring against significant odds. One is reminded of Albert Camus's interpretation of the Sisyphus myth: that in rolling the rock up the hill, "the struggle itself . . . is enough to fill a man's heart." Her tenacity intrigued me. I suspect the roots of her commitment to teaching are to be found in her early experience, for she was raised by idealistic parents—young people disillusioned with the Vietnam War—who had dropped out to start a school with friends. Thus in her early years Susan had been essentially home-schooled, joining the public education system when she was ten. That was in Virginia. "We lived out of the mainstream," she explained, "so from the beginning I have looked at teaching and learning a little differently than my peers." Those formative years have bred true: in her caring, insightful approach to teaching, she illustrates the power of early experience in shaping our intuitive behavior as adults.

James Heckman, the distinguished economist and Nobel laureate, is in agreement. In early childhood, poverty of parenting is more powerful than material privation. Heckman has demonstrated that approximately half the inequality of lifetime earnings among individuals can be accounted for "by factors determined by the age of 18." He faults U.S. public policy in promoting predominantly cognitive measures to track student performance in school. Such measures miss the essence of the problem. America's "testing mania," as *The New York Times* has described it, where Congress requires states to give annual math and reading tests for middle-grade students, ignores social skills and the development of responsible self-command, providing a poor index of what it takes to succeed in the real world. Heckman puts it well: "life-cycle skill formation is dynamic in nature. Skill begets skill; motivation begets motivation . . . and they cross foster each other." If a child does not, through parental and adult guidance, become motivated to learn and engage early in life, it is likely that as an adult he or she will fail both socially and economically. Rather than the carrot-and-stick approach of competitive testing and the manipulation of federal support based on test results, public policy would be better served by repealing such laws and supporting teachers in building relationships with their students and their parents, one step at a time. Susan Corbin has discovered this power of attachment from her own experience, and it is a similar approach that has proved successful in Finland.

One impediment to adopting such a people-intensive educational strategy and supporting America's teachers is the size, diversity, and economic disparities that exist within the nation. A critical stumbling block is that children receive a qualitatively different education depending on the state in which they are born, and the school district to which they are assigned. This is because the funding of the public school system in America is heavily dependent on local property taxes, with state and federal resources often making only minor contributions. In some states, wealthy school districts may invest twice that of the poorer ones, and in other instances, as in California, the ratio can be three to one. It is estimated that this leaves 40 percent of public school students being educated in districts that are seriously underfunded.

For a nation as rich as America, such inequity is disturbing, especially when we recall the finding of the McKinsey study that an equitable quality of instruction is necessary for high student performance. With one-third of American students studying in relative poverty, thus compromising the quality of instruction and the material resources available to them, we place ourselves in double jeopardy. Not only are we restricting the potential to develop independent, skilled citizens, but in so degrading the nation's future workforce we also are saddling the economy with an unnecessary long-term burden. Should such circumstances prevail, what threatens America's future economy is not the slowdown in college attendance but the number of individuals capable of benefiting from it.

The decline in student performance has prompted vigorous political debate in the United States and Britain. The disagreements run deep. Conservative forces, particularly in the United States, have argued that the educational system can be salvaged only by privatization and competition. At the other end of the spectrum, powerful teachers' unions oppose any such intrusion, defending their own self-interest and the democratic ideal of one system for all.

The charter school movement has emerged as a controversial attempt to straddle this divide, especially for the disadvantaged. Charter schools—and in Britain the recently championed "academies," which are now replacing the old grammar school concept—are publicly funded but independently managed, giving greater control over curriculum and teacher selection. This shift in policy potentially offers smaller class sizes and an opportunity to build basic trust among teachers and students. It is a formula that is popular with parents in both countries, despite the politics, and the number of such independent schools is growing.

In the United States in 2013, there were estimated to be more than six thousand charter schools, teaching some 2.3 million children. However, although widely spread across the nation, this effort accounted for only about 4 percent of the total number of children enrolled in public education. Research into the achievements of the charter program is patchy in quality. The most credible studies come from the Center for Research on Education Outcomes (CREDO) at Stanford University, which uses information provided by the participating states to create a student data set—with observations in 2013 from 1,532,506 charter students—matched with a comparison group of traditional public school students. In a 2009 sample, across sixteen states, CREDO found approximately 17 percent of charter schools to be performing better than the public schools in the same region, while 37 percent were trailing behind. One consistent finding of significance, however, is that the charter schools particularly benefit black and Hispanic students from disadvantaged families. For example, the KIPP movement (Knowledge Is Power Program), established in 1994 and operating in poor neighborhoods across America—in Washington, D.C., some 44 percent of the publicly funded system are charter schools—has shown that disadvantaged children can perform well and achieve college entrance when given opportunity, good teachers, and the necessary resources. These outcomes were confirmed in the survey reported by CREDO in 2013, in which 54 percent of the sampled students were living in poverty across twenty-six states.

DISCUSSION OF WHAT we now know about the brain's maturation and its impact on the learning process has been largely absent from the political debate surrounding education. And yet our advancing knowledge of brain and developmental psychology is of great practical importance. As children grow into the latency and teen years, the major maturational challenges they face are sharpening the capacity for focused attention and strengthening self-regulation, especially learning how to control immediate emotional impulses in favor of future opportunity.

The classic work on delayed gratification by the distinguished psychologist Walter Mischel highlights the long-term importance of mastering these challenges. From a series of studies beginning in the late 1960s, Mischel discovered that the ability to defer reward not only varied among young children but also correlated with success later in life. In the now-famous "marshmallow test" young subjects around the age of four were offered a marshmallow, with the opportunity to receive two if they postponed eating the treat until the experimenter returned from being out of the room. Around 30 percent of the kids held out for the fifteen minutes of the experiment, usually by employing various mental tricks that diverted their attention, such as closing their eyes or looking away. Years later Mischel found that these children had greater academic and social achievement. Indeed, those who had been successful in postponing their reward for fifteen minutes had SAT scores that on average were 200 points higher than those who could wait only thirty seconds.

Not everybody is endowed with the same capacity when it comes to self-command. The good news, however, is that persistence and skillful schooling can enhance the ability to delay gratification. Walter Mischel explored this with his young "marshmallow" subjects and found that by teaching them to "reframe" the candy—literally by imagining it to be a picture and thus inedible—or by focusing their attention upon another thought or object in the room, their self-control was strengthened. The further challenge is for the child, the parent, and the educator to turn these tricks into habits that become intuitive. The charter school movement—Teach for America and Teach First in Britain are examples—strive to go beyond the parroting of Gradgrind facts and statistics as measures of outcome, working hard to find teachers committed not only to winning the students' trust but also to enhancing their academic and social achievement by fostering self-control and good interpersonal skills. David Levin, one of the founders of KIPP, is collaborating with Mischel to embed such skill training into the curriculum. Using peer-modeling techniques similar to Mary Gordon's Roots of Empathy program in Canada, children aged four to eight swap strategies in class, among themselves and together with a tutor, on how to refocus attention in the presence of short-term distraction.

Although the brain reaches approximately 90 percent of its adult size by the age of six, it takes another two decades to achieve functional maturity and for the neuronal highways to become fully myelinated—myelin being the fatty layer of insulation around the axons that is necessary for efficient nerve conduction. This process of myelination follows a varied time course across different brain regions. Of particular importance is that in the executive cortex—specifically the prefrontal cortex and its most lateral, inhibitory region—maturation lags behind the limbic system, where the ancient emotional centers of the brain are seated. Also, during late puberty, the plasticity of the brain increases with a burst of development in nerve cells and synapses, later to be sculpted by pruning in response to meaningful environmental interaction. Because of this pruning the prefrontal cortex again matures at a different rate from that of the limbic brain and particularly from the nucleus accumbens, which is the brain's pleasure center.

These shifting alliances of different brain regions influence the capacity for self-control. In a series of studies the developmental neuroscientist B. J. Casey, the Sackler Professor at the Weill Cornell Medical College in New York, has provided evidence that it is precisely because these old and the new brain regions mature differentially that the adolescent years are so complex. In a laboratory study Casey and her colleagues compared self-regulation in children, adolescents, and adults who were undertaking a task designed to test impulse control, with regional brain blood-flow being assessed concomitantly by fMRI scan. The adolescents, in comparison to the children and the adults, and in association with poor impulse control, were found to have increased nucleus accumbens—the pleasure center—blood flow. In contrast, the blood-flow activity of the executive cortex in these same adolescents—specifically the orbital-frontal region—appeared closer to that of children than adults. This suggests that in its maturation the brain's capacity for self-command lags behind that of the ancient pleasure center's expression of emotion, biasing adolescent behavior toward choosing immediate reward over the delayed gratification that serves long-term advantage.

It is generally accepted that an important mark of maturity is the ability of an individual to suppress impulsive or inappropriate behavior, especially in the presence of a compelling incentive. Such abilities are acquired only slowly, however, and with much practice. Thus gaining intuitive social understanding and mastering skills in numeracy and literacy—the essential goals of education—requires a long-term perspective, including forgoing the pleasured excitement of risk-taking and impulsive behavior that is so attractive to the adolescent mind. The teenage age years and young adulthood are thus a paradoxical time for the educational mission. The brain retains the extraordinary plasticity of childhood with its heightened capacity for rapid learning and memory, but self-command remains elusive, especially in times of emotional stimulation. Thus education during adolescence should be purposeful, focusing upon the strengthening of meaningful self-examination and disciplined exploration guided by a trusted tutor, be that a principal, teacher, or parent. This quality of instruction is hard work and challenging. With such guidance, however, the complex maturational stage of adolescence can assemble the flexible toolkit that will best serve future opportunity.

Thus the lesson from developmental neurobiology reinforces the common wisdom and the findings of the McKinsey studies, which I described at the beginning of this chapter: what works in education is a mix of high-quality instruction, made consistently and equitably available to every child, by engaged, dedicated, and well-rewarded teachers. As Susan Corbin commented during my afternoon with her in Torrance, "seasoned teachers continuously draw upon their intuitive skills." Each semester, each class, each student is different. "You must be willing to change gears, which is the challenge and the fun, but it also makes teaching to multiple choice tests and to a federally mandated curriculum extremely difficult." There is economic evidence supporting Susan's opinion. The National Bureau of Economic Research, investigating a data set that spans two decades, has recently shown that gifted, experienced teachers have a significant "value-added" long-term influence upon student performance and subsequent employment.

IDEALLY, FORMAL EDUCATION is an extension of early parenting. It is a process that should harness the young student's maturational drive to forge and hone the adaptive skills that will serve lifelong autonomy and self-directed growth. We describe this collection of skills for resilience, empathic understanding, self-control, and prudent planning as *character*, from the Greek word *charaktêr*, meaning "mark," as in the markings of a coin. Hence in common parlance character implies the distinctive behavioral marks of an individual—a person's qualities and habits that are stable and that define his or her behavior within a social context.

Marks of character are commonly labeled "good" or "bad," with these labels becoming the basis for others' "moral" judgment of that person. There is substantial agreement regarding the cross-cultural consistency of how such judgments emerge, a subject known as *intuitive ethics*. In close parallel is the concept of virtue. Thus the virtue of *compassion* is a reflection of empathic understanding; the capacity to defer gratification is the virtue of *prudence*; the skills of attentive concentration and dedication to a task translate into the virtue of *perseverance*; and a balanced ability to manage life's vicissitudes is the virtue of *self-command*.

These are the skills of self-tuning that enable each of us to flourish in society—intuitive habits of mind that foster the individual talent of being a good teacher, a responsible citizen, or a fine craftsman. Rather than being fixed in quality, these intuitive skills provide the practical, everyday wisdom that underpins tranquillity and well-being, the quality of mind that in the Greek language is called *ataraxia*. These too are the skills of resilience, interaction, and caring that sustain the common courtesies—the social manners—that facilitate everyday living. It is the quality of these social skills and how we employ them that determine whether the culture in which we participate is enhanced or degraded. In short, individual character is the backbone of vibrant human society.

The development of character in the young is a collective enterprise. As has been evident in my discussion, in the first few years the burdens and the opportunities of the effort fall disproportionately on parents and family. But the execution of these responsibilities is intimately entwined with the commitments that the rest of us make in the structural and cultural supports provided to young households. For example, while in 2011 almost 60 percent of American women were working outside the home, the United States is one of the few rich countries that do not require paid maternity leave. And yet most of us are aware of the importance of fostering a healthy and stable attachment between parent and infant child, recognizing that nurturing the first steps on the maturational ladder is an investment in the future.

On the other hand, as a culture we seem entirely comfortable with the commercialization of children's lives from the earliest age. The typical American toddler can recognize the logos of its favorite foods by eighteen months of age, usually from watching television programs, and will ask for them consistently by the third year. And that is just the beginning. In 2009 total direct advertising to children was estimated as between $15 billion and $17 billion. The purchase of children's toys tells a similar story. Although the United States has only 3.1 percent of the world's children, U.S. families annually purchase more than 40 percent of the toys "consumed" globally, with total retail sales of some $20 billion.

As Americans we take pride in being child centered, but today our behavior goes suspiciously beyond pride to consumerism run amok.

Beyond doubt we have been overindulging our children. But the damage goes beyond the material. Such profligacy is rapidly eroding our collective responsibility when it comes to the teaching of good habits and the building of character. It would seem that as a culture America has now perfected the art of the mixed message. While we gain satisfaction from being a nation of can-do individuals—taking few vacations and committed to a vigilant around-the-clock, technology-saturated work ethic—our overindulgence of our offspring does little to prepare them for the challenges of the workaholic world that we have created. The educational calendar, for example, is still true to its agrarian roots. At thirty-two hours the school week in the United States is one of the shortest in the world: at the other end of the spectrum is Sweden at sixty hours. Long afternoon hours and a three-month summer recess, designed around the farming life of decades ago, are now time frequently spent with little adult oversight. For the adolescent mind this is not only an invitation to mischief, drugs, and losing oneself in cyberspace but potentially also the gateway to anguish and significant personal conflict.

Ironically material indulgence appears to play a disproportionate role in these challenges. Suniya Luthar and Shawn Latendresse, both from the Teachers College at Columbia University, have found in a series of studies that children from high-income families, attending an affluent suburban high school, had significantly higher use of tobacco, alcohol, marijuana, and hard drugs than did their matched inner-city neighbors. In these groupings of wealthy children, isolation from adult role models, pressures to perform on academic tests, and a lack of family routine all contributed to low self-esteem and poor performance in school.

A further irony is that being poor in America offers little protection against this onslaught of consumerism, which has become pervasive in all socioeconomic groups. Indeed, the affluent society—where affluence is defined, you will recall, as a continuous flow of novelty at ever decreasing cost—increases the jeopardy. Not only do low-income families suffer from the poverty of opportunity and choice that comes with being disadvantaged, but also they are frequently burdened by a poverty of understanding, having little awareness of how corrosive the cacophony of consumerism can be to the development of character-building skills.

When it comes to education and the development of character, America has been running a social experiment on a grand scale. After three giddy decades of celebrating immediate gratification, self-indulgence, and profligate spending, we find ourselves wondering why social manners, patience, and self-control are becoming such rare American qualities. As a society in myopic pursuit of a dream made material, we have forgotten how clever we are in imitating others, especially when it comes to the intuitive development of habit, be that virtuous or otherwise. The culture of affluence is eroding prudence and the capacity for self-directed growth, thus undermining the brain's capacity to achieve self-command.

It is clear that we have much to do. As the number of people making poor decisions increases, so do our social, economic, and environmental challenges. As we work to retrieve a sense of cultural balance, reinvesting in the human side of education would be a good place to start.

Chapter 8

Habitat:
Made to Man's Measure

> The more living patterns there are in a thing—a room,
> a building, or a town—the more it comes to life as an
> entirety, the more it glows, the more it has this self-
> maintaining fire, which is the quality without a name.
>
> It is a process which brings order out of nothing; it
> cannot be attained, but it will happen of its own accord,
> if we will only let it.
>
> Christopher Alexander, *The Timeless Way*
> *of Building* (1979)

THE SMALL ITALIAN TOWN of Sabbioneta, like some Hollywood film set, rises abruptly from Lombardy's fertile northern plain. Built in the latter part of the sixteenth century, this exquisite fortified enclave reflects the ambition of one man, Vespasiano Gonzaga, a noble mercenary, military engineer, and patron of the arts who in his dreaming had sought to construct a Renaissance city of perfection.

The visit that bright Sunday in late July had been my first. Our traveling companion and guide was Hans Wirz, the architect and expert in urban design who makes his home in Basel, Switzerland, and has been a friend over many years. In hope of completing the two-hour journey before the heat of the day, we had left early from the Villa di Monte, an ancient manor house perched high in the hills some thirty kilometers from Florence, and the summer refuge of Hans and his wife Anna, a prominent neuroscientist.

The initial drive had been delightful. When it comes to considering human habitat, Tuscany provides instruction beyond its physical beauty. Man's hand has touched every inch of the landscape. Bridges and tunnels—plus wayside herds of freshly shorn sheep, bells clanking as they jostled in protest of our disturbing presence—dominated the weaving, sinuous road that morning. Evident beyond the immediate highway were small farms that over the centuries had tumbled together into villages, nestled now among manicured hills ribbed with orderly vineyards and a patchwork of harvested fields. But swiftly, within the hour, as we connected with the Rome autostrada, such pastoral scenes were behind us. Leaping forward, released and unimpeded, we were soon heading into the shimmering haze of the great Po valley and toward Italy's industrial north.

The summer had been unseasonably hot, and Sabbioneta made no exception for our early start, greeting us with heat of furnacelike intensity. Built upon sandy shores—*sabbia* is the Italian word for sand—and cradled within a generous meander of the River Po, this tiny town's formidable fortifications remain intact. The simple stucco-faced dwellings that crowd its cobbled streets shelter some seventeen hundred families. Indeed, take away the parked cars and the streetlights hanging from overhead cables, together with the occasional plastic chair, and one has the sense that the architecture of the place, and even the size of the populace, has changed little since Sabbioneta's creation some 450 years ago.

The Gonzaga family, known for their horse breeding, military prowess, and political maneuverings, dominated the Po valley for over four centuries, from 1328 until the early 1700s. Although despotic in the early years of their climb to power, during the Renaissance the family discovered its gentler side, seeking prestige and status through patronage of the arts, humanities, and architectural innovation. As a result, in the sixteenth century Mantua, the family seat, emerged as a prominent cultural center in northern Italy. Sabbioneta, just thirty kilometers to the southwest and one of the smaller city-states ruled by the extended Gonzaga family, similarly reflects the aesthetic strivings of the period. A town in miniature, today it stands witness to Renaissance values in art, architecture, and urban planning.

Vespasiano Gonzaga (1531–91), the mastermind of Sabbioneta, was by all accounts an intelligent, cultured fellow with close ties to the Vatican on his mother's side. Vespasiano had grown to manhood under the tutelage of Phillip II and the Spanish Court and in his maturity had been the king's viceroy in Navarre. As a celebrated soldier with a passion for the classical architecture of Rome, Vespasiano had a singular vision. This was to rebuild Sabbioneta, a small township inherited from his family, as an impregnable fortress while adhering to Renaissance ideals. He sought to construct the perfect city for his time—over which he would preside as duke and patron—complete with palazzi for aristocratic friends, an academy, an art gallery, public theater, and a summer palace for his own retreat. Vespasiano undertook this challenge with unwavering personal dedication: in just over thirty years, within the span of his own lifetime, an old castle and a tiny village were turned into a utopian dream.

In keeping with the best military engineering of the day, combined with the techniques of ancient Roman urban design, Sabbioneta has a star-shaped plan with the town entirely enclosed within defensive walls. Inside, a right-angled grid of streets—essentially a labyrinth of T-traps within which we were quickly lost—is served by two imposing gateways and two central piazzas, with the main public buildings distributed between them. It's a city perfect in its human scale: even Disney, I mused, could have learned something from such precise attention to detail. Indeed, the classical symmetry of many buildings I found reminiscent of Georgian London. As Hans reminded me, that should have come as no surprise given that the duke's designs were greatly influenced by the Venetian architect Andrea Palladio. Palladio was Vespasiano's contemporary, and his elegant constructions, combining function and beauty, were to become an article of faith in the eighteenth century, profoundly influencing European architecture and even inspiring Thomas Jefferson in his conception of Monticello.

Not surprisingly, therefore, despite Vespasiano being a successful professional soldier of stoic disposition, Sabbioneta is no bare-bones military encampment. Informed by the Renaissance ideals of rational humanism, the duke was a perfectionist in his passion and drew strength from the ancient world. In this creed visual harmony was to be found in the mathematical proportions of the buildings and in the whole-number ratios reflected in the divine proportions of the human body—as is most famously represented in the image *Vitruvian Man* drawn by Leonardo da Vinci. But in distinction to the family seat of Mantua, which was adapted slowly over centuries from its Roman origins to embrace a Renaissance vision, Sabbioneta represents an entirely new town planned and built within one generation. Thus while the architecture of the little city precisely reflects the planning conventions of the time, it is an image framed almost entirely by the aspirations of its inventor. Vespasiano sought the advice of some of the leading architects of his day, but the design, scale, and placement of the ducal and public buildings is his own, inspired by Roman principles. As a result their facades, while simple and imposing, are strikingly uniform in presentation.

When it came to decorating his palaces and public buildings, however, Vespasiano sought out and employed the best artists from across Lombardy, including Bernardino Campi, who established his own school in Sabbioneta. Many of the frescos survive, and especially the ceilings have retained their original appearance. Within the public spaces trompe-l'oeil architectural illusion is repeatedly featured amid traditional depictions of Greek and Roman mythology. Complementing the prominent display of Gonzaga ancestral figures and heraldry, the glorious heritage of Rome, and Vespasiano's personal exploits as a soldier are also images revealing a puckish sense of humor. One mural that caught my eye—while glancing up at the lavish, domed ceiling of Vespasiano's private study in the Palazzo Ducale—depicted the daily passage across the sky of the chariot of the sun. Perhaps in reference to Phaeton, who in attempting to drive his father's chariot lost control and set the world on fire, a precariously balanced charioteer is depicted wrestling unsuccessfully to control the flight of two powerful horses; his cape and tunic balloon above him to reveal, exquisitely rendered by the muralist, the intimate details of a naked torso.

Undoubtedly Sabbioneta's most celebrated building, however, and deservedly so for its design and many murals and statues, is the Teatro all'antica. Constructed between 1558 and 1560 by Vincenzo Scamozzi, Palladio's pupil and illustrious successor, this freestanding and roofed public theater was one of the first to be built in Europe. In its innovation it included practicality, with a special entrance for the musicians and performers, fixed scenery of an urban landscape, and a sloping stage for greater audience visibility. Finished just before the duke's death, it represents the pinnacle of his architectural achievement. In the creation of Sabbioneta—true to his passion—Vespasiano crafted a Renaissance gem.

SO WHAT CAN THE urban planner of today learn from the little town of Sabbioneta? This was the question I posed to Hans Wirz when late in the afternoon, dusty and parched, we sat down for a beer in the shade of the Palazzo del Giardino, beside the long gallery where Vespasiano once kept his collection of Greek and Roman sculpture.

"One immediate lesson," Hans replied without hesitation, "is that top-down planning rarely works. For all its classical beauty and attention to detail, Sabbioneta has no *genius loci*, no spirit of place. The town reflects one man's will: the duke's will, the soldier's will. Vespasiano planned Sabbioneta with accomplished architects and artists but essentially ignored the people who lived and labored there. So beyond the vision of the duke, nothing grew organically."

During the duke's lifetime, Hans went on to explain, the town worked as a fiefdom, but after his death, when the control of the city passed to his son-in-law, rioting ensued. It soon became clear that the people of Sabbioneta no longer felt a special relationship with their ruler, and Vespasiano's daughter decamped to Naples as a quieter, safer place to live. The sixteenth century was a dangerous period in Italy's history. Whereas both England and France became unified monarchies, Italy remained a patchwork of city-states and warring factions. The duke, as an intellectual and a military man, had risen to the challenge. Sabbioneta's fortifications, which Vaspasiano had designed, served brilliantly and together with a large garrison of troops kept the townspeople safe. But when it came to filling in the details that make up the verve of city life, things hadn't worked so well.

"As we have seen, the plan of the town is rigid and hierarchical," observed Hans. "It proved difficult for the duke to create a community that worked beyond his beautiful buildings. He was determined, for example, to construct a theater that rivaled that of the Duke of Mantua, but when it opened there was no natural audience. So Vespasiano dressed up his soldiers and his farmers and they came and they clapped, but it was contrived. There was no spirit of place.

"So after the duke was gone, Sabbioneta rapidly became a sleepy backwater," he went on, "and it so remains today, which is why it is architecturally so well preserved. And the town's location didn't help: that's the next lesson. Sabbioneta, even in its years of glory, sat apart from major trade routes—even from the river—so there was no vibrant merchant exchange with other communities, such as that which fueled Mantua or the great city-state of Florence."

Hans contrasted Sabbioneta's prevailing circumstances with those of the Tuscan towns and villages through which we had passed early that morning. There among the pastoral hills, in his opinion, were to be found examples of how landscape, architecture, and economic necessity can come together to sustain a natural synergy, "with the right buildings in the right topography." Over generations the talent essential to securing human habitat took advantage of both landscape and climate: to exploit a water supply, to command the best pastures, sometimes for defense. But always, in distinction to the creation of Sabbioneta, there was a *functional* imperative behind the buildings constructed, usually in the service of sustaining individual families and community.

Our conversation lapsed. The shadows were lengthening across the square, and the air felt decidedly cooler. I realized we were facing north, shielded from the worst of the summer heat by the stone walls of the garden palace. Clearly, I mused, our conversation was not giving Vespasiano sufficient credit: here in the shaded garden we were enjoying some of the exact same architectural principles that Hans had been describing. I was reminded too of the old New Hampshire farmhouse that has long been my home in America, a perfect example of habitat constructed with materials at hand. Built in the late 1700s, it sits facing south on a protected knoll halfway up a larger hill that overlooks a brook and open fields. An old maple tree on the southwest corner shades it from the summer sun and provides the air conditioning. A massive chimney built of fieldstone and brick stands at the core of the house, providing central heating for the winter and affording each principal room a hearth. Timber-framed and clapboard-sided from wood that was cut and milled locally, it is an example—just one among many—of houses constructed during the European settlement of New England, from materials at hand, as the climate allowed, and within the technology of the time.

I reflected aloud upon the ingenuity of such New England homesteads, and Hans nodded in agreement. "As in any vibrant economy, a spirit of place is created and sustained by the needs and actions of ordinary people," he observed. "That's why autocratic, top-down planning rarely works." Vespasiano had ignored this principle because he could, through his wealth and power as a duke, and Hans believed that modern technologies have the capacity to promote a similar blindness. "Just because we are able to construct something without restriction, technically speaking, does not guarantee people satisfaction or sustainability. Today we have the capacity to drop a box, literally by parachute, to any spot on the planet's surface, with heating and air conditioning available at the touch of a switch. But that's not a marriage with topography. It's not a sustainable symbiosis of man and nature."

"Swept away by modern technology, as we frequently are, it's important to recognize another reality," Hans continued. "Using modern sophistication, we can build houses and urban centers that possess the same unifying qualities that are found in the old villages. All you need are talented architects, flexible urban designers, and creative engineers working in harmony with the real people who will be living there. Then technology becomes a tool and not an end in itself. Many little Tuscan towns are just as desirable to live in today as they were two centuries ago. They are adaptable to today's uses. Flexibility is the essence of sustainability."

Beers finished and thirsts quenched, we faced a long drive ahead, and it was time to leave Sabbioneta. The setting sun had disappeared beyond the fortifications and most of the day's visitors with it. As we walked to the car, Hans was summing up, energy undiminished, much as he might do before his students in London, Paris, or Basel. "So in architecture and urban planning," he explained, waving his hand in the direction of Vespasiano's long gallery, "to say that something is sustainable doesn't mean that it is fixed in time, as are these monumental buildings." In Hans's mind sustainability depended on how intelligently a project was conceived. "In modern analogy think of it as a question of hardware and software. The hardware is the brick, the marble, and the concrete of the construction itself; the software is human need and the differing viewpoints held by those whom the structure will serve, both as individuals and through time." Over a succession of generations needs and interests change: the software of life adapts. And in a sustainable building the hardware also has the capacity for functional change, while retaining its integrity. The old house changes from a dwelling to a farm; it turns into office space or becomes a shop. But through all these different uses—these different twists and turns—fundamentally the same structure remains. "So it's integration of the shifting patterns of people and place that create the *genius loci* that is essential to human habitat," Hans concluded. "Vespasiano missed that on his first pass: but he was an intelligent man. Who knows—if he had lived another decade or two, such integration might have happened here."

IT IS THROUGH THE PATTERN of events that we experience—through events that repeat themselves—that we discover and remember the character of a place. Many of these happenings are mundane and repetitive, occurring over and over again, but collectively it is the habits of everyday life—breakfasting in the kitchen, catching up with the news, preparing for work, returning home, eating supper, going to bed—that define the built environment. It is these patterns, anchored in time and space, that give the human world its structure.

Thus it is through memory and habit formation that the structures in which we live come to shape the way we think about habitat and its relationship to the natural world. We each have our own points of reference. So for me one image of the old New Hampshire farmhouse that is etched in my memory is of the kitchen, where in the chill of early winter the woodstove is crackling and the supper is being prepared. And another image, this time of Italy and summer, is the light of the late evening sun reflected in the pines and the olive trees at the Villa di Monte, a tranquillity played out against a cacophony of motor horns as an endless stream of cars, their occupants eager for supper, wind up the long hill to the town of Arcone.

An awareness of place and the ability to creatively express that self-awareness is something that starts early. Remember the games of childhood, of playing house? For Nancy, my partner, who grew up on a farm in Michigan, the favored location for such games was the granary at her grandmother's or an empty corncrib, which had the added advantage that looking out between the slats, you could see those approaching. "We preferred dimly lit places," she says. "We swept away bugs and grain and cobwebs—real acts of bravery and tasks into which we would need to be coerced, had we been at home." Old utensils, jars, towels, rags, tin cans—whatever the grown-ups might not notice—were smuggled in. "Tables were made from stacking grain boxes. This also worked for chairs. Our rags were our tablecloths. We picked flowers, made mud pies and milk shakes and weedy salads. We hung things on make-believe windows—though we never wanted a real window, for someone might actually see us. It was our own pretend world, and we wanted no adult to shatter the illusion." Secret, intimate, and memorable places were created within that corncrib, places for pretending and for fantasy with imagination being the essential ingredient. "But rarely did we make a bed," recalls Nancy. "There was never time for sleeping."

Christopher Alexander, a celebrated architect and tireless advocate for connecting human values to home construction and to urban planning, believes that it is through such memories that we first understand the true relationship between our surroundings and ourselves. The urge to build, he argues, is a fundamental human drive, as much a part of human instinct as the begetting of children. But to master the language through which such instincts can be expressed in design, we must first build a generative grammar. Alexander has described this intuitive sense as *pattern language*. Just as language gives us the power to create an infinite variety of sentences, through pattern language we have the capacity to design an infinite variety of spaces that are vibrant and alive. How are family patterns of interaction served by the layout of a home? Where is the window best placed in a room so that the light may enter and the eye be drawn outward? What is the most comfortable place to sit near that window, so that one may enjoy the outdoors from the warmth of the house? In answering such questions Alexander believes that an understanding of pattern language offers an infinite supply of practical solutions. The focus upon need, memory, and imagination in the development of human habit, he asserts, is a "timeless way of building. It is a thousand years old, and the same today as it ever was."

SOME WOULD DISMISS Christopher Alexander as an incurable romantic. However, his focus upon improving the architecture of place—of facilitating through design the natural patterns and spontaneity of human interaction—has increasing resonance for those planners involved in meeting the challenges of the modern world. In large part due to the dominance of the automobile, life in the affluent society today has become centrifugal—that is, far-flung, time expensive, and disruptive of family patterns and community engagement. Alexander has not been alone in being disturbed by such trends as destructive of human caring. For example, in New York City, as early as the 1960s, the pioneering work of William Whyte and Jane Jacobs offered visionary insights into the nature of big city life and how an understanding of behavioral patterns is essential to the favorable design of public space.

Jane Jacobs, the American-born Canadian activist, first became fascinated by urban life when living in Greenwich Village in the 1950s. Working as a freelance writer, she found herself intrigued by how the dynamics of small market interaction—routine shopping and other mundane chores—often assumed greater social meaning and helped frame acceptable behavior. Particularly she noted that adults working and shopping in neighborhoods where they lived would take responsibility for the safety and disciplining of children playing in the street. Over time, she suggested, it is this interaction and sharing of experience that helps shape the character of community members, creating a sense of pride, belonging, and social coherence. At a time when cities worldwide were bulldozing "slums" and replacing them with high-rise dwellings remote from economic life, Jane Jacobs was arguing for the exact opposite—for greater density, cohesion, and human diversity— as the essential bedrock of urban living.

William Whyte, sociologist, author of *The Organization Man*, and an early mentor of Jane Jacobs, helped validate much of Jacobs's thinking through his own meticulous observation. In 1969, while working for the New York City Planning Commission, Whyte began a decade long, camera-based study of public spaces in the city that culminated in the publication of both a documentary film and the now-classic volume *The Social Life of Small Urban Spaces*, first published in 1980. These were not surveys of community life but rather the study of specific public squares and other gathering places tracking the behavior of local residents and that of transient urbanites, through time. What makes an inviting public space? Whyte asked. How are they used, and by whom? What makes them work or fail? What is the importance of ambience; of seats, and trees, and fountains; of sunshine and shade? What of location, the surrounding streets, and the abutting buildings: what role does the space play in creating and sustaining a vibrant community?

The pioneering work of Whyte and Jacobs offers insight into the behavioral patterns that emerge in communities when individuals have the freedom to interact and to choose their own preferences. But the flip-side lesson of their work is that the strength of a community is significantly dependent upon the *character* of the people who live there and, furthermore, that successful urban development is by necessity an expression of that collective character. Thus, as in city planning in general, the design of public space without "bottom-up" engagement is unlikely to be successful.

There is a living example of this truth just a few blocks from where I live in urban Los Angeles. While it is a green and sunny city, we have few neighborhood parks, and a well-meaning local council in recent years has been determined to change that. Unfortunately, in my neighborhood at least, the plan was carried forth apparently in ignorance of Whyte's principles, with little local consultation and even less interest in the activity patterns that a new public space might foster. Thus, even though the local library is not far away, when a vacant building site sandwiched between a drugstore and a parking lot suddenly sprouted trees and a surrounding fence—to be locked at night against vagrants—there was little neighborhood interest or enthusiasm. The lesson again is that top-down planning doesn't work: it didn't in ancient Sabbioneta, and neither does it in contemporary Los Angeles.

But a lack of forward thinking is only part of the problem. There is another variable that helps explain the failure of my neighborhood park. Los Angeles is not a walking city: life is unthinkable without a car, and Angelinos drive everywhere, even to the neighborhood library. It was not always so. In 1920 metropolitan Los Angeles had the longest streetcar network in the world, established at the turn of the century by tycoon Henry Huntington. At the time, to build the tramlines had been in his best interest as a real estate developer. Indeed Huntington's streetcars survived, somewhat diminished, until the 1940s, when the system was purchased by a conglomerate of automobile, oil, and tire manufacturers led by General Motors, again in their own best interest. That was essentially the end of efficient public transport in Los Angeles. We had nothing but buses and cars until—in a twenty-first-century reawakening—light rail has begun to make a comeback.

Nonetheless in Los Angeles urban life remains totally dependent on the automobile, not only to get around but also economically. Some 38 percent of the downtown area is devoted to parking, and private lots are a $5 billion-a-year business. For over half a century much of the city's landscape has been designed for and by the automobile, and yet traffic congestion is the worst in the nation, with the average commuting time on weekdays being over an hour. Living in an apartment close to the university where I teach, I manage to avoid all that, but I'm probably one of the few who walk to work. Indeed, when I first arrived in the city, kindly folk would occasionally stop to ask if I needed help, so ingrained is the habit of the motorcar.

My assistant, on the other hand, drives each day from Valencia, a planned suburban community some thirty miles north of the city. If one uses the Interstate 5 highway, the travel time is pegged by Google Maps at thirty to forty-five minutes, but that figure rises by 50 percent in the morning rush hour, and in the evening, her homeward journey is frequently doubled to over ninety minutes. And there is irony here. Victor Gruen, the architect who designed Valencia and who in the 1960s invented the shopping mall and did much to shape suburban America, was a man who hated cars. It had been his vision—he was an Austrian immigrant who had fled the Nazi occupation of Vienna with little more than the clothes on his back—to recreate the vibrancy of a pedestrian-friendly, market-driven European city center—reflected in the dense urbanism of the shopping mall Gruen designed—together with a series of supporting neighborhoods interconnected by walking paths. Valencia would be, as an early enthusiast described it, "an island of reason in the path of metropolitan sprawl."

In comparison with many other suburban areas in America, Valencia has done well, especially for young families. Until the collapse of the housing bubble in 2008 the planned-community neighborhoods had continued to grow, with light industry and small businesses keeping pace. In 1987 Valencia merged with several neighboring communities to create the city of Santa Clarita, with a population of some 150,000 persons and an annual family income approximately double the U.S. average. But Valencia, despite the presence of the Six Flags theme parks, is still unmistakably a suburban enclave. Single-family homes dominate, and while the Spanish-style city center is safe and tidy, complete with fountains and landscaping, a cinema and restaurants, there is little *spirit of place*, as Hans Wirz described it. Public transport is absent, and despite the many bike paths, most people drive—some 50 percent of them, including my assistant, commute each day to work in Los Angeles. For five decades the motorcar has been the American way, and old habits are hard to break.

BUT TIMES ARE CHANGING. While Valencia fared better during the Great Recession than many suburban areas in California, housing prices dropped 35 percent from their peak in 2007. Early in 2014, as I write this, while prices are again rising, some three hundred homes are on the market, with approximately a third of them bank-owned or in various stages of foreclosure. This is not good news, except when compared to such fringe communities as the Franklin Reserve neighborhood close to Sacramento in central California: there of the ten thousand suburban homes that were built between 2003 and 2006, many now stand empty and abandoned. In 2014 home ownership in these areas is at its lowest since the 1970s. This blight is continuing to spread. Some estimates suggest that by the third decade of the new millennium, there may be a surplus of some twenty million family homes in suburban America.

It is tempting to ascribe this upheaval in the suburban real estate market to the collapse of the housing bubble, the recession that followed, and higher gas prices. Growing evidence, however, suggests otherwise—that while this "perfect storm" may have been catalytic, a structural shift in sentiment is also under way. While for sixty years American families have been moving to the suburbs with the expressed intent of freeing themselves from urban blight, the trend now seems to be in the opposite direction. Car-dependent suburban sprawl may have reached its limits. With an increasing number of Americans now living alone, busy, walkable, and densely knit urban centers, especially those served by rail-line transport, are becoming increasingly attractive to both young and old. This movement is reflected in real estate sales, where home prices have dropped particularly in those areas that necessitate a long commute. Space in urban residential neighborhoods now costs 40 to 200 percent more than in suburban areas that are isolated from shopping, work, and entertainment. Similarly suburban towns with walk-about urbanlike centers, such as Valencia, are more desirable than those lacking such attractions. Suddenly it seems that when given the choice, folks like lively spaces, varied shops, and busy pavements, just as William Whyte predicted.

This shift in the American spirit suggests that some deeply ingrained habits are being called into question. It was in the compelling embrace of the shopping mall and suburban living that the American Dream first became manifest for many middle-class families. Beginning in the post–World War II period, and fostered by generous tax incentives, the march of the mall into suburbs and exurbs became unstoppable, with destructive consequences for the economy of many town centers. But today, as urban living has begun a renaissance, the ability to recreate the suburban enclave into a pedestrian friendly and more interactive environment is challenged. With approximately 23 square feet of box store retail space per capita, the United States leads the world by a long way, and with some discomfort. Our nearest rival, Canada, manages only about 60 percent of that, and in Europe Sweden heads the pack with just over 3 square feet per capita.

Furthermore for the automobile, the matchmaker in this suburban romance, the bloom is also off the rose. While the recession and high gas prices have taken their toll, there appear to be longer-term factors in play here too. Young Americans are neither buying cars nor driving as much as did their parents' generation. With shopping online and home delivery, why fight the traffic to the mall? And when it comes to just hanging out, social media help keep us in the swing. America is not alone in this trend: car use, whether measured by trips taken or distance driven, is also declining in Britain, Sweden, and France. And with transportation and housing costs now eating some 50 percent of the typical family budget, it is not only the young that are looking for alternatives. Why not move back to the city, dump the car, invest in a smartphone, use public transport, and stay connected at half the cost? And if you really need to travel to odd, out-of-the-way, places there is always a car rental service or the convenience of Zipcar, the world's fastest growing car-sharing company, with close to one million members.

IN 2010, 82 PERCENT of Americans lived in an urban environment: it is estimated that by 2050 that figure will have risen to 90 percent. When we consider that cities are responsible for some two-thirds of the energy we use and 60 percent of the water, and produce about the same proportion of greenhouse gases, the technological challenges to achieving a sustainable, balanced future are enormous. But so too are the opportunities for enhancing human habitat. The "new urbanism," as it has become known, is also a potentially healthy development, in every sense of the word, promoting both exercise and social interaction in the individual and efficiency in energy consumption. Change will not be easy, however. The task of developing such new habits and the infrastructure to support them will be particularly difficult in the freeway-sprawling, car-focused, metropolitan areas of the Sun Belt such as Los Angeles, Phoenix, Atlanta, and Houston. But other, smaller cities—Portland, Oregon, is the poster child—have already taken giant steps toward the goal of establishing a "progressive" urban culture where most people bike or take the train to work, recycle materials, and generally live closer to the organic cycles of the natural world.

If this shifting sentiment sounds like a trend toward a European lifestyle, adapted to American frontier ways, it is because it is. Portland frequently compares itself to the little town of Freiburg im Breisgau, in Germany, or to Zurich in Switzerland, where the citizenry share the Portland dweller's love of trams and dramatic views of distant snow-capped mountains. Hans Wirz, the Swiss urban planner whom you met earlier in this chapter, knows both cities well, and on a recent visit to London I sat down with him to gather further insight.

Hans teaches from time to time at University College London, in the renowned Bartlett School of Architecture, which promotes itself, modestly, as a "world-leading faculty for multidisciplinary education and research for the built environment." On this occasion, appropriately, Hans had just finished an introductory student lecture on "What is good urban design," which I attended. And not without a certain sense of nostalgia, I might add, for I had been an undergraduate at the college in the 1960s before going on to study medicine at the university hospital across the street.

Hans agreed that Europe and the United States were indeed experiencing similar cultural shifts. "It's all about density," he explained. "Density is the key word. You need a minimal density, of so many inhabitants per square hectare, to justify and sustain tramways or an underground system. Suburbs are just not dense enough: then inevitably comes dependency on the motorcar. And that is not the future," he added emphatically. Hans believed there were ten or twenty towns in Europe that had found the right mix. "When you get it right the advantages are rapid and real," he asserted. "You still have your own dwelling unit, a maisonette or terraced house, with all the privacy that offers, but in addition you enjoy convenience and choice—walking to get your groceries or go to restaurants, coffee houses, theater, health services, and so on—each within easy distance." The challenge in modern urban planning therefore is to take old towns of a certain density, or to build new communities within them, while artfully shifting the emphasis away from the built environment per se to seeing it as the backbone to creating a first-class quality of life.

While the ideal is that this new vision comes together in happy confluence, in reality it usually takes good political leadership to initiate such change. "In all the successful cases that I know, there is a mayor— and that includes Sam Adams, the mayor in Portland, Oregon—and a municipal council that has ambitions to go in this direction," said Hans. "There has to be a reservoir of community talent, the right kinds of engineers and architects who know how to do it, and the population has to be ready, sufficiently enlightened to support this kind of social change. At the personal level motivations vary—perhaps to reduce personal costs by consuming less energy, maybe not even to have a car, or simply to broaden social opportunity and increase excitement. And of course, the business community must be in on the plan too, especially in the housing market, with committed developers who are willing to use modern technologies like photoelectric paneling, heat pumps, and so on. The whole culture must change."

As Hans had described in his lecture earlier that day, urban redesign is not something that is accomplished overnight. The conception and management of a large project is usually a process to be counted in years rather than months. And it is a rigorous one, with clear indices to be considered when measuring the outcome. *Function, order, identity,* and *appeal* are the hallowed objectives of any design effort, and it is the collective judgment of those who live the experience day by day that determines the success or failure of any gestalt that is created. Just as we perceive the world at large through the five senses—feeling, seeing, hearing, listening, and smelling—so do we appraise the built environment and act accordingly, in the classical action-perception brain cycle of Joaquín Fuster, which I described in Chapter 4. A subjective sense of balance, of an engaging ambiance, is key. Such moments come when the pieces fit together in the mind of the participant, and to maximize that potential, much research is required at the front end of any project. Urban design is by necessity an interactive, iterative, and democratic process. Investors, residents, merchants, and the public authorities all must be involved in defining the project's objectives and ultimately in reviewing and choosing among the proposals created. Only then does construction begin.

Hans considered that in Europe the best examples of such successful change are in Germany, agreeing that Freiburg im Breisgau was indeed one, and Tübingen another. He himself had been working for some time with the city of Saarbrücken, once an industrial and transport center that is now seeking to reinvent itself. It was, as Hans observed with characteristic self-effacement, a process "that takes much persistence and some patience." Then he added quickly with a smile, "But when brownfield sites have been converted into fantastic residential areas with lots of colorful, interesting architecture and many smiling faces, you don't need a questionnaire to measure the outcome." And such renewal is not limited to new construction: such success, Hans assured me, can be achieved equally well in historical towns and established urban centers. I knew that to be true for I had witnessed it myself in London's Marylebone, a district just one mile west of University College. That afternoon, with time to spare, Hans and I stepped out to check on progress.

AS A MEDICAL STUDENT, during my clinical years, I lived in Marylebone High Street, now a fashionable shopping area that sits below Regent's Park and runs parallel with Baker Street to the west. In those days, however, Marylebone was far from fashionable. Indeed, *seedy* would have been a better description. It was dangerous at times, with some fairly shady characters lurking in the backstreets. But that, of course, was how I could afford to live there. For five pounds a week I found a room over a music shop right next to a little graveyard, which is all there is left today of the church where Lord Nelson and Lady Hamilton christened their illegitimate daughter, Horatia, in 1803. The place was full of history. My room, on the third floor, was tiny. Quite literally I could stand in the middle and touch everything that was in it: my sway bed, a little writing table, an electric cooking ring, a miniature hand basin, and a small gas fire that took shilling coins. It was an efficient space. The only downside I recall was the loo, the lavatory, and its placement. It was at the back of the building, on the second floor, and cantilevered out over a schoolyard, like some limpet mine. But I was happy there at number sixty-five on the High Street, and the little place served me well.

After graduation I returned to Marylebone occasionally. The music shop became a place for sandwiches and then a café, and the gravestones next door grew a little more moss, but otherwise little seemed to change. I moved to America: decades passed. And then in the late summer of 2005, while participating in a workshop organized by London's Central St. Martins College of Arts and Design, I met Patricia Michelson, who had been born in Marylebone and owned a cheese shop, La Fromagerie, just off the High Street. However, as I soon learned, this was no ordinary cheese shop, but one considered by experts to be among the best that England had to offer. It was my introduction to the reinvention of Marylebone as a dynamic, thriving, and eclectic urban enclave.

The renaissance began, as Patricia described it, around the new millennium, when the leadership of Howard de Walden Estates embarked upon a ten-year program to upgrade the High Street. Some history is necessary here. London is an unplanned city, and the "estate holdings" by old aristocratic families are an idiosyncratic part of its development. Howard de Walden is one of those "estate holding" families and owns some ninety acres of prime real estate across London's West End, including Marylebone High Street.

What is called the district of Marylebone today is part of London's great expansion during the eighteenth century, when the city moved west and north to gobble up residual farmland and what remained of noble hunting grounds. The architecture is Georgian, with a Palladian flavor, although the facades are not uniform as in Sabbioneta. Indeed, far from it, as many great architects contributed over decades to create a varied and pleasing townscape. Beyond the High Street itself, which in its lower portion follows the meandering path of what was once the Tyburn River, is found a grid of streets and landscaped squares that now host a mix of residential and commercial properties, churches, small colleges, and at least one celebrated recital hall, all contributing to the richness of the community. Although most of the property is designated as historic and "conserved," this has not detracted from the continuous renewal and reimagining of the functions behind the facades. Hence, while the Georgian character of Marylebone has been retained, the use of its buildings has evolved in dynamic synchrony with the changing needs of those who live and work in the neighborhood. Beyond their beauty, these venerable old buildings—evoking Hans Wirz's definition—have a sustainability that is timeless.

It was against this backdrop that in the year 2000 or so the de Walden Estates began their effort to revitalize Marylebone High Street, which had grown tired and dowdy, just as I experienced it when a student. The plan was simple enough: by attracting the right mix of merchants, retailers, and artisans to bring energy, novelty, and value to the commercial heart of the district, they sought to create a villagelike atmosphere that would serve local residents while being worthy of London's reputation as one of the world's great destination cities. This was, in a phrase, "bottom-up" urban planning. After anchoring the north and south ends of the street with an upmarket furniture retailer and a fine grocery store, the leadership focused upon leasing the many smaller shops. Consciously rejecting the major chain brands, even though that would have produced greater immediate revenue, they targeted the recruitment of independent, entrepreneurial small business owners who believed in the transformation, offering them highly competitive leases and a responsive management. It was, as Patricia Michelson described it, "an opportunity to grow with the High Street" in a mixed-market environment—with butchers, bakers, and even candlestick makers—supported by an appreciative, closely knit community of local residents and a strong carriage trade of international visitors.

The turnaround was dramatic. Marylebone is well served by public transport, and within three or four years the foot traffic tripled. Not only were revenues up in the retail marketplace, but the income from the surrounding residential and commercial properties soared as Marylebone become *the* desirable place to live and to work. This spirit is evident every year at the Marylebone summer fair, which attracts upward of thirty thousand visitors, and in the farmers' market that is held each Saturday throughout the year. An active retailers' association similarly encourages cooperative activity and organizes special events, further supporting *genius loci*—the spirit of place. *The Marylebone Journal*, a bimonthly magazine, covers topics of local interest, including commerce, medicine (the London Clinic is part of the Harley Street community), food, and drink, together with highlighting the arts and local history.

AND THERE'S PLENTY of history to celebrate in Marylebone: many notables, and some scoundrels, have made their home in the district. Charles Dickens, for one, was living on the High Street when he came up with the idea for *A Christmas Carol*. What fascinates us about Scrooge, of course, is that in his misanthropy he is a species outlier. As social creatures, we are not by nature isolates but thrive on being together; and we are good at the game. On crowded evenings in Marylebone the street is thick with a mixture of bustling, hurrying, laughing, and high-spirited people, but there is little jostling to be felt. There is no bumping into one another: humans are too clever and adept for that. We intuitively read subtle body cues and glances, even when moving in crowds, and plan a path accordingly. In the modern world living together in cities has become our adopted habitat. We now need to get smarter at designing the city, preferably with the focus on accommodating people rather than the automobile, which implicitly has dominated our planning over the last century.

Slow progress is being made: urban living has the potential to be healthy. Taking London as an example, controls on the burning of fossil fuels are now firmly in place; gone are the acrid, choking fogs of my student days. But there is much left to do. The transformation of our urban environment must be in harmony with our need for a sustainable future, leaving room and flexibility for individual projects and personal expression. The generic challenge is that which I have been emphasizing throughout these pages: we must fight our affluence-primed, instinctual myopia and look to the long term. Today, as an example, in the face of the obesity epidemic (Britain sits just behind the United States, with 64 percent of its population being overweight or obese), we urgently need an urban environment that encourages physical activity, with broad sidewalks, safe bike lanes, public recreation areas, and interesting exercise opportunities built into it. With a little creativity it's an achievable goal. That exercise can be made fun, for both children and adults, is exemplified by the experimental musical staircase built at the Odenplan entrance to the metro system in Stockholm. Step on the treads, and they play notes just as do the keys of a piano. Within hours of its opening, apparently, there was a 66 percent increase in those choosing to use the stairs rather than the adjacent escalator.

Striving to create vibrant city communities also makes economic sense, as is evident in the Marylebone experience. People of all ages wish to live in such places. We know that those engaged in active urban lives, walking, cycling, and using public transport, are healthier and happier than those who must fight traffic to drive into the city each day. The demographics reflect this trend: well-educated young people—college graduates between the ages of twenty-five and thirty-four—are migrating to inner city neighborhoods at twice the rate of those choosing to settle in the outlying metropolitan areas. Similarly, at the other end of the age spectrum, retirees are increasingly opting to "age in place," to remain in the city and in close proximity to lifelong friends and familiar shops.

But most critical in fighting the scourge of obesity is revitalizing our relationship with the food we eat and where it comes from. The intertwining of settlement and food production is as old as human history, with the city melding "dining room, market and farm." The built environment of the city and the farmer can still intersect in mutually beneficial ways when planners, designers, and architects work together. Fostering a renewed awareness of this natural cycle is already revitalizing communities across America and in Europe. Indeed, evidence of that spirit of renewal is there in Marylebone High Street, a few doors down from number sixty-five, where I lived as a student.

Started in 2008, the Natural Kitchen is the partnership of two successful food men, Andrew Jordan and John Bartlett, chef and butcher respectively, with half a century of experience between them. With a first-floor café, food to go, a delicatessen, and an organic butcher's shop on the premises, it aims to bring locally produced food back into the city center. "Healthy choices that are easy, affordable, and engaging," as Harriet Burwood, the general manager, describes their philosophy: and where possible, choices made with humor it seems. As Hans and I passed by that evening, a delivery of produce was being taken inside. It was difficult to miss the bold labeling on the boxes: "Warning: Real Food. Side effects may be elevated energy levels, increased sex drive, rejuvenated sense of productivity and glowing skin." It's just part of a habitat made to man's measure.

Chapter 9

Food:
The Staff of Life

Husbandry is, with great justice, placed at the head of human arts, as having a very great advantage over all others, both with regard to antiquity and usefulness. It had its birth with the world, and has always been the genuine source of solid wealth, and real treasures; for it will furnish the people with everything necessary to render life happy and desirable.

The Complete Farmer (1777)

Agriculture is surely the most important of all human endeavors—by far the main source of our food, by far the world's biggest employer, with by far the greatest impact on our fellow creatures and the fabric of the earth itself. It is the foundation of everything that we might aspire to achieve, from good health to world peace to wildlife conservation. It is the thing we absolutely have to get right. To succeed we must treat farming as an exercise in applied ecology.

Colin Tudge, "Small Is Beautiful," *Literary Review*
(December 2013)

FOOD AND EATING are essential to all living creatures, yet in the human experience they are so much more. The sensual pleasure of eating is the most accessible of the instincts and the one that is infused most readily with social meaning. From the earliest strivings of our species the task of feeding ourselves has been a collective effort, one that fosters social interaction and primes curiosity.

The history of food is the history of human cultural development. In retrospect we see agriculture as the civilizing force, as the invention that broke our dependency upon the variable offerings to be gleaned from the natural world through hunting and gathering. It is in such husbandry—in the artful cultivation of plants and the domestication of animals—that we have sought to overcome the seasonal limits of our food supply. In complement, in our curiosity, we became fascinated with fermentation and used it to our advantage in making bread, cheese, beer, and wine. But when it comes to innovation in what and how we eat, it is in *the cooking of food* that we are truly distinct. Among the earth's creatures it is man, and only man, who exploits fire to cook. It is through cooking that we translate nature's offerings into something entirely different and uniquely human.

In our ingenuity we have transformed the pain of hunger and privation into the pleasures and celebration of the harvest. The annual feast days found in each and every culture stand in evidence of our artistry. What we grow, gather, and herd remains a singular link with the natural world, while what we eat and how we prepare it is shaped by the culture in which we live. As the historian Massimo Montanari has described it, "Food is culture."

When we eat together, we strengthen the bonds we have both with each other and with our culture. But in the helter-skelter modern world, such communion is becoming an increasingly rare event. In the closing decades of the twentieth century life around the table changed in America and even across Europe. A hectic lifestyle and the prepackaged processed meals of the "Western" diet now threaten traditional mealtime practice and also public health. A time famine has enslaved us to speed, disrupting the rhythm of life and the social resilience that has been built around food and its preparation. Today in America, more often than not, we eat alone.

As great a change is that we are no longer close to the source of what feeds us. Food production, from tillage to table, has become industrialized, driven by profit rather than palate. Across America the preponderance of what we eat comes from the same few food conglomerates, selling essentially the same products through the same vendors in the same megastores. As an example, Wal-Mart, not generally known as a grocery store, accounted for about 25 percent of food sales across the United States in 2013, a sum amounting to a staggering 55 percent of its American business. Just a handful of supermarket retail chains, led by the United States and Europe, dominate the world's food markets, accounting for approximately 30 percent of all global trade. Even for those in constrained economic circumstances preprocessed food is now so cheap and so calorie rich that obesity is emerging as a primary public health problem across the globe.

It is a paradox of achievement that we now find ourselves facing an age of food abundance with a brain programmed for scarcity, as did Henry the fabled pheasant. For us Americans, this challenge goes beyond biology, however, for it is confounded by our cultural relationship with food and with the food industry. Producing more processed calories than we should consume as a citizenry, we have become ignorant and wasteful, perhaps even disrespectful toward what we eat. In the 1700s it was generally known—so I am informed by my friend Patricia Michelson, proprietor of La Fromagerie in Marylebone—that cows should be encouraged to graze on wild grasses, for then the milk made better cheese. Sadly, two centuries on and divorced from the natural ecology, most of us have lost the ability to judge such particulars. Guidance about eating and the intuitive pleasures of taste discrimination are no longer schooled in the local market, from the experiments of mother's kitchen, or through lively discussion around the table. Indeed the average American family now spends more time driving around in the car together than gathering for a family meal.

In today's fast-food culture we have exchanged the poverty of physical hunger for a poverty of self-understanding. We have confused frenzy with efficiency, trading quantity for quality and losing sight of the broader pleasures surrounding food and its consumption. Food's traditional cultural role in society has been distorted and in some instances overwhelmed by aggressive marketing. Eating together is an antidote to stress. The daily sharing of good food can offer cohesion and solace when the workaday experience no longer provides personal meaning and space for reflection. It's a reminder that what makes us human is not just physical survival and individual success but also the pleasures that flow from empathic bonding with others. The cultivation and sharing of good food serves the greater function of helping cultivate ourselves: in a disparate world the table becomes a place of gathering and reunification. And it is here too—through a greater knowledge of the food we eat and where it comes from—that we can rediscover our connection with the natural world.

I believe such rediscovery is essential to the future health of our nation. In Chapter 1 I detailed how Americans have the dubious distinction of being among the fattest people on earth, a circumstance explained in part by the high-stress, demand-driven lifestyle that we have adopted. But there is also much to suggest that the disruption of local food sources and the relentless industrialization of our food supply—especially in supplying the cities where most of us now live—has helped foster our present plague of type 2 diabetes, heart disease, and some cancers. Inadvertently we have made ourselves sick. As Michael Pollan, the journalist and activist, has whimsically observed, it is as if we Americans have "ushered a new creature onto the world stage: the human being who manages to be both overfed and undernourished."

Driven by growing concern over this epidemic, of late Americans have taken a renewed interest in what they are eating. In the United

States approximately 50 percent of meals and snacks are prepared out-side the home. People have begun asking questions: What goes into those meals? Where does the food come from? How is it prepared? What are the ingredients, and who is providing them? What are the links between the nation's health and the increasingly shrink-wrapped "food" that we consume?

To date such questioning has not inspired any noticeable change in the staple American diet of hamburgers and fries. But it has fos-tered citizen-based movements seeking a return to traditional, locally grown food sources and greater social responsibility on the part of the food industry. As a result, farmers' markets, community networks, and grocery stores devoted to "organically" grown food have seeded them-selves across the country. In the media the selection, preparation, and cooking of food has become something of a popular sport, with spe-cialized magazines, trendy restaurants competing to offer novel cui-sine, and celebrity chefs holding forth on television. Americans are not alone in these efforts, as is exemplified by the Slow Food movement that began in Italy in the 1980s and now has chapters across Europe and the United States. In 1999 the initiative was extended to the Slow City—a place where the inhabitants celebrate the slow course of the seasons and their relationship to local taste, health, and custom with-out excluding social and technological advance.

I believe we are on the cusp of social change in America. Our awareness of food is shifting, moving beyond a mere commodity of consumption to a place once more at the center of human culture and human health. It is the genesis, pitfalls, and promise of this shifting cultural awareness that I examine in these next pages.

IT WAS THROUGH EXPERIMENT—from trial and error—that humankind first distinguished what is edible from what is to be avoided. In the care of the body, Galen's principles of medicine, which dominated Western thinking for two thousand years, were based on balancing the elements of the universe, two by two, as hot and cold, dry and moist. A man was healthy when the four elements of the body—air, fire, earth, and water—were paired off in harmony. Cooking followed these principles through the skillful combination of ingredients to achieve an appetizing, nutritious diet.

Medicine and cookery evolved from the same body of wisdom, where pleasure and health were considered mutually reinforcing around the consumption of good food. We once knew nothing about what today's biochemistry tells us regarding antioxidants, for example, and their ability to mop up those molecules in the body that might otherwise damage cells. But instinctively we are drawn to such foods, as are other creatures. Much as we may now enjoy the sight and taste of blueberries—high in antioxidants—on breakfast cereal, Martin Schaefer, a scientist at the University of Freiburg, has found that the European blackcap, a small bird of the warbler family, also enjoys them, using the color and taste of fruits high in antioxidants as a guide to foraging.

Prior to the modern-day technical revolution in medicine, instruction in dietetics was the primary therapeutic intervention for most ailments. Pick up any medical text from the nineteenth century or visit the apothecary shop at Colonial Williamsburg, and you will see what I mean. Later, as medical science came of age, the focus turned to "deficiencies of nutrition," something that I remember from my own days in medical school: a shortage of vitamin D causes rickets, an inadequate intake of vitamin C produces scurvy.

In contrast to these "deficiency" diseases, it would appear today that the pendulum has swung, and the major challenge for the health sciences is to understand excess. We are getting fat simply because we eat too much and the wrong stuff. The seductive onslaught of a processed diet rich in animal fat, sugar, and salt—constituents that we crave, for they were scarce and hard to come by in Paleolithic times— has hijacked our culinary tastes. This is part of the story, but suspicion is growing that we are losing something vital to our health through the industrial "processing" of food, which frequently has the prime objective of increasing shelf-life in the grocery store. Perhaps those reassuring lists of "nutrients" found on the back of the cellophane packaging are not a substitute for what the body receives when we eat food fresh from the garden. Perhaps dietary deficiencies persist; perhaps indeed we are both overfed and undernourished.

It is well to remember that the deficiencies driving rickets and scurvy were of man's manufacture. The blackened skin and bleeding gums of those who had been too long at sea were familiar scourges for centuries before scurvy was recognized as a deficiency of the ascorbic acid that is contained in fresh fruit and vegetables. Scurvy was an illness of circumstance just as was, and is, the bone softening that marks the rickets of childhood, driven by a lack of vitamin D. Malnutrition can precipitate that deficiency, but so did the sun-blocking, smoke-filled atmosphere of England's northern cities during the long transition from an agrarian economy to the Industrial Revolution.

With hindsight it all seems so simple. But what are the deficiencies that we may be facing now with the industrialization of our food supply? The evidence there is not yet clear. But slowly, in the face of ignorance, an awareness of the distinction between nutrition and food is returning, reinforced not by science but by the simple intuitive sense that we know a tasty vegetable when we meet one. And as in the stories of scurvy and rickets, science is beginning to catch up in aiding our understanding. Even in diseases such as cancer evidence is accumulating that a diet rich in fresh fruits and vegetables plays an important role in combating the recurrence of illness, switching off genes that promote rogue cells and encouraging those metabolic processes that inhibit them.

Compared to our ancestral hominid diet, to which we became genetically attuned over five to seven million years, the coming of agriculture—just ten thousand years ago—ushered in profound changes in what we eat and how we live. The ancient mixed diet of plants and some meat, which had varied dramatically with local climate and geography, shifted toward uniformity, especially after the cultivation of grains. The staple crops that have supported the growth of civilization since—barley and wheat in the Mediterranean and the Middle East, millet and rice in Asia, and maize in the Americas— were not discovered by chance but selected and propagated by early farmers in parallel with hunting and gathering. Subtly at first and then more rapidly as livestock was domesticated, the shifts in diet have fostered genomic discordance, promoting a mismatch between our ancient evolved experience and the novel culture.

Through natural selection we strive constantly to adjust to these changes, sometimes with success. A good example of where we now understand the underlying human biology is the story of lactose—the sugar present in milk—for which the necessary digestive enzyme lactase diminishes rapidly after weaning in childhood. For the majority of the world's peoples this is a normal metabolic shift that in adult life makes the digestion of animal-milk products difficult, inducing the syndrome of lactose intolerance. However, in some minority populations—like those European farming cultures where the consumption of dairy products has been the norm for many generations— lactase persistence has emerged through the natural selection of genetic variation.

Doubtless there have been many such adaptive shifts in the genome that we are yet to understand, but in general it is safe to say that our cultural evolution has dramatically outstripped our capacity to cope, both behaviorally and physiologically, particularly since industrialization and the advent of advanced technology. Some 70 percent of the total daily energy typically consumed by Americans—the dairy products, cereals, alcohol, vegetable oils, and the ubiquitous refined sugars, particularly fructose, contained in cookies, cakes, crackers, soft drinks, and snack foods—would have contributed little or none of the calories present in the preagricultural diet. In consequence, having replaced the plant foods that once sustained us with a highly processed dietary intake, we must now juggle rising blood glucose levels, changing fatty acid composition, shifts in chemical balance, a reduced level of fiber, and the challenges of chronic metabolic stress. Collectively these shifts in body chemistry drive our modern-day "diseases of civilization." While it has been fashionable to seek unitary explanations for these disorders, for example, that cardiovascular disease is related to excessive fat intake, the mounting evidence is that in our postindustrial diet multiple factors play their part—both what is in it and what isn't—and together conspire with lifestyle to generate disease.

While in the United States we no longer believe in the humoral theories of Galen, humankind is still hungry for securing the balance that promotes health, as evidenced by the billions spent on such wellness "enhancers" as ayurvedic supplements, exotic grains, and herbal teas. Is this some preconscious attempt to return to the natural world, to tap again into the intuitive power of phyletic memory? Does such striving reflect our estrangement from the land that feeds us? If so, why has that happened? What drives the industrialization of our food chain? To answer these questions, we must further consider the role of the city, where most of us now live.

THERE ARE ESSENTIAL LINKS between the growth patterns of a city and how it eats, as Carolyn Steel has described in *Hungry City: How Food Shapes Our Lives*. Carolyn lives in London and is a practicing architect—one with a passion for food, I might add—who also teaches the principles of sustainable urban design at Cambridge University. "Feeding cities," she explained to me when we first met in 2009, "arguably has a greater physical and social impact on us and our planet than anything else we do. Think of it: for a city the size of London enough food for thirty million meals must be produced, imported, sold, cooked, eaten, and disposed of *every single day*. And something similar is happening each day for every city on earth."

Framed in this way, it seems self-evident, given the gargantuan nature of the task, that supplying and satisfying the appetites of the modern city shape our relationship with food. "Historically it was grain production, essential to the baking of bread, that first fed the hungry city," Carolyn explained. "A navigable river and fertile lands in close proximity were essential if an urban center was to thrive: that in the beginning was London's strategic advantage. And open, central markets provided the necessary infrastructure in managing food delivery."

Indeed, I knew that truth for myself. The great, specialized markets of central London—Covent Garden for fruit and vegetables, Billingsgate on the river for fish, and the Smithfield meat market—were all still operating in their original locations when I was a student in 1960s London. Today, for the moment Smithfield remains on site, but both Covent Garden and Billingsgate have moved out of the city center to cheaper land and better transportation. Supermarket supplies to London, as in other metropolitan areas, now arrive mainly by truck in the dead of night from someplace unknown and far away.

Cattle that once arrived on the hoof and later by rail now are slaughtered remotely, and it is the refrigerated carcass that satisfies the daily demand of butcher's shops and restaurants for "fresh" meat. Indeed, the majority of modern city dwellers live thousands of miles from the landscape that feeds them. In the urban setting we no longer have an emotional connection to the source that provides what we eat, yet the production and merchandising of food still shapes the way we live. Carolyn put it to me succinctly: "those vital activities that were most visible in the life of the preindustrial city have become essentially invisible."

Perhaps most startling is that this profound cultural shift has occurred comparatively swiftly. For Adam Smith agriculture formed the basis of a nation's wealth, but he considered interdependence with the city as necessary to drive continuous improvement. "The great commerce of every civilized society, is that carried on between the inhabitants of the town and those of the country. The country supplies the town with the means of subsistence, and the materials of manufacture. The town repays this by sending back a part of the manufactured product to the inhabitants of the country. The gains for both are mutual and reciprocal," he wrote in *The Wealth of Nations*. But less than a year later *The Complete Farmer*, my much-thumbed leather-bound compendium of 1777 from which comes the epigraph to this chapter, records in detail how rural life in England was already breaking from its ancient agrarian roots.

A century earlier Parliament had encouraged the enclosure of common lands, replacing them with the hedged, privately owned rectangles that we now consider to be the typical landscape of Britain. This refinement in farming increased crop yield, as a greater proportion of solar radiation reached the open fields. It was just the beginning. Subsequently the discovery and harnessing of fossil fuels dramatically reduced the traditional dependence on the annual organic cycle of energy renewal. In parallel, thanks to the likes of the Lunar men, science-driven innovation proceeded apace. Mechanization and a canal system for transportation significantly enhanced agriculture production and distribution. By the mid-nineteenth century the advent of the steam locomotive brought the emancipating spread of the railways, and the need for physical proximity between city consumer and country producer began a rapid decline.

But the city's demand for food was growing. A population explosion in the industrializing urban centers and the specter of Malthusian catastrophe shifted the focus of attention. In feeding the hungry hordes, now the economic objective was to produce agricultural goods as abundantly, cheaply, and reliably as possible. In achieving that goal, the vagaries of nature had become the chief enemy. The massive and unprecedented growth of industrial centers—towns that could no longer reliably feed themselves from the surrounding countryside—demanded new farming methods. So began the transition from Adam Smith's time-honored, sustainable "agri-*cultural*" practice to what today is known as industrialized "agri-*business*."

In driving this transition, biological chemistry was to play an essential role. In the early nineteenth century Justus von Liebig, in Germany, and Jean-Baptiste Boussingault, in France, both made pioneering contributions to agricultural science. Comparing the nitrogen content of animal manure, blood, bones, and fish in 1836, Boussingault discovered that a fertilizer's effectiveness was directly proportional to its nitrogen content. Plants need many nutrients to thrive—phosphorus and potassium among them—but they are particularly dependent upon nitrogen, which in the natural order of things is taken from the atmosphere and fixed in soil by microbes living in certain legumes and in manure. This is the process that provides the basis for sustainable soil renewal through crop rotation. However, the natural reservoirs of reactive nitrogen are limited.

Liebig was one of the first to recognize this limitation and propose the direct application of nitrogen-based agents such as ammonia as artificial fertilizer to plant roots. Then in 1908 the German chemist Fritz Haber patented a process where, in the presence of iron oxide, under pressure, and at high temperature, three atoms of hydrogen and one atom of nitrogen could be combined into the pungent gas that is ammonia. Rapidly industrialized by Carl Bosch, this "fixation" of nitrogen from the atmosphere had many uses, but principal among them was the production of explosives and artificial fertilizer on a massive scale. In regard to the latter, because of Haber's discovery, it is estimated that the yield from one hectare of arable land more than doubled, from supporting 1.9 persons in 1908 to 4.3 persons today.

This was an astonishing achievement, but it was not the result of artificial fertilizers working alone. By the middle of the twentieth century the search for increased yields had become the stimulus for plant breeding and new crop-growing methods. Most famously Norman Borlaug, an American agronomist working for the Rockefeller Foundation in the 1940s, began using hybridization methods specifically to develop grains that would benefit from readily available nitrogen. The result was a series of high-yield dwarf varieties of wheat and rice that after 1970 rapidly swept across the world. By 2000 these carefully bred seed varieties accounted for an astounding 86 percent of the wheat grown in Asia, 90 percent in Latin America, and 66 percent in the Middle East and Africa. Similarly the new breeds of rice accounted for 74 percent of that staple being grown in Asia and 100 percent of that in China.

But there is paradox here, as Carolyn Steel made plain during our discussion. In step with the triumph of feeding billions of people, the rush to industrialized farming has had a dark side. Blind to the longer-term view, we have been interfering with the cycles of nature on an unprecedented scale, promoting the use of poorly tested fertilizers and weed killers, plus a conveyor belt approach to animal husbandry. The devastating drought that turned the great plains of America—the breadbasket of the world—into dust during the 1930s gave us pause and sparked early debates that continue today regarding the merits and limitations of organic and industrialized agriculture.

"The great Dust Bowl certainly was a wake-up call," explained Carolyn. "I think it inspired the rigorous, ecologically designed soil experiments undertaken by Lady Eve Balfour here in Britain, those which she described in her classic book *The Living Soil* published in 1943. And of course there was Rachel Carson's *Silent Spring* in 1962, which exposed the destructive use of DDT and changed America's pesticide policies. These were the pioneers, but I fear their insights have had little impact on the average city dweller. Our industrialized approach to feeding ourselves remains pretty much beyond general awareness. It seems that the closer we live together, the further we get from an appreciation of nature."

There is truth here. The "green" revolution, as some have labeled Norman Borlaug's postwar success in chemical agriculture and plant hybridization, has been essential in feeding the seven-plus billion human beings now on the face of the earth. The world output of cereal grains tripled between 1950 and 2000 although the area of cultivation increased only by 10 percent. However, partnering with such extraordinary yields have been unintended consequences, and most are not environmentally friendly. Many of the new grains have proved less resistant to disease than anticipated and therefore require pesticides to sustain their growth. Agents developed in wartime to kill lice on soldiers will certainly kill bugs in the field, but slowly they destroy other things too, including birds, insects, and other creatures essential to biodiversity.

Also the new varieties of high-yield seeds require not only artificial fertilizers but also large amounts of water, creating both shortages and unforeseen problems. Nitrogen run off from fields has poisoned fish and shellfish in many coastal regions by reducing the oxygen in the water and encouraging the growth of algae and weeds. In India—specifically in the Punjab, the cradle of India's "green" revolution—the heavy drawdown of the region's water through deep wells has caused a dramatic fall in the water table, lowering it fifteen feet in just the decade between 1993 and 2003. Indeed the depletion of groundwater has become so severe that many farmers in the region are unable to satisfactorily irrigate their crops, with yields dropping in consequence. And India is not alone; the Great High Plains Aquifer that lies beneath the vast midwestern plains of the United States, stretching from South Dakota and Wyoming to the Texas Panhandle, is also failing. A half-century of center-pivot irrigation—the deep wells and rigs that create the patterned circles of crops so evident when flying over the territory—has dramatically reduced the available groundwater, drying creek beds and endangering this vital agricultural region during periods of drought.

The lesson is familiar. In our zeal to solve an old problem—in this case hunger—we create a new one. It is increasingly apparent that the "green" revolution, relying as it does on fossil fuels together with massive fertilizer and pesticide campaigns, disrupts biodiversity and the capacity of the living soil to maintain the ecological balance essential to the production of healthy food. This is potentially counterproductive, increasing the risk of rapidly evolving pests and destructive crop diseases that will further disrupt the world's food supplies. The processed and fast-food conglomerates that dominate in feeding the masses of the hungry city, but which are heavily dependent on industrialized farming and cheap transport to reduce their costs, perpetuate and exacerbate these potential pitfalls.

"We are as dependent on food conglomerates as ancient city dwellers were on their king or emperor," ventured Carolyn during our discussion. "Yet unlike them we have no direct relationship with those feeding us—apart, that is, from when we hand over the cash at the till. Supermarkets supply eighty percent of our food in Britain. In the name of efficiency we have streamlined nature itself. Even more ironic is that we city dwellers have been sold the idea that food is cheap," she continued. "Nothing could be further from the truth. The only way to sustain that illusion is by externalizing and hiding costs. So in reality a third of the globe's greenhouse gases are derived from industrialized food production, which also consumes some seventy percent of the water we use. The American diet takes ten calories of energy to put one calorie of food on the table, so buying a hamburger should cost around two hundred dollars. It is a system both expensive and wasteful: Britain throws away 6.7 million tons of household food a year—one third of all that we buy. Clearly the prevailing economic model for feeding ourselves is unsustainable."

For Carolyn Steel life is full of fascinating puzzles. How we sort through them helps shape the way we think, and urban food distribution is one such puzzle. Thus it follows for an individual with a flair for urban design that if the places where we live are shaped by food, then food is potentially a creative tool through which to build better places. The logic goes something like this. With industrialization, civic centers built around vibrant food markets are largely a thing of the past. Food no longer comes to the urban center but to peripheral megastores: we drive out of the city to buy what we eat. Within the city itself the "good" food goes were the money is, while the poorer city districts become "food deserts": de facto commerce is designing our cities.

But food is culture. Food is a shared necessity and frames a shared way of thinking. Food goes beyond what is on the plate to show us that the mundane elements in life are connected: food carries meaning and values. So when we pause to see the world through food, we come face to face with the kind of world we are creating. In short, for Carolyn Steel thinking about food gives permission to think again about big ideas. "What kind of society are we trying to produce?" she asks. "When we talk about food systems, we ask *how are we going to feed the world? We be should asking *what sort of world do we want to feed?* We've got the question the wrong way round."

The implication of such thinking is that we need a second green revolution and a real one this time, one less dependent on industrialized agriculture and the heavy use of fossil fuels. We must balance a blind faith in the technology of monoculture with organic fundamentalism. Fortunately this shift is already in process for we are wiser now. When singularly pursued, industrial agriculture and organic farming both fall short in the feeding of billions. What is needed is a third way, combining ancient wisdom with modern technology. A dynamic network of local farms supported by strong infrastructure must supplement the globalized food chain. Such is the philosophy of the Slow Food movement—a system where the consumer and the producer once again have a dynamic relationship such that production more closely equals demand and waste is reduced. But in the twenty-first century where are those knowledgeable local farmers to be found?

OJAI IS A SMALL TOWN some ninety miles north of Los Angeles. Nestled up against the mountains, it remains a farming community growing mainly citrus fruit and avocados. It has also become a haven for prep schools, artists, and entertainment industry refugees from big-city life. The main street has a park and an arcade of shops with Spanish-style facades. There is also a small movie theater tucked in next to the post office; the theater looks back to the heyday of Hollywood before it was harassed by televisions and electronic tablets. In the foyer they still sell popcorn from a glass cabinet framed by mahogany columns, and on the walls are photographs of bygone stars.

One bright afternoon in the fall, just days before Thanksgiving, I attended the screening of a new documentary made by one of the townspeople, a woman who is enthused about organic farming but also deeply moved by the tragedy of war. *Ground Operations* was the film's simple title.

The theater was packed. As the film opens, two shadowy figures, wrapped in armor and clutching heavy weapons, cautiously pick their way through a blanket of fog. Slowly the mist clears, and two young men, now in T-shirts and jeans, are walking down a farm track in bright sunshine. The camera pans outward over the mountains to reveal a sun-blessed valley, spectacular in its autumn foliage. Focusing down, we find ourselves standing in front of a herd of curious cows, who are solemnly investigating the camera and quietly chewing.

Then with a crash the silence is broken: the screen is leaping toward us. Suddenly we are back at war, as amid the whickering of gunfire a massive explosion craters the road in front of our vehicle and spins it sideways. . . .

"It's ironic," declared Delanie Ellis, the film's producer, when we met the next morning at breakfast. "Rural America has sixteen percent of the population and yet provides forty percent of our military personnel. Disproportionately kids from the farm belt are fighting our wars in the Middle East. And many are coming home to no jobs. Returning veterans need real opportunities—to heal, to pay bills, take care of families, to start a new life. They're not complaining. They will tell you they chose to serve. But to be roughed up in war and to come home to a void is to me a double tragedy. That's where I know farming can help."

Delanie is a woman of passion and energy, while at the same time intensely practical. Those who know her well say that it has always been so. As a girl growing up in the San Fernando Valley before it was overrun by the urban sprawl of Los Angeles, she loved horses and open space; that ended abruptly when her father changed jobs and moved the family into the city. After college her filmmaking career began promisingly in Hollywood but sputtered and slowed in one of the industry's many economic downturns. In self-defense she retreated to a small family-owned beach house in Ventura County, only to fall in love again, this time with the village of Ojai and with gardening. "I taught myself from books," she declared unabashedly, "and I made lots of mistakes. But they were good mistakes. Failure teaches you how complicated and difficult growing real food can be. It makes you appreciate the product." She was hooked. Even when the economy rebounded, she did not go back to L.A. "My daughter and I," she added proudly, "have been gardening and cooking together since she was two."

Inspired by her new passion, Delanie returned to directing films, focusing on documentaries. The first was on preserving farmland. "The short answer to that challenge is better urban planning," she quipped, "going up, as in Europe, not going out." Next was a film about farmworkers; another focused on land stewardship. Then she met Michael O'Gorman, the founder of the Farmer Veteran Coalition, a nonprofit organization dedicated to rejuvenating small farms by strengthening the network of veterans in agriculture. For Delanie it was a project made in heaven. "As a filmmaker, I was on to the idea immediately, much as a hungry flea jumps on a dog." *Ground Operations* was the product.

A series of screenings across California and the Northwest followed, connecting returning veterans to one another, to local food producers, and to businesses. "We always start with food—with a supper of local produce—then the veteran speaks, and then the film," explained Delanie. "It's a prescription that's memorable. The stories told by these young men and women are heartbreaking and inspiring in the same breath. It's living testimony to how the scars of war—the traumatic stress, the damaging effects of concussion—can heal and joy can return, not to mention the real goods that they bring to the table. In Santa Monica recently one young artisan brought mead wine made from his honey; another was making ketchup from his heirloom tomatoes. The audience couldn't get enough of them: from warrior to farmer—from bayonets to pruning hooks—and with business savvy too."

America needs battalions of such artisans. Of the more than 320 million people who live in the United States, less than 1 percent consider themselves farmers, and they are an aging group. There are eight times as many farmers over sixty-five as there are farmers under thirty-five. Production is increasingly concentrated in the industrialized sector of our farming enterprise. In the 2007 census taken by the U.S. Department of Agriculture, a mere 187,816 of the 2.2 million farms registered in America accounted for 63 percent of all agricultural products sold. America's vital base of small farms, those with incomes between $100,000 and $250,000 that supply local markets, has been eroding for decades. And perhaps most important is that the transgenerational knowledge base of seasonal husbandry, of sustainable crop rotation and other organic practices, has been eroding with them.

"To feed the growing demand for local markets, it's estimated that we need one hundred thousand new farmers each year for the next ten years," Delanie explained during our conversation at breakfast. "That's where veterans can make a difference. It's a great union. Small-scale farming needs a mix of talents and the ability to make do with what you have. That's something the veteran understands and has practiced repeatedly, frequently under fire. They know machines: they know what it takes to make something run and to keep it running. And they understand risk and strategic thinking. These are the people we need in local farming—people who don't give up when things get tough. And for the sixty-year-old seasoned farmers doing the training, it's an opportunity: they love the eager energy that the young people bring. Yes, it's a great union: the kids from the farm belt are coming home."

When it comes to educating young farmers, such apprenticeships follow an organized tradition in America. The 4H clubs—pledging head, heart, hands, and health—have been in the game for a century or more. Supported by state colleges, county agents, and enthusiastic families, the movement remains strong in the Midwest and in rural areas. I speak from experience: my two daughters Kate and Helen, growing up on a small farm in rural New Hampshire, reared enough heifers between them to help pay their way through college; Kate ended up a large animal vet, and Helen is a sheep farmer.

Indeed, it has been suggested—as a twist to the story—that American agriculture's pursuit of biotech innovation, yield, and profit has its roots in the aggressive promotion of novel farming practices by the land grant colleges and their 4H extensions during the settlement of the Midwest in the late nineteenth century. From the start, compared to many European countries, the United States has treated the growing of food as a commodity to be maximized and traded rather than an extension of culture, cuisine, and conversation. So if a hybrid seed outgrows the seed corn saved from last year's harvest and increases yield, then more to the good. It's a different way of thinking. Perhaps such thinking helps explain the industrialization and bifurcation of American agriculture into large- and small-scale farming during the later part of the twentieth century?

I asked Delanie what she thought. "That's possibly true," she replied swiftly, "but it's not an either-or proposition. We will always need some big agriculture," she said. "We're not going to be growing wheat or soybeans on a five-acre farm. And cattle need big areas for grazing, so there's always going to be a place for that. But we need a balance between big and small. A major problem at the moment is that big agriculture has a grip on farm legislation in America. Originally the farm bill was set up during the Great Depression to keep farmers on the land—because there was no food—and to save people from starvation. But that has changed: now the farm bill is essentially a subsidy for the 'agri-business' with minimal assistance to the small 'agricultural' farmer. For example," Delanie continued, "did you know that you can't use food stamps at the Ojai farmers' market? Does that make sense with the obesity problem we have in this country? Essentially federal policy dictates that the poorest people can use food stamps only to buy processed food."

Delanie paused. "We need better balance between industrialized monoculture and diversified, sustainable local farming. The inner city is a food desert: why not bring real food production to within sight of the city walls and improve the health of those who live there? Our returning veterans can help do that: impact ten to twenty percent of the market, and the politics will follow. The teenagers have no summer jobs—we can change that. Many in America are suffering from poor nutrition—we can change that too. So my work with veterans is just a small contribution to solving a much larger set of problems. But the bottom line is that for reasons of both economy and health we must reestablish a direct relationship between farmer and consumer."

TO REESTABLISH SUCH a relationship in America may now be possible. After more than half a century of federal subsidies that have favored intensively farmed monocultures fostering overproduction and low prices, food costs again are rising. Among the factors driving these increases are that China has doubled its appetite for meat; the movement to develop domestic biofuels is consuming one-third of America's annual maize production (filling your gas tank with ethanol requires about as many corn calories as does feeding an individual for a year); the cost and availability of water for factory farming is rising; and fossil fuels are increasingly expensive to extract. Paradoxically these increasing costs offer an economic opportunity for small-scale producers interested in developing a sustainable business model through supplying fresh food to their local city neighbors.

Several elements are in place to encourage such entrepreneurship. First, approximately 80 percent of small farms selling at the local level are situated in metropolitan counties or close to them. Research also suggests that 30 percent of shoppers will change where they buy their food in order to purchase local products. It's a classic case of back to the future. City leaders, as of old, are learning that they can improve a region's economy by facilitating strong relationships with local farms and at the same time, as a bonus, potentially improve public health.

And the influence goes further. The greater interest in locally grown and organic food is changing not only the habits of customers but also in turn the habits of the groceries that serve them. In Los Angeles Whole Foods, which trades on "providing food that is good for you," is growing against its traditional competition. In response Safeway Stores and other established grocers, including Tesco—an upstart from Britain—have launched small neighborhood stores that sell fresh produce. The avowed goal in typical Madison Avenue jargon is to offer the shopper a "new lifestyle experience." Even Wal-Mart, the world's largest retailer, is developing a smaller grocery chain known as Marketside—purchasing from local suppliers—which goes to affirm, as Delanie Ellis believes, that ideological movements at the social margin can change not only consumer habits but also established market practice.

These new city stores offer convenience by reducing the number of choices in each product category—too much choice confuses: few shoppers need fifteen varieties of ketchup—making it easier for the individual to buy wisely when pressed for time. Hence such stores carry only about 15 percent of the inventory found in large grocery chains with about half of the items on display being fresh fruits and vegetables, local meats, cheeses, and healthful pre-prepared foods. Some of the stores are hybrids, preparing and serving food on the premises, as typified by the Desert Rain Café in Sells, Arizona, which is run by the Tohono O'Odham Nation. The goal is to return locally sourced, nutritious indigenous foods to the Pima diet as a first step in combating the obesity epidemic.

Other stores have emerged from the opposite direction, being developed by the farmers themselves. Some of these are backed by established resources such as the Blue Hill restaurant at Stone Barns in the Hudson Valley, while others have grass roots. The Farmer and the Cook, run by Steve Sprinkle and Olivia Chase, is such an example in Ojai. Here a simple restaurant and market garden shop are the backbone of a program in "community-supported agriculture," where subscribers pay $100 a month to take home freshly harvested vegetables, sustainable fruits, and varieties of herbs throughout the year. With sixty subscribers it has a waiting list and reflects the extraordinary enthusiasm for locally grown produce that is emerging across America.

But enthusiasm does not necessarily equate with sustainability. Objectively the challenge in remaking a viable fresh-food system is formidable. Certainly the consumer and the farmer are the critical elements of such a system, but they must be knit into a dynamic whole by an infrastructure that makes it possible for farmland to be preserved and farms to be run effectively as a business while at the same time large institutions within the city can purchase regionally produced fresh food directly and efficiently. In simple terms we need unfettered local markets that work.

As my friend and colleague Michael Smith of Gypsy Meadows Organic Farm in Plainfield, New Hampshire, has described it, the mechanics of local farming separate into two parts—the growing of it and the getting rid of it. "The growing is hard work," says Michael, "but in some ways it is ridiculously easy: plants grow. I don't mean to diminish it, but it is simple. If you know what you're doing and pay attention to things, you grow better plants and so on. But selling it—how you market the stuff—that's not so easy, especially if you have the old-fashioned idea that the cost of purchase should reflect the cost of production. To hold down costs, an efficient infrastructure is essential, and in most communities we don't have what's needed. Sustainable fresh-food economies are not built on the backs of local farmers' markets."

In California, three thousand miles to the west, Larry Yee would agree with Michael's assessment. Cofounder and president of the

Food Commons, a national think tank dedicated to a new economic paradigm for sustainable farming, Larry has worked tirelessly for over three decades, both nationally and through the University of California Cooperative Extension, to develop innovative practices in local food marketing. Establishing a networked infrastructure of physical, financial, and distributional support is a central challenge in remaking any local fresh-food system. To do so is not easy. Success requires a combination of local leadership, community and political support, and consistent financial investment, often including philanthropy to serve as a pump primer.

The Philadelphia-based Common Market is one shining example of achieving such success. When Tatiana Garcia-Granados and Haile Johnston, both graduates of Wharton, the University of Pennsylvania's school of business, set up home in the Strawberry Mansion district of North Philadelphia in 2002, they soon discovered that they were living in a fresh-food desert. Working initially with neighborhood groups to establish a farmers' market, the couple quickly realized that the problem ran much deeper. With no stable customers and no delivery system, the connections that had once existed between Philadelphia and its surrounding farmland atrophied. For lack of customers local farmers were rapidly going out of business.

Tackling the problem at its source, in 2008 Garcia-Granados and Johnston founded the not-for-profit enterprise Common Market as a distribution link between threatened farms and Philadelphia's fresh-food-deprived urban communities. Troubled by the health disparities clearly evident in many poor neighborhoods and recognizing the role healthy food plays in enabling young children to succeed, the pair focused Common Market's initial efforts on cultivating institutional customers, particularly schools and hospitals. This strategy had the double advantage of adding freshly picked produce to the meals fed to those most in need of it while at the same time stabilizing the market for local producers. With a $1.1 million development grant from the Kellogg Foundation and a generous credit line supplied by the Rudolf

Steiner Foundation program for social finance—to pay farmers rapidly and fairly, thus shielding them from institutional tardiness—the Common Market has moved forward quickly.

In 2011 Common Market's customers included more than fifty public and charter schools in Philadelphia and New Jersey in addition to local groceries and hospitals. And the statistics are compelling: working with Common Market, the farmer on average earns 76 cents on every food dollar compared to less than 12 cents when working with conventional food distributors. And the food is indeed fresh, traveling less than 200 miles from farm to table compared to an average of 1,500 miles for conventional food sources. Thus Common Market's locally grown fruits and vegetables are picked to order and usually sold within seventy-two hours of being harvested. It's all part, as Haile Johnston describes it, of establishing from birth to death a "whole life–good food" continuum.

PETER FORBES, MY SON-IN-LAW, has long asserted that good food starts with good land. "What we eat and drink is our most important daily relationship to the land," Peter observed as he carried a skillet of freshly prepared home-reared lamb to the table. "The marinade is yogurt and ginger," added Helen, "and Wren scrubbed the potatoes and made that beautiful salad."

The occasion was suppertime at Knoll Farm a year or so ago: excited voices, the dog barking, the enticing sizzles and smell of the lamb, and the clatter of cutlery. It was late summer. That particular evening we ate in the small solarium just off the kitchen, looking out at the pond and the massive old barn. The farm chores were complete. The sheep had been gathered up from the field for the night. It was a precaution against the coyote: with the llama having recently died, they had lost their protector. The chickens were returned to their coop, enticed by fat cuttings from the lamb and by their grain. Wren had set colorful napkins and name tags around the table, except for her own place because she knew where she would be sitting. Fresh cucumbers in rice wine, shallots, red greens, and new potatoes complemented the lamb. The salad of three varieties of heirloom tomatoes—red, green, and saffron yellow—finished the spread. "It's all from Knoll Farm," Wren whispered to me proudly as we sat down. I nodded and smiled in appreciation.

This was a special meal. I rarely miss an opportunity to visit my daughters and their families, but on this particular occasion I had gone to Vermont to learn from Helen and Peter about their decade of farming experience. I wanted to get beyond the nostalgia and romance of covered bridges and the fall colors to learn about what it takes to build an economically viable farming enterprise in a rural community. Fayston lies close to Waitsfield in Vermont's Mad River Valley, a picturesque tourist area in the summer months and a destination for serious skiers during the winter. I was curious. How much did local farming fit into what was increasingly a transplanted city culture? Was the production and marketing of fresh food taken seriously?

"It depends on who you ask," Helen explained. "Those who have lived here for generations always grew their own food, so to them it's no big deal. People who have summer homes or have moved here recently from urban areas find it a complete revelation to start eating locally. They seize on the idea that good food brings good health; and it's also about neighborly support, getting together and learning new skills. It's a new culture for them: it's exciting, it catches on, and it's good for us. Farmers' markets are a huge trend in Vermont. The amount of money generated by farmers selling directly to the public is three or four times that of most states. That's one index of local interest. And of course it's an entirely different community experience," she added. "That's probably why it is so appealing to the newcomer. There's far more human interaction in buying fresh food from a local farmer than there is in picking packages off the shelf in a chain store."

In the first decade of the twenty-first century, farmers' markets grew rapidly across the country. "All states have seen huge increases," said

Peter, "perhaps multiplying tenfold to some ten thousand in all." Peter considered that the trend was about rediscovering relationships, not only with food but also with each other. "That's why Michael Pollan's books have sold so many copies; that's why sustainable agriculture is blooming. In this technology-saturated world the local food movement is about human connection. Cynically one might consider it romanticism, but here in Vermont it's real. And it's happening in other parts of the country too. Local farming is cheaper and healthier, and it's more fun for both producer and customer."

As the name implies, Knoll Farm is a hill farm, 140 acres of hillside pasture and sugar maples that has been farmed since 1804. The land and buildings are on the National Register of Historic Places and are conserved by the Vermont Land Trust. Central to the farm's economy is its herd of purebred Icelandic sheep, known for their fleece and mild flavored meat. Each spring forty to fifty lambs are born and raised by their mothers on milk and grass until about eight months of age. The best animals are sold for breeding or kept to strengthen the flock, and the rest are purchased as meat by local restaurants and individuals. In complement eight varieties of organic berries are grown for local markets and sold to farm visitors picking their own. A shop, situated at the farm and open between June and October, offers the berries, other produce, jams, eggs, grass-fed lamb, wool, yarn, blankets, and sheepskins. The enterprise turns a profit but would need to get larger to support the family as the sole source of income. Hence as for many small farms, the family income is supplemented by outside activity, with Helen working as a writer and editor and Peter lecturing widely on land conservation and leadership. Workshops on sustainable farming practice and summer retreats in collaboration with the Center for Whole Communities, which serves environmentalists and social activists around the country and makes its home at the farm, complete the picture.

Both Helen and Peter enjoy the diversity of what they do, believing that the way they farm and approach the stewardship of their land—

with the next generation in mind—is more important than any one aspect of the business. "Some people might criticize our work here as being at the margin," Peter said, "but it is at the margin that change occurs." And it is true: Scott Nearing had been at the margin—as had Eve Balfour and Rachel Carson—but Nearing's example helped catalyze the land trust movement decades after his death.

In Peter's mind, reengaging with why, how, and what we feed ourselves can return a sense of meaning even to the busiest of lives. So for the soccer mom from Annapolis "who has got debt up the wazoo and two kids she's trying to raise," going to the local farm to pick up the week's vegetables becomes a meaningful moment in an otherwise hectic life. The kids get to see what a carrot looks like, and the mother gets to connect with her neighbors. "That's when stuff begins to change," asserted Peter. "Such little moments are happening across the country. In the age of the Internet the food movement offers *real* connection to who we are as social beings. What started at the margin in small towns in Vermont and on the coasts is beginning to have national impact. And not just in the rural areas. Think of Just Food in New York City, Growing Power in Milwaukee and Chicago, and People's Grocery in Oakland. There's something like twenty-two hundred CSAs—community-supported farms—in the United States right now, and the numbers are growing fast."

I reminded myself once again: food *is* culture, and it runs deep. Within the subcultures of America there are great traditions around food and food preparation. Those shared family memories of cooking with grandmother, of chatting, of savoring the soup are real and pervasive. The cultural experience is bigger than food alone: it's a collective memory that conjures ethnic identity and ancestry to live again in the immediate moment.

Taking the long view of history, the era of industrial agriculture is just a tiny blip in the farming experience. But as Helen remarked during our supper together, "industrialization has become so pervasive that the last two generations in America have no memory of how to get

a tomato out of their backyard." So to succeed, the "real food" movement must go beyond privilege, romantic images, and glossy picture
books to reeducate and to reorient the next generation of children—
and do so early, forging lifelong habits of healthy eating and good
food. During World War II many American communities and families
supplemented their local food supply by planting a "victory" garden.
By 1943 there were more than 20 million such gardens—at homes,
in parks, and in the schools—producing more than 8 million tons of
fresh food. This is now happening again with school garden programs
across the country, driven in large part by the obesity epidemic and a
growing concern for long-term public health. It is the beginning of a
cultural reawakening. Through such programs children are learning to
make different choices, seeding islands of hope for the future.

Peter reminded me during our evening together of the geological
term *terra refugere*, which refers to those fragments of land that were
untouched as the last ice age moved south, small pieces of the earth
that were sometimes a quarter acre, sometimes less, where plant and
microbial life survived. Today much of our natural world, including
the habitat that sustains us, derives from those conserved islands of
refuge. The return to sustainable practices in agriculture seeks to further preserve that refuge, both to retain the legacy of a way of life that
honors the complexity of our planet's ecology and to refine that understanding in the future interests of human health and thriving.

Chapter 10

Imagination: The Playful, Creative Brain

My shaping spirit of imagination . . .

Samuel Taylor Coleridge, "Dejection: An Ode" (1802)

I am enough of an artist to draw freely upon my imagination. Imagination is more important than knowledge. Knowledge is limited. Imagination encircles the world.

Albert Einstein, in *Saturday Evening Post* (1929)

THE MUSEUM OF JURASSIC TECHNOLOGY can "really mess with your head," as one spindly adolescent described it to me during a recent visit. Even its location along a disheveled stretch of Venice Boulevard, at the edge of Culver City in Los Angeles, seems incongruous. Sandwiched between a carpet shop and a real estate office that appears permanently closed, and surrounded by gas stations, mini-marts, and automobile body shops, the Museum of Jurassic Technology (known fondly as the MJT by devotees) is in the last place where one would expect to find "an educational institution dedicated to the advancement of knowledge and the public appreciation of the lower Jurassic."

Even the museum's name is enigmatic. "The lower Jurassic—isn't that something to do with dinosaurs?" I asked the friend who introduced me to the place. "No, not a dinosaur in sight," she replied. And that, I was to learn, is the point. The MJT is designed to keep you off balance: it's a place of not quite knowing.

Later, when I met the founder and proprietor, David Wilson—who won a MacArthur "genius" award for exceptional creativity in 2001—I began to understand. A soft-spoken, bespectacled, and mild-mannered man with a gray-peppered, Abe Lincoln–style beard, David is quietly passionate about his work. In its original meaning a museum is dedicated to the muses, he explained, as a place where the mind can stand apart from everyday affairs. The early vehicles for such mental transportation were *Wunderkammern*, or wonder cabinets, collections of curiosities first accumulated by the wealthy in seventeenth- and eighteenth-century Europe. The MJT, in seeking to be a haven for the curious mind, draws from that tradition.

Perhaps in harmony with those early collectors of natural history, David Wilson was first a student of etymology—of the urban variety: bedbugs, carpet beetles, and similar pests—before studying film at the California Institute for the Arts. Both subjects have inspired him. Indeed, the meticulous construction of the museum's exhibits reflect that for a decade animation and special effects provided the bread and butter for David and his wife, in addition to supporting the nascent MJT. It was, as he described it to me, no easy task. Indeed, perhaps the museum would never have come into being but for dedicated friends and colleagues—the true collaborators—who "got stuck on the idea." With no fixed entry fee the "economics of the place are at best a miracle." The ideal is that of the Fields Museum in Philadelphia, founded in 1802, "open to all people, including children and the fair sex"—a place where the learner is led always from the familiar object to the unfamiliar, guided along "by a chain of flowers into the mysteries of life."

Initially, before the museum settled on Venice Boulevard, the "MJT traveled to any place that would have us," Wilson explained, "adding more and more material—heavy glass cases, etc.—until it got to be ridiculous. Then we decided we must bring the people to the museum rather than the other way around." In those early days of settlement, often the good proprietor could be found playing his accordion in the street outside the museum, to pass time but also in hope of luring the public into his labyrinthine world of dimly lit rooms and astonishing brain-teasers.

Within the walls of three modest townhouses, the MJT now fosters an experience unique in Los Angeles and beyond. The exhibits, although cloaked in history and formality as in a traditional museum, invite a different state of mind, provoking first curiosity and then a playful unease, as the storytelling unfolds in ways that challenge credulity. From the miniature painted image of Pope John Paul II, sculpted from a human hair, to the stink ant of the Cameroon, dead from the fulminating fungus growing from its head; from the "vulgar knowledge" of past generations that dead mice (on toast) may solve bedwetting, to the ingenious entrapment of the *Deprong Mori*, the piercing devil, a bat that is thought to penetrate the solid walls of buildings—each exhibit employs strangeness as a probe for thinking. Today in our information-saturated, technology-driven world, where mystery is fast being relegated to crime novels and horror films, it comes as a challenge and a surprise. As the spindly adolescent colorfully observed, "It messes with the head."

Gregory, the anthropologist friend who was with me that afternoon, commented as we left the MJT that "probably the most terrifying insight from the many exhibits is that, with attention to detail, you can make anything seem significant to the human mind." He reminded me that four volumes on the life of barnacles by Charles Darwin had been the groundwork for *The Origin of Species*. "Beyond what many may hastily dismiss as ridiculous," Gregory added, "there emerges a compelling aesthetic quality—an example of what the mind can achieve stringing single grains of truth together on the thread of one's own imagination. Perhaps the real genius of human intelligence is to create the story that enables the threading." I found that to be true. It is the brain that spins the tale. But also true is that after a while the mind becomes restless and curious, striving for closure. There is a compulsion to lift the curtain—to discover the Wizard of Oz. This, I believe, is the playful magic of the MJT. In promoting what appears to be reasonable, David Wilson adds a pinch of madness that disrupts the comfortable habits of everyday life, much as the proverbial grain of salt keeping reason from spoiling. The MJT, in its ingenious spinning of stories, leaves us hanging between wonder and disbelief. Breaking the hard shell of certainty, it is a museum devoted to celebrating the creative power of the human imagination.

A SENSE OF *WONDER* is what comes from the intellectual rummaging that curiosity induces, but in our search for understanding it is the act of *imagining* that fills in the gaps of mental knowledge. Imagination offers the capacity to distance oneself from the surrounding world and then to reconstruct that world, bringing to mind something not wholly present. It is a unique ability of the human animal, and it underpins much of the everyday behavior that we take for granted: storytelling, hoping for a better future, the fantasy play of childhood, the empathic concern for another's circumstance, the visceral engagement felt when reading about Harry Potter's exploits—all are dependent upon the capacity to conjure images in the mind. Imagined reconstruction is the mental projection through which art is created, religious beliefs are sustained, scientific hypotheses are explored, and material technologies are advanced. In short, imagination and creativity are the brain's kissing cousins and the wellspring of cultural vitality.

The seeds for imaginative thinking are planted in infancy. Comparing the early intellectual development of our closest living relatives, the great apes, with that of the human infant, it becomes apparent that there are intriguing similarities—such as facial recognition, imitation, and rough-and-tumble play—but also major differences, particularly in the complexity and progression of social interaction. For example, young children from about the age of eighteen months are helpful to others—witness my granddaughter's fascination in assisting with the sheep herd. Young chimpanzees raised by humans will demonstrate similar altruistic interests, although not reliably.

In the few laboratory studies that have directly compared children between two and four with chimpanzees and bonobos in the same age range, developmental differences—particularly in the pace and pattern of social engagement—are readily apparent. By the age of four, children are substantially ahead of the young apes in attentive capacity, and many have become adept in figuring out the motivation and needs of others. For example, the majority of children quickly solve the puzzle of fitting together three pieces of plastic pipe after the experimenter has "failed" to do so, whereas most of the young apes seem pleased to receive what they consider to be a new plaything—examining, throwing, and banging the pipe lengths together but rarely seeking to join them.

The challenge of the puzzle is instructive in dissecting how the young mind works. Problem solving demands close attention, but the young participant must also be able to imagine what the experimenter is attempting to achieve, and it is here that the human infant excels. Indulging in such guesswork is the beginning of what later will emerge as empathic understanding—the ability to imagine oneself in another's place—but it starts with the capacity to watch, listen, and imitate the behavior of others. Both apes and humans are capable of imitation—such as copying sticking out the tongue—shortly after birth, but in humans such crude "hardwired" responses recede as the capacity for play evolves. The solitary activities characteristic of the infant soon give way to a preference for peer interaction, with both species consistently using facial expression to communicate and build alliances.

In tracking and engaging the social interaction going on around them, however, human infants rapidly outstrip young chimpanzees. As I have noted in earlier chapters, infusing objects with meaning and sharing them with others in pretend play is a distinguishing feature of human infancy, one that places us apart from our primate cousins.

This capacity for imagination, which is central to the game of pretend, strengthens further as language evolves. Charades are the alternate, imaginative world in which we practice navigating the complexities of human society—learning about the emotional idiosyncrasies of others, juggling multiple perspectives, and distinguishing fact from fantasy. The child is "mummy" to her teddy bear, while remaining herself. The distinction is clear to the youthful mind: at one and the same time Teddy is a real live friend in whom secrets may be confided while also being just another stuffed animal, albeit a special one. It is through Teddy's exploits, and those of other imaginary friends, that the young child first invents narratives and comes to appreciate a causal chain of events: Teddy loves to sit down and have tea, but in his excitement he frequently spills his cup because he's clumsy. So it was in my own childhood. In my early forties, when my mother died suddenly, a scruffy, eyeless bearlike creature with a broken leg was discarded from her house by unknowing relatives: many of my childhood fantasies went with him.

It is through imagination and such make-believe that we first learn to think in parallel, on two levels at once, a practice that is fundamental to human cognitive development and one in which children quickly become skilled. As the eminent developmental psychologist Paul Harris has documented in *The Work of the Imagination* and *Trusting What You're Told*, children weave together what is learned from their own observation and imaginative exploration with information gathered from others whom they consider trustworthy—much as Susan Corbin described to me how she first learned to read by crawling into her father's lap with a book in hand. This highlights a special talent of the human animal: we love to educate each other, and we delight in shared understanding. Unlike other species we learn from what we are told and the testimony of others. Being taught by those we trust locks in rapid cultural progress: as individuals we do not need to discover everything anew for we are willing to defer to others and to their knowledge. The veracity of that commonsense knowledge is then personally ascertained by distilling it through our own imagination and cross-checking it with what we have previously experienced—which parenthetically is why after an hour or so at the Museum of Jurassic Technology one begins looking around for the proverbial Wizard of Oz.

Make-believe games are the harbinger of a lifelong propensity to consider alternatives to given assumptions. It is the human advantage that in our individual development we build not only on imitation but also upon imagination to embellish the knowledge acquired by previous generations, an evolving talent that is clearly evident in human rituals, technology, cooking practices, and attempts—both good and bad—at engineering the natural environment. In contrast, other primates do little to advantage themselves and to shape their habitat. The ape may learn adaptive tricks and the use of primitive tools from parents and peers, but rarely does that knowhow persist beyond one generation.

PRETEND PLAY, AND THE storytelling it evokes, may be considered the childhood training ground for later problem solving and creativity—a prelude to "imagining the future," as Joaquín Fuster described it to me—reflecting the uniquely human capacity to gain insight and invent novelty through the melding of abstraction and distilled memory. These are talents in continuous use: within the fast-moving, dynamic world of the subjective self it is imagination that writes the screenplay, making each of us whole as a person. But one may ask, where in the brain's mental workspace do we conjure such magic?

Let's consider music as a way into the question: what is it about a series of transient sounds that can be so engaging that we call it music? For most individuals the stimuli of the individual "musical" notes are abstract, having—in distinction to language—no inherent meaning. And yet on the physiological level we know that music can evoke definitive and impressive responses in mood and in thought, even for those of untrained ear.

That music has no self-evident function troubled the precise mind of Charles Darwin. And yet, he mused, music is more powerful than the spoken word in its capacity to unify the emotions of great crowds, "making heaven descend upon earth" or stirring up "the sense of triumph and the glorious ardour for war." In *The Descent of Man*, published in 1871, Darwin ruminated upon this conundrum. "As neither the enjoyment nor the capacity of producing musical notes are faculties of the least use to man in reference to his daily habits of life, they must be ranked amongst the most mysterious with which he is endowed . . . [and yet] . . . they are present . . . in men of all races." The human attraction to music, Darwin tentatively concluded, might best be explained as an instrument of courtship and propagation—the romantic arts of singing and of dancing, and of poetry too, having similarly "arisen during the earliest ages of which we have any record."

Perhaps one source of Darwin's difficulty was that while "music expresses itself through sound, sound in itself is not yet music," as Daniel Barenboim, the celebrated pianist and conductor, has perceptively observed. Music, a ubiquitous but culturally diverse activity, has its natural place alongside abstract thought and language: it is a function not of sound but of how the brain works. As in language, the brain imposes its own organization on the pitch and sequence of the sounds we perceive. At its most evolved, the shaping of this order is the craft of the musician, acting upon perception to create the rhythm and harmony of the singing voice, or that of instrumental music. In short, music—both in its creation and in its appreciation—is an exquisite example of the brain's perception-action cycle at work, the dynamic core function of the adaptive brain that I explored in Chapter 4.

With this insight we edge closer to engaging my question. Music, in its riches, has universal appeal because it engages the perception-action cycle in a special way, bonding through imagination the immediate stimuli of the notes themselves with the reflexive understanding of the intuitive mind. A well-shaped musical theme—in its capacity to evoke half-forgotten thoughts, images of persons or places, a familiar fragrance, the echo of a past passion—draws upon intuitive memory to initiate a dialogue between emotion and reason, which in turn gives rise to further association. This capacity of music to bind the identity of nations is the stuff of anthems, but in private we each have our familiar themes. For me, as a single example among many, I find J. S. Bach's suites for the unaccompanied cello to be deeply moving. I need only those early sonorous notes of the first prelude to be immediately transported back in time. Once again I can feel the sticky heat of London on a late summer's evening, and the sweet taste of cheap Greek wine, and relive my youthful desire to one day reliably produce such all-embracing sound.

That talent never emerged, despite my longing. But now, as a neuroscientist reflecting upon that imagined moment—in my mind's eye as real as any stage set—and coupling the experience with the knowledge gathered from recent brain-imaging studies, an understanding of the networks that delineate the brain's imagination workspace comes a little closer.

As we all know from personal experience, musical sounds can evoke a range of emotion, including distinct discomfort in response to dissonance. Stefan Koelsch of the Max Planck Institute for Human Cognitive and Brain Sciences in Leipzig, Germany, has taken advantage of this truth. In a study of individuals without musical training, employing pleasant and unpleasant music to evoke emotion while measuring the brain's response, Koelsch has used fMRI technology to track the temporal shifts in blood flow across anatomical regions. It will come as no surprise that the amygdala—the brain's sentinel of emotion—is activated by both pleasant and dissonant music. In addition, the hippocampus—playing a critical role in memory processing and recall—and also the associated cortical areas that surround these core brain structures, were found to have increased blood flow. In complement, the basal ganglia, important you will remember in the acquisition of intuitive habit, appear to be essential to following the musical beat.

Experiencing pleasure in music heard, however, recruits other brain networks beyond these core activities, including the medial prefrontal region that monitors pleasure and the executive and planning areas of the frontal cortex. In addition, because the blood flow in these areas increases as the pleasant music progresses and is appreciated, the results suggests that these are brain regions intimately involved in processing the structure and sequencing of the music that is heard. If, by now, you have the impression that there is a lot going on in the brain when music stimulates the imagination, you are correct. It is clear from these studies that when listening to music—as when J. S. Bach transports me back to my youthful love affair with the cello—that the brain is a busy place. Similarly in reading a novel—as when the child (or adult, for that matter) is engrossed in a Harry Potter story—the emotional imagery evoked in the mind commands the brain's full engagement. Thus we may conclude that when the imagination is at work, the mind is actively connecting and exercising the whole brain.

But the evoked imagery from listening to music or reading a book is distinct from coming up with a new tune, writing a story, or deconstructing the image of a violin to create a cubist painting. It is in witnessing such achievements that we find ourselves face to face with creativity, the kissing cousin to imagination. Of course, just uttering a unique sentence, which we do hundreds of times each day, is creative: but what of "when, from the sight of a man at one time, and of a horse at another, we conceive in our mind a Centaur," as Thomas Hobbes observed in *Leviathan*, written in 1651? How do we create such novel visual images from familiar or abstract forms? What are the brain networks that support the inventive facilities of mind?

Peter Ulric Tse and his colleagues at the department of psychological and brain sciences at Dartmouth College, in Hanover, New Hampshire, are honing in on these questions through a series of studies designed to better define what they call the brain's "mental workspace." To do so the researchers employ a synthesis of fMRI techniques, neuropsychological challenge, and network analysis. First, to explore the brain's network patterns when involved in a creative process that can be studied in the laboratory, the team developed one hundred abstract images. These serve as visual stimuli that can be imaginatively manipulated in the mind of the experimental subject, while simultaneously the brain's regional cerebral blood flow is being measured in an fMRI scanner.

During the experimental sessions the fifteen participants are asked to mentally combine these abstract stimuli to create novel, complex shapes. Subsequently, in a second phase of the study, the shapes generated are either mentally dismantled back into their parts or are simply maintained in the mind's eye, depending on instruction. The researchers conjecture that to process the abstract visual cues, and to support the mental gymnastics required in imaginative thinking, coordination among the brain's distributed networks would be essential. This has proved to be so. A multivariate analysis of brain blood flow, Tse and his team reported, confirmed a "widespread and interconnected information-processing network . . . that supports the manipulation of visual imagery," with the dorso-lateral prefrontal cortex of the "executive" brain and the posterior parietal region taking the coordinating roles.

Taken together, Tse's studies and those investigating the perception and appreciation of music suggest that the workspace of the brain employed in mustering imagination and creativity is extensive and varied, drawing upon the network of dynamic, interdependent systems that support emotion, working memory, the reasoned sorting of information, and choice. These identified networks are comparable to the *cognits* described by Joaquín Fuster, as when the reflexive, intuitive mind and the conscious, reflective mind come together in the functional harmony of the perception-action cycle. Imagination reflects this continuous exchange but transcends immediate experience to craft stories of the past and assemble future dreams, all refracted through the tinted lens of subjective meaning. Creativity—demanding a prodigious and disciplined memory, plus the courage to break old thinking habits—extends the imaginative manipulation of abstract concepts in the brain, translating them into ideas and actions that become appreciated and validated by others. This is the zenith of human intellectual achievement, a special wisdom that is anchored in the biology of the human brain and uniquely expressed in its most mature mode of operation.

IMAGINATION IS THE MENTAL capacity that sets us apart as a species, and not only in our biology. It is also the pervasive driver for many of our social and cultural achievements. In hindsight the Enlightenment is commonly considered the Age of Reason, when the writings of Isaac Newton first held sway and the scientific revolution made possible thinking about the material world without reference to a divine power. But this is simplification. In the eighteenth century both David Hume and Adam Smith recognized the essential nature of imagination in making it possible to think about things not immediately present, be they mundane, of science, or in the arts. This "shaping spirit of the imagination," as Samuel Coleridge described it in 1802, fills mental gaps in perception and provides coherence to experience. From childhood onward imagination is the glue that helps hold us together both as individuals and as social beings.

Imaginative thinking sets us apart from other animals because it releases us from attending exclusively to the immediate. Whereas the dog can attend to, see, hear, and smell a horse, as can we, and can similarly perceive a man, in the awareness of the dog's brain these are distinct information files. Most certainly the normal dog's brain does not combine the two and image Hobbes's centaur: such confusion would not serve the animal's survival. For the dog *unimodular attention* is essential. The human brain, in contrast, has evolved the capacity for *cross-modular attention,* where distinct information files not only can be cross-referenced against other networks but can also be integrated with them to create novel, symbolic forms, as we first do in the fantasy play of childhood. To quote Peter Tse, "It is not simply that there is more connectivity in the human brain, it is of a different kind."

So when did this difference in the thinking capacity of *Homo sapiens* first become evident—setting us apart from *Homo erectus* and *Homo neanderthalensis,* our forebears in the hominid line? Richard G. Klein, the Bass Professor of Anthropology and Biology at Stanford University and a leading authority on the tools and artifacts created by early humans, sets the date at 40,000 to 50,000 years ago—that is, in the Upper Paleolithic, also called the Old Stone Age. It was during this period, notes Klein, that a dramatic shift is found in the fossil record, a transition from the long-standing and widely spread use of archaic stone implements to "the burgeoning of unequivocal art and personal ornamentation," suggesting the emergence of a "capacity for abstract or 'symbolic' thought."

In the archeological record of western Europe this mushrooming of creative talent is reflected in the ancient cave paintings of France and Spain, the oldest of which date back some 30,000 or 40,000 years. This time frame coincides with the period when early modern humans, migrating out of Africa with new social skills and novel tool making to their advantage, arrived in the Iberian Peninsula. The migration brought them into close proximity with the Neanderthals, a stone-tooled, cold-adapted hunting-and-gathering people who had lived in the region and across much of Eurasia for more than 200,000 years. The invaders—commonly referred to as Cro-Magnon man, a name derived from the cave in southwestern France where in 1868 their remains were first discovered—appear to have lived in organized settlements, clothed themselves, carved bone ornaments, and chipped flint to make weapons. The archeological evidence suggests that their numbers grew rapidly. Indeed Klein, among others, has proposed that it was this explosion in the Cro-Magnon population and their superior creativity that contributed—despite some cross-breeding—to the ultimate extinction of the Neanderthals, approximately 30,000 years ago.

What promoted this sudden explosion of innovative practice in the Cro-Magnon? In primate and hominid evolution previous advances in adaptive behavior had been tied to brain growth (you will recall the work of Robin Dunbar in Chapter 6), but judging by the size of the skull's cavity the Neanderthal brain was as large as or larger than that of early modern *Homo sapiens*. In Cro-Magnon the relationship between brain morphology and behavioral advantage shifted. Does this imply a neural rewiring—a move toward cross-modular thinking and flexibility of attention—perhaps driven initially by a fortuitous mutation in the genome? If so, was this change comparable in its impact to the slight variation in base pairs found in the human FOXP2 gene—which I discussed in Chapter 6 and which appears to have been the critical variable in the development of sophisticated language? Is this the epoch in the evolution of human biology that heralded the birth of our prodigious imagination?

The 30,000-year-old cave paintings of France and Spain are spectacular but also sophisticated in their aesthetics. Principally the images are of the large animals that then roamed Europe; bison, stags, mountain goats, horses, mammoths, and ancient auroch cattle, interspersed with abstract renditions of the vulva and stencils of the human hand. Judith Thurman, after making a personal visit to the caves of Ardèche in south-central France in 2008, described the collective impact as "a bestiary of such vitality and finesse that, by the flicker of torch-light, the animals seem to surge from the walls." That these images are reflective of nascent human imagination, there can be little doubt.

But, one is compelled to ask, is symbolic *meaning* embedded in these glorious creations? It's a subject of continued debate. Were the caves simply a practical refuge from a brutal, shifting climate for a nomadic, hunting people? Or did they serve as temples for ritual cele-bration of religious, shamanlike beliefs at the interface between worlds tangible and intangible? The role of the shaman—extrapolating from the beliefs of today's remaining hunter-gatherer societies—was to travel between these worlds, to visit the ancestors, to commune with spirits, past and future, and to return with wisdom relevant to the challenges of the moment. So did the cave paintings play a role in these worlds of the imagination, with the shaman as the mystical guide? To some, that the artwork is largely remote and clustered around passages or fissures in the rock face supports such claims. Similarly, it is argued that the many hand stencils—the hand is placed against the wall and paint is blown around it, such that the image blends with the rock—may reflect ritualized efforts at communication with the gods of the underworld.

Setting aside the specifics of such speculation, Maurice Bloch, pro-fessor in anthropology at the London School of Economics, believes that the very existence of the cave paintings of the Upper Paleolithic has broad social significance. He believes these artifacts are a bell-wether, signaling a radical shift in human ingenuity and the social order. "Religious-like phenomena," he argues, "are an inseparable part of a key adaptation *unique to modern humans . . . the capacity to imagine other worlds . . .* an adaptation that lies at the very foundation of modern society." In other words, it was the fluidity of their imag-ination—of which the cave paintings stand as early evidence—that distinguished Cro-Magnon, the early modern humans, from their forebears.

Human society, Bloch asserts in harmony with Adam Smith, exists as a system of social order because of the interactions among the people who live within it. In this sense human social organization is little different from that of the great apes, the closest of our surviving relatives. Chimpanzees, for example, create long-term coalitions, as do we; they are self-centered but solicitous of kinship; they sometimes share food; and they are not beyond a little Machiavellian politicking when necessary, another behavior that we hold in common. Bloch describes these social interactions in anthropological terms as "the transactional social," as in the behaviors essential to Smith's concept of barter and exchange. These behaviors, however, are to be distinguished from "the transcendental social," which is fundamentally the product of imagination and pervasive in the determining the complexity of human culture. Neither chimps nor any of the other great apes exhibit such behaviors.

In human societies the transactional and the transcendental are inextricably intertwined. This is readily apparent in the organization of the market society, where in concept the *transaction* of goods is central. The abstract ideas of money, value, and transgenerational possession that make the market viable, however, are the products of imagination: these latter are *transcendental* concepts. Fundamentally, transcendental social behaviors reflect the human search for order and meaning. Life is characterized by its transience, proceeding through birth, development, reproduction, aging, and death. So what is the larger purpose? Human self-awareness drives such questions and the continuing quest for explanation. In our imagination we can construct processes of transcendence that help answer such puzzles—creating worlds and social roles that order existence beyond the determining biology of the life cycle. As a compassionate physician, as a good mother—even in death, and beyond—it becomes possible to see oneself as transcendent of time and mundane interaction to become part of a larger, all embracing, transgenerational social network.

Through these transcendental behaviors—like the spiritual trans-world communications of the shaman—imagination has traditionally provided stability and meaning in a changing world. Thus in navigating a multifaceted social order, imagination serves as a touchstone. The adaptive logic, Bloch argues, is simple enough. If human beings can simultaneously entertain fact and fantasy—the transactional and the transcendental—and do so from an early age, then doesn't it make sense that society will be similarly layered? What begins as role-play, and is acted out in childhood, continues as a culturally franchised reality that is complementary to everyday experience—one that can be lived in, that others can be drawn into, and through which forebears can be celebrated. As contemporary stereotypes assert: "I am an American: I live in a land of opportunity and freedom, made possible by the vision and sacrifice of the Founding Fathers"; or "As a Christian, I am in communion with the Son of God, who is my savior." Such sociocultural structures—secular and religious—create time-resistant, stable networks of complex social relationships that transcend and complement the immediate. This is the historical contribution that imagination makes to stability and to the sustaining values of human culture.

TODAY, HOWEVER, THE SUSTAINING values of human culture are changing. An invasive "technology of the intellect" is eroding the traditional role of imagination in society, particularly in the gadget-driven, time-starved, rich world. Neil Postman, the American author and cultural critic, writing in 1992 described this new society as a "technopoly," the implication being that the master narrative framing the human story has shifted. We are now in the thrall of our machines.

On May 11, 1997, the chess grand master Garry Kasparov, the reigning world champion, sat down with IBM's Deep Blue. It was a rematch, played under classical tournament regulations. A little over a year before, Kasparov had beaten the computer and its retinue of human assistants by four games to two. This time it was different: the supercomputer, which had been "upgraded" and was now programmed to systematically evaluate 200 million possible moves per second, ultimately won three and a half games to Kasparov's two and a half, by "brute number-crunching force." It was an impressive achievement by the IBM team, although whether the victory had anything to say about the nature of human imagination and creative intelligence is another matter. Deep Blue, as Kasparov himself pointed out, is intelligent only in the way that a programmable alarm clock is intelligent—"not that losing to a ten-million-dollar alarm clock made me feel any better," he added ruefully.

Deep Blue's symbolic victory nonetheless promotes important personal and cultural questions. In this era of intellectual technology, if brute-force programming can deliver the best chess, why labor to become a grand master? Why strain the mind and memory? Why bother with all that work? And yet Garry Kasparov, as a human being, has little doubt that learning to play chess is an effort inherently worthwhile. As he described it in his 2007 book, *How Life Imitates Chess*, the noble game offers "a unique cognitive nexus, a place where art and science come together in the human mind [to be] refined and improved by experience." Chess, the fifteen-centuries-old war game of strategy and skill—and a game symbolic of human thought—is an unparalleled laboratory for the training of memory and imagination and the evaluation of risk.

By comparison, despite the impressive technological triumph that Deep Blue represents, its inanimate number-crunching capacities fall far short of human ingenuity. Its achievements in winning the game of chess against Grand Master Kasparov are not to be equated with the intelligence of the human mind. If indeed Deep Blue "thinks," then it does so in a linear fashion: it does not understand process. It has none of the intuitive, cross-modular sensibilities that in human terms offer the brilliance and satisfaction of a chess game well played or of a life well lived. By contrast, as Kasparov has emphasized, when we set out to master in our mind the intricacies of chess, the game becomes a teacher of such sensibilities.

One does not need to be a chess grand master to experience the Deep Blue effect and the impact that technology now has on how we think and process information. Relatives from the Deep Blue family are hard at work in society and have pervasive influence in structuring many elements of daily life. I have come to find the laptop computer on which I write these words extraordinarily valuable, indeed indispensable, especially when formatting and editing. Similarly the new voice recognition computer software that I use at times to improve my typing speed is more helpful, and makes fewer mistakes, than the last version that I purchased some years ago. Of course, neither of the programs, nor those that went before them, understand a word of what I'm saying in a conceptual sense. Rather, in "typing" the letters and words that appear on the page as I speak, my voice detector is merely stringing together phrases that are common in everyday language, programmed to key on phonics. The system is impressive, and these are now standard technical tools of the writing trade, but they do not think for themselves.

Not so when reading the words that I have written, as you are now doing: reading remains an ancient art. Your mind continuously imposes an unseen order: an intuitive set of rules—as familiar to you as are the rules of chess to Garry Kasparov—enable you to link the ink marks that you see on the page to words that you can hear in your head. Your brain perceives these little marks and, drawing upon intuitive memory, acts to give them meaning through which you, as the reader, then come to understand my intentions. The brain collects information, sorts it, chooses from among its elements, and through imagination claims it for its own. It is something that only the human brain knows how to do, and our attempts to technically duplicate the process remain far behind. This is both good news and bad. On the good side of the ledger, we can reassure ourselves that we remain in charge of our machines, if we choose to be so. But on the negative side it is clear that when it comes to processing the massive volumes of information that today's technology-driven society generates, the human brain can be a limiting factor. That in a nutshell is how Deep Blue can win at chess, without understanding the principles of the game.

The written word has been around for a long time—even the printing press has been with us for six hundred years—but it is computer technology and increasing access to the World Wide Web that have precipitated the tsunami of information that now floods everyday experience. As an index of that assault, *Bloomberg BusinessWeek* has estimated that the average person processes 63,000 words of new information each day, which in volume is approximately equivalent to the words contained in a good-sized novel. Information has moved from the local market and the coffeehouse, the television set and the newspaper, to reappear in digital form on the laptop and the smart phone. Today we do not seek information: it confronts us, traveling with us wherever we go.

Worse than that, the relentless flow of information is a powerful, distracting force. The Pew Research Center's mobile technology fact sheet for 2013 informs us that in that year 90 percent of American adults had a cell phone and 58 percent owned a smartphone. Some 44 percent of individuals reported sleeping with their phones to avoid missing calls and other updates during the night, and 29 percent "couldn't imagine living without" the convenience. Perhaps even more surprising, the technology is evenly spread across all age groups and shows little variation based on household income or ethnicity. Three-quarters of smartphone owners use their devices as a memory bank for telephone numbers, for e-mail and street addresses, and for directions (even in their hometown), while of the 55 percent of those who go online, some three-quarters are discontented with the speed at which it happens. For the majority a personal connection with the Internet has become "essential." This reflects a massive cultural shift in how we communicate and how information is processed and received. Nor is America unique: the statistics for other industrialized nations are comparable.

Today, in airport lounges and coffee shops, there is a disturbing absence of voices and of conversation. We receive our information not by word of mouth but through e-mail, Facebook updates, Google searches, unsolicited advertising, and a blizzard of other trivia. We each have a physical presence in the world, but life is increasingly conducted elsewhere, through the touchscreen interface of our electronic gadgetry. Technology dominates the cultural environment, and we are beginning to feel the weight of its presence. Characteristically, with technology having created the problem, it is through technology that we mindlessly seek a solution. So why not, as *BusinessWeek* has boldly championed, get a new app for your smartphone—with the attractive name of Cue—that will scan your e-mail, social media, and other communications, collecting them together in one simple, searchable in-box? In that way you can receive all 63,000 words that constitute the novel of the day in a unified dispatch. But of course, the words will still need to be read.

THE PROCESSING OF INFORMATION has been industrialized, much in the same way as previously we industrialized farming and food processing and perfected the assembly-line production of the automobile. The motivating philosophy behind those earlier innovations was economic efficiency, maximum production in the minimum of time, as first popularized by the work-management theories of Frederick Taylor, at the turn of the twentieth century. An increased profit margin was the principal goal, while reducing cost to the consumer. These objectives remain primary in the business of technical innovation. But it turns out that enhancing human muscle power, or increasing the efficiency of making a journey, is rather different from helping humans think, especially when selling product remains the key motivation. Purchasing a snowblower to help with winter's chores, or buying a ticket on a train, does not invade one's privacy or decision making, but it is becoming increasingly evident that shopping online certainly can.

The Internet, from its beginning as a bunch of cables and net-worked servers, has become an ideology influencing how we think, behave, and live day by day. At the end of the first decade of the twenty-first century, essentially four intensely competitive and wealthy companies—Google, Apple, Facebook, and Amazon—dominated the consumer Internet. From the data they have amassed—the personal data sets that have made their corporations rich—each of them has more knowledge about all of us than we have about ourselves. Ironically much of the information that these businesses gather we first offer willingly. Online social media encourage us to collect our own data and publicly advertise them to friends, to recommend the restaurants where we eat, the music that we listen to, and much more beyond. These are the data we give away, to then have them given back. When we search a question on Google, the now-familiar warning appears: "Cookies help us deliver our services. By using our services, you agree to our use of cookies." Buy things from Amazon, and a similar but cryptic warning emerges. Cookies are the secret to one-click shopping and those personalized, ubiquitous recommendations that visit us each day. That's how Google makes money: click on an advertisement, and Google's cash register rings. I book a flight to New York, and a host of energetic supplicants instantaneously appear seeking to rent me a car, find me a hotel, or become my escort for the evening.

It appears sometimes that I'm more welcomed online than at my favorite restaurant. Every foray has uncanny relevance to what I have purchased or thought of purchasing; similar online greetings are evoked by places I have visited or those I have merely considered visiting, frequently only in fantasy. Suddenly, it seems, without realizing it was happening, I have outsourced not only my memory but also my curiosity and my imagination. Add to that the publicly available information that appears to be regularly vacuumed up from the corners of the Web—age, race, educational level, children, house, cars, political contributions, and magazine subscriptions—and one may forget worrying about the surveillance tactics of the National Security Agency: one's profile is already there on the Internet. To live in the electronic world today is to live in the public eye. This is Neil Postman's technopoly made manifest.

So what is this new culture doing to the way we think? Nicholas Carr, the author of *The Shallows: What the Internet Is Doing to Our Brains*, believes that the impact is profound. From both his personal experience as a writer and from a careful review of the research literature, Carr sees the world online as "chipping away [at the] capacity for concentration and contemplation." As a seductive gateway to just about everything, the Internet encourages "cursory reading, hurried and distracted thinking and superficial learning." While "it's possible to think deeply when surfing the Net," Carr contends, "just as it's possible to think shallowly while reading a book, that's not the type of thinking that the technology encourages and rewards." Drawn in by hyperlinks, video clips, and inviting sidebars, the mental modus operandi becomes one of switching rapidly from reading to watching to listening—garnering along the way a trove of information but building little insight or lasting knowledge. Living close to the Internet, Carr suggests, fosters a "juggler's" brain.

The juggler's brain has much in common with what in the past has been labeled the multitasking brain—when in a delusion of enhanced efficiency we undertake several chores at once, as in answering e-mail and listening to the radio while speaking on the telephone. In reality such efforts degrade our mental ability, dividing our attention and interrupting the brain's smooth processing, encoding, and storing of information. Yet as I know from my teaching of medical students, such practices are now commonplace in the classroom, with significant impact on student learning. Indeed careful, well-controlled multitasking studies suggest that Web-connected laptops or other devices, to be used ostensibly for note-taking, offer a powerful temptation during lectures—even for the most disciplined scholar—distracting not only the individual involved but also those sitting in close proximity.

So is the playful, creative human brain in jeopardy of being hijacked by the Internet? Perhaps *hijacked* is not the right word, but the Net is certainly seductive and potentially addictive. It must be remembered, also, that as a migrant animal, we are predisposed to such seduction: we are by nature distractible and focused on the short term. It is part of our survival kit: we are constantly vigilant, on the lookout for threat, opportunity, and social reward. Thus in many ways, by feeding our fascination with novel information and the delights of shopping, the Internet taps into our ancient proclivities as chance-driven hunters and gatherers—much as our ancestral cravings for salt, fat, and sugar have helped stoke the obesity epidemic. Compelling and powerful, the interactive technology of the Internet offers the consumer immediacy of information and the illusion of innovation and knowledge. Despite spreading confusion at times, as startup companies come and go with the speed of meteor showers, the Net is nonetheless steadily reshaping the way we live.

In Silicon Valley and Seattle there is no confusion. There the story is all about market share. Through their dominance of the information economy, the big four of the consumer Internet have developed a business plan that works, especially for themselves and their shareholders. Indeed, as the cultural historian Michael Saler, a professor at the University of California, Davis, has observed, "Information only *appears* to be free on the Internet. In reality, ordinary users provide personal information to companies, and receive services in return: a form of barter. The monetary value that people provide to the information economy is both 'off the books' and in the pockets of the Internet corporations." We're trading privacy for product.

As these corporate data-collection systems grow ever more powerful, the information we leave behind us—the so-called "digital exhaust" of Web searches, credit card purchases, mobile phone activity, and the like—is increasingly swept into analytic commerce. This exploitation of what is called Big Data is considered the next wave of opportunity in the tracking and quantification of behavior. In this hyperconnected world, what we think, feel, and desire has moved from the intimate security of one's own head into the online glare of the public arena. For the first time in human history we are outsourcing to machines, and to the whims of others, our habits, our thinking, and ourselves.

AS IN THE LATE 1990s, in the final, fulminating years of the dot-com bubble, once again we are in danger of becoming blind to our own future. The invention of the World Wide Web goes beyond brilliance to being both a splendid convenience and a life-enhancing tool: *but it is not, in itself, a way of life*—unless we choose to make it so.

Thus it may seem that kids have a natural fascination with electronic gadgets. And indeed, the kaleidoscopic and interactive nature of the touchscreen is inherently compelling, particularly to infants. In reality, however, what children are fascinated by is what their parents are doing, which in truth is spending an inordinate amount of time with similar gadgets. Inadvertently, so do we teach children habits that constrain them in exploring the larger world. Similarly, if we no longer make eye contact when speaking with them because we are checking our e-mail, then with frightening speed that socially isolating habit will be adopted. As in the obesity epidemic, the child will be drawn along by an addictive compulsion comparable to that of reaching for a sugar-laced soda.

The ability to focus attention consistently on something of interest, to hold it in memory, to dissect it in reflective, conscious, awareness, and further to analyze its meaning is a talent of mind that the modern human has built over millennia. Today, in thrall to the Web's "technology of the intellect," we are busily dissipating such capacities. When reflexive habit and imitation replace memory and imagination, much is lost in the reflective realm. The smartphone, for example, is a handy depository for memory, but in relying on it exclusively, we risk losing not only a data bank of telephone numbers should we misplace the instrument, but also the facile function of the brain's working memory. Increasingly we make connections on the touchscreen but fail to do so in the brain: the Web's connections are not to be confused with those of the mind.

Do you remember the telephone numbers of your closest friends when the cell phone battery dies, or even your own number, for that matter? Can you be sure that you have been given the correct change when the restaurant's cash register is on the fritz and credit cards are useless? In its role as the body's chief processor of information, the brain requires constant engagement and practice. Proximity in time to emotion, memory, and repetition of experience are important strengtheners of the brain's networking activities. When the processing stops, just as when one stops exercising a muscle, the brain loses its tone. It's simple enough: the human brain sustains high performance by continuous vigilance and interaction with the real world, not by Web surfing and outsourcing. Thinking with the tips of your fingers doesn't work.

In our blind pursuit of technology, we also risk compromising other talents—a practical understanding of the world and the pleasures of craftsmanship being among of them. It is through diligent attention to the crafting of skills, broadly defined, that imagination, creativity, and technical understanding come together. The American sociologist Richard Sennett, in *The Craftsman*, argues that such skilled practice provides an anchor against the rising tide of materialism. Being skillful in body and mind builds and sustains a sense of mastery and individual accomplishment. Before industrialization this was easier to understand as a concept, and to achieve, than it is now. Then the majority of people knew how to make the few things they used. The exact opposite is true today. Now few of us have a working knowledge of the tools we use every day, let alone how they are made. In the presence of our automated machines, most of us are now passive observers. The servant has become the master.

And yet for each of us, the drive for our own mastery remains. One of the privileges of being human is to have a mind that can be explored, tuned, and refined over a lifetime of experience. The brain is an extraordinary instrument, and when well tuned, it offers extraordinary reward. Garry Kasparov knows that, as did J.S. Bach before him. Slowly, as I have described in these immediate past chapters, as the mind matures and we grow comfortable in who we are, we learn to refine our sense of self and come not only to appreciate the talents that are vested within us but also to value and celebrate the many achievements and caring concerns of others—those social investments that collectively make society whole.

Imagination plays a critical role in this ongoing personal and cultural tuning. Imagination is not something mysterious that is occasionally unearthed during the education of a particularly gifted artist, or a talent confined to the ruminations of business entrepreneurs. Rather, as I have explained, imagination is the melding of diverse brain talents—of perception, emotion, memory, habit, and choice—in a way that is uniquely human and broadly shared among us. The sense of wonder that feeds imagination is with each of us every day and in every moment. But competing now, as our imagination must, with a seductive materialism and a global industry that is manufacturing novelty on a massive scale, that sense of wonder must be fostered beyond the market.

There's no need, however, for the commercialized, technical fix of an electronically programmed brain gym: rather, make use of the mundane, and you will rediscover the living world. Look in on the "being," on the presence, of things around you. Rekindle the art of paying attention. Such a life-view costs nothing in the material sense but offers an infinitely rich opportunity to engage both curiosity and imagination. Rather than being frustrated by the queue in the grocery store, wonder about the life of the person in front of you, and per-haps start a conversation; take a child to the park—without your cell phone—and watch what they do when you let them wander; compare the facades of the buildings around where you work and see if you can figure out when they were built, without succumbing to Google; read a good novel, in a quiet, well-lighted space in a comfortable chair; take up tennis, gardening, or chess; perhaps learn to tune the harpsichord; and if all else fails, visit the Museum of Jurassic Technology. In the modern idiom, be mindful.

WHETHER IT IS IN the service of survival or a product of attentive curiosity, a fertile imagination has been at the foundation of adjusting to change and creating new knowledge since the days of Cro-Magnon man. It is particularly important now, as many of the familiar dimensions of everyday life shift around us, that we do not abandon our sense of wonder—we must continue to affirm that complexity and not knowing are the prelude and stimulus to knowing. Given today's challenges, it is imperative that we willfully harness our imagination.

Imagination is a valuable tool of exploration, for the individual, for science, and for society, blending as it does the reflexive and reflec-tive elements of mind. But as also is clear, what engages the imagina-tion is for each of us both distinct and varied. As the personal stories recounted in these pages illustrate, for one it may be the excitement of creating a local food distribution system: for another, seeking to map the social brain, or creating a novel approach to teaching, or under-standing the brain's internal market, or designing an efficient trans-port system—in the larger world the list is infinite. In envisioning the future it is not the subject itself but the focus, the commitment, and the skill—the self-tuning—that an individual brings to a subject that ultimately determines the power of the imagination to create change. Essential, too, in this mix, is the self-discipline and strength of character to step back from, and to question, the habit-patterns of everyday life, together with the cacophony and demands that feed them.

Change is not easy, and changing our social behavior is especially difficult. It takes a collective effort—the melding of the imagination of many people. Also, as any creative individual knows, even the most brilliant insights, backed by sound and detailed analyses, rarely lead smoothly to the "right" solution. At some juncture a courageous but informed leap often becomes necessary. We call this wisdom: the vision to reach beyond the immediacy of the moment, better to embrace the history and realities of the larger world, so to reimagine them.

Wisdom: Retuning for a Sustainable Future

Mankind achieved civilization by developing and learning to follow rules that often forbade to do what his instincts demanded.... Man is not born wise, rational and good, but has to be taught to become so. Man became intelligent because there was tradition [habits] between instinct and reason.

Friedrich Hayek, *The Fatal Conceit* (1988)

Gross National Product does not allow for the health of our children, the quality of their education, or the joy of their play. It does not include the beauty of our poetry or the strength of our marriages, the intelligence of our public debate, or the integrity of our public officials.

Robert Kennedy, University of Kansas, March 18, 1968

LET ME RETURN to where I began this book. Besides reimagining progress and regaining balance within the natural ecology, there is another important piece of the puzzle to be considered. In our social evolution as a species, biology and culture run on parallel tracks, but they do so at different speeds. Thus biology, quickly and disruptively, can be outpaced by cultural change. As I have detailed, a significant number of the challenges that we face in the developed world are rooted in this mismatch.

To better grasp how this puzzle comes together, I take you back to a primary source of knowledge about evolution. In the Pacific Ocean, straddling the equator approximately six hundred miles off the coast of Ecuador, is found the Galápagos archipelago. This remote collection of volcanic islands, as Charles Darwin described them when he traveled there, is "a little world within itself." Today it remains so, thanks to the vigilance of the Ecuadorian government and the Galápagos Conservancy. Located at the confluence of three ocean currents, and with the volcanic and seismic activity that formed the islands eight to ten million years ago still ongoing, the Galápagos is the ecosystem—unique in its vegetation and wildlife—that emboldened Darwin in his conception of the principles of evolution.

Hence in the summer of 2013 I was pleased to help organize a special meeting of the Mont Pèlerin Society (MPS), *Evolution, the Human Sciences, and Liberty*, on the island of San Cristóbal, at the Galápagos campus of the Universidad San Francisco de Quito. Our topic was in keeping with Friedrich Hayek's founding vision of an association broadly invested in the natural sciences—one that would advance "the principles and practice of a free society."

The most easterly island in the archipelago, San Cristóbal, is where Darwin's ship, the HMS *Beagle*, first made landfall on September 17, 1835. Indeed, just a short walk from the university study center, to commemorate the spot where Darwin stepped ashore, there is an unflattering statue of the man. A mile or so to the south now exists Puerto Baquerizo Moreno, the administrative center of the Galápagos and a thriving town of more than six thousand people, but otherwise one's first impressions are remarkably similar to those Darwin recorded in his diary.

The rocky shoreline of the island is black volcanic lava, twisted and buckled. Scarlet, scurrying crabs visibly mottle its surface, in contrast to the black marine iguana—"imps of darkness," was Darwin's description—that lurk among the rock crevices. Today there is no litter of giant tortoiseshells, as Darwin observed. The surviving descendants of these ponderous creatures—once preyed upon by visiting whalers as a ready source of meat and terrapin soup—are now a tourist attraction, living protected lives. Sea lions, however, remain ubiquitous and when resting from fishing are usually found sunning themselves on public benches along the promenade.

The *Beagle's* epic voyage was well into its fourth year when Darwin reached the Galápagos. The idea that common principles underlie nature's order was already forming in his mind, and the five weeks of land expeditions, specimen collecting, and sailing among the nineteen islands only strengthened these thoughts. Darwin found the natural history of the archipelago to be "eminently curious," with subtly different flora and fauna inhabiting the individual islands. Created by volcanic plumes thrusting up from the earth's core, and with the major formations thirty to sixty miles apart, it was unlikely that the existing land mass had ever been united above the ocean. The flightless cormorant; the iguana; the blue-footed booby; the hawks; the giant tortoises—Darwin's fascination grew as each new encounter revealed to him that "the different islands to a considerable extent are inhabited by different sets of beings." Almost against his will, he wondered whether he was witnessing accommodations by living creatures to a varied environment. This disturbing thought called into question the stability of individual species, which in Darwin's time were considered immutable categories, with each unique plant and animal being the product of divine creation.

To complicate things further, there were the Galápagos finches. As Darwin confessed in his *Journal and Remarks* of the *Beagle's* journey—published in 1839, after his return to England—at first he failed to recognize the significance of a "most singular group of finches, related to each other in the structure of their beaks, short tails, form of body and plumage." I find such oversight easily understood. Despite their fame in scientific circles, Darwin's finches are unassuming birds. The small hostelry where I was staying overlooked the harbor. With a fresh breeze off the ocean, and the weather being what it is on the equator, there is little need for window glass, so every morning the finches were in eager attendance at my breakfast table. Just as Darwin described them, the birds have a short tail and scruffy black plumage and are about the size of an English sparrow. The variations in beak size and shape are readily apparent. So too, regardless of beak size, is their preference for scrambled eggs.

Upon Darwin's return to England, with careful study of the finch specimens at the Zoological Society of London, thirteen distinct Galápagos species were identified. Evolved from a common ancestor, probably a ground-dwelling seed eater of South American origin, over millennia, the survivors of this generic stock had adapted to fit the varying and differing habitats of the individual islands. "One might really fancy," wrote Darwin perceptively, "that from an original paucity of birds in this archipelago, one species has been taken and modified for different ends."

In all birds the beak is a vital life-supporting tool. Pecking away at scrambled eggs, of course, is easy. But for seed-eating birds, small variations in beak formation and strength can make a big difference, especially during times of drought. With some kernels harder to crack than others, the deeper and stronger beaks provide an advantage. The principles of such adaptation have been validated by the research of the British evolutionary biologists Peter and Rosemary Grant, both professors at Princeton University, who have spent decades in the Galápagos. The Grants have demonstrated that changing climatic conditions do indeed dramatically alter the nature and quantity of the finches' food supply. Under changing circumstances, variations in beak structure of individual birds then determine survival through natural selection, confirming the fundamental principles of evolution that Darwin set forth in *The Origin of Species*. Published in 1859, this groundbreaking work was to change the course of human thought.

BIOLOGICAL EVOLUTION, in its essence, is a gradual process of variation, selection, and replication whereby living things, in the service of survival, find adaptive fit with changing environmental circumstances. Friedrich Hayek, in *The Fatal Conceit: The Errors of Socialism*, professed his great admiration for Darwin, "as the first who succeeded in elaborating a consistent theory of evolution in any field." Hayek was quick to add, however, that the dynamics of Darwin's understanding had deep roots in earlier *sociocultural* writings, including those of Thomas Malthus and Adam Smith. Indeed, by 1838, within two years of the *Beagle's* return to England, and when a comprehensive theory of evolution was beginning to occupy him, it is clear from his notebooks that Darwin had read Smith's *Essays on Philosophical Subjects* and *The Theory of Moral Sentiments*.

In their ideas Smith and Darwin, and Hayek too, are much in accord. The common conceptual thread binding together an understanding of the social order and evolutionary biology is that *complex social and biological systems, interacting freely with their circumstances, inherently organize, adapt, and find balance.* As John Kay, the British economist, described it, reflecting upon the MPS Galápagos meeting in the *Financial Times*, evolution is a generic process through which "designs of extraordinary complexity and efficiency can be achieved without the aid of a designer."

Hayek described such spontaneous, self-organizing, and self-correcting designs as *systems of extended order*. In the biological world, environmental circumstances *naturally select* from a range of physical attributes and behaviors to foster the optimum fit for survival of the living organism. Similarly, in the social arena, including market systems, adaptive strategies emerge from the behavior of many individuals *selecting options* that best fit individual opportunity and their collective needs. In each instance, it is through the dynamic dance of variation and selection—without the aid of an omnipotent designer—that systems of extended order emerge and evolve. There are also differences, however, between the biological world and human society in the dynamics of how these systems organize and are perpetuated, two of which are particularly important as we strive to regain our place in the natural order.

First is the divergent time course of adaptation, as I noted in opening this chapter. In simple terms, in the biological evolution of any organism, including us, it is spontaneous mutation that drives genetic variation and environmental fit. Thus, when it comes to human biology, we can no more determine the course of our evolution than can the Galápagos finch or any other living creature. Human biology, given the length of time between individual generations, evolves slowly.

On the other hand, social and technological advances evolve at a comparatively rapid pace. Each generation transmits valuable knowledge and behavior to the next, powerfully shaping cultural inheritance. Since the Enlightenment and the harnessing of fossil fuels, in particular, our sociocultural evolution has run ahead of biological adaptation.

The second important difference, as Hayek recognized, is that while a free society is dynamic and open in function, it is not freely self-organizing. Beyond kinship and familiar neighbors, he asserted, what holds societies together as they grow in size and scale is not just self-interest and attachment but also the cultural rules and rituals that we learn from one another and that are passed down over generations. In Hayek's words, sitting between instinct and reason, it is "tradition"—what, in this book, I have described as intuitive habit—that holds the social order together. In cultural evolution, aware of it or not, the habits we acquire play a role in cultural design. But as we shall find, traditions are at times rigid, confining our ability to adapt appropriately in times of need.

*   *   *   *

IT IS THROUGH HABIT that the brain is tuned to prevailing circumstances. Or more precisely, I should say it is in acquiring habit that the brain tunes itself. This preconscious tuning, you may recall, is in the service of reflexive efficiency and essential to daily living. But beyond the mundane, depending upon the resilience of the tuning achieved, habits may be a blessing or a curse. Without deliberate and reflective self-appraisal, it is frequently difficult to know the difference between those habits that are adaptive and those that are impediments. This is because tradition and habit intuitively bind us to past experience, making behavioral change difficult.

As animals, our evolved biological propensities reinforce these circumstances. Evolution has no plan; rather the process is one that selects the best available fit from strategies that have worked in the past. This can be particularly maladaptive when, for example, the evolving cultural narrative reinforces our innate, instinctual, proclivity to seize upon short-term opportunity, regardless of the longer-term consequences. The result—as is evident in the affluent society—is a Faustian alliance that in the myopic pursuit of reward can kindle epidemics of obesity, financial excess, and the denial of future challenges.

Today one of the habits disruptive to a healthy and sustainable cultural narrative is how we conflate measures of economic growth with the idea of progress and social well-being. That has not always been so. Defined in the *Oxford English Dictionary* as the act of journeying and moving forward, or advancement to a better state, *progress* has been the animating idea of Western civilization since the Enlightenment. The concepts of liberty, tolerance, equality of opportunity, and social order emerged then as expressed human aims, and it was accepted that society's common purpose was to realize these goals. Each technical advance, each gain in knowledge, each improved utility would bring us closer to perfection and to happiness; progress was dependent upon freedom and the human will. This powerful lodestar is now waning. Increasingly, the word *progress* is framed in economic terms and is becoming synonymous with increased production of goods and services.

Within this construct the objective measure of progress is the gross domestic product (GDP), which seeks to quantify the growth of a nation's annual domestic economy. That well-being will improve with money available to secure the necessities of life makes sense, of course, and studies from across the world suggest that as income rises to the equivalent of approximately $10,000 per year, that is exactly what happens. Beyond that yardstick the picture is mixed. Hence in 2013 the GDP of the United States was $15,800 trillion, yielding a per capita GDP of $53,143. More than 70 percent of the total expenditures, $11.501 trillion, were accounted as personal consumption. Nonetheless, despite this growth in income and expenditure, indices of subjective well-being, such as personal happiness, have been stable in the United States since the mid-1960s, when the average American's income was approximately one-third of that achieved in 2013.

In America shopping is a tradition. Objective evidence that money does not buy happiness has little effect on shopping behavior. Consumer spending has driven U.S. economic growth for decades, climbing to 75 percent of GDP in 2007, just before the global financial crash. Furthermore, as the subsequent recession tightened its grip and credit was squeezed, a growing social inequality was revealed. American society was splitting into the haves and the have-nots. This was no news. For a decade a majority of the American citizens surveyed had been telling the pollsters from NBC News and *The Wall Street Journal* that the nation was "on the wrong track." The main result of this protestation was the hardening of political ideology. "What happened to our country's stride and spirit?" asked the *New York Times* journalist Frank Bruni in the spring of 2014. Although the United States, at that time, remained the world's wealthiest nation, as measured by the GDP, two-thirds of Americans already believed that China was the world's leading economic power. Also becoming evident, as I have documented, was the bad news that in Europe social mobility was increasing, while the performance of the American school system lagged behind that of many other rich countries. Washington, for its part, amid partisan bickering, was encouraging a return to home-based manufacturing and greater consumer confidence. The Tea Party was in its ascendance. Nostalgia was in the air.

I caricature the situation to illustrate my point. The GDP's faithful indexing of the goods and services produced no longer serves to reflect the growing discomfort of many middle-class American families; nor can it document the future challenges we face. GDP accounting makes no distinction between the quantity and quality of growth, as is evident, for example, in the escalating level of U.S. health care spending compared to that of other rich countries, despite the poor outcomes achieved in many illnesses. Nor are environmental factors and issues of sustainability and waste considered: when a farmer preserves seed from which to grow next year's crop, it does not register; a living forest contributes to GDP growth only when the trees in it are logged; and the value of fisheries is measured in the tons of fish caught, as if their supply were infinite. Similar questions pertain to water and soil conservation, together with the extraction of the earth's raw materials, and the list goes on.

The accounting of GDP has become dissociated from the social currency and natural resources that will be necessary to sustain us in the future. The United States is in the grip of a tradition-driven mythology, one where it is assumed that the future is best defined by the past, with economic growth remaining the fundamental strategy, and GDP our measure of success. Within an evolutionary framework, our circumstances are best described as a decline in adaptive fit—a growing mismatch between what we do and the sustainable well-being of ourselves and the planet. And yet our behavior does not change.

* * * * *

SO IS THIS A MORAL ISSUE? I think not, at least not at its foundation. Rather, it is a problem that grows from the human's rigidity of habit—another mismatch between biology in its broader context and the speed of our cultural advances. From the behavioral perspective, given our intelligence, it is a failure of rational accommodation to changing circumstances. Hayek was correct in identifying tradition as the guardian of culture, but equally tradition can impede the dynamic evolution of cultural adjustment.

In the developed world, as measured by product, for over two hundred years we have been adapting triumphantly to what once appeared to be an infinite supply of natural resources and easily accessible energy. Having discovered this treasure trove—this unusual niche of environmental opportunity—ingenuity and hard work have led to phenomenal growth in human societies and to our numbers on this planet. It is this experience that frames our cultural habit, and it is the framework to which the developing countries aspire.

Assuming leadership of the Industrial Revolution from Great Britain in the late nineteenth century, with less than 5 percent of the world's population the United States now consumes approximately 25 percent of the world's resources. Indirectly the nation's major investments in infrastructure, in technology, in economic growth, and in living standards are all tied, in one way or another, to consumption of fossil fuels. Diligence and cultural tradition have reinforced opportunity to reward the United States with extraordinary material wealth. With brains long tuned to abundance, we Americans are inclined to deny the future and its forebodings. In our cleverness and flourishing, we have transformed the planet's ecosystem by ignoring it. This is the dark side of our success. But as the global economy has grown and the world's population has exploded, it is a reality that can no longer be ignored. We are hoisted by our own petard. In alliance with the brain's instinctual reward systems, intuitive habit now holds reason hostage.

It was Darwin's dynamic theory of natural selection, and his brilliance as a thinker, that first gave weight to the idea that new organisms could appear and old ones disappear, with different creatures populating the earth at different times. It has been estimated that there have been five mass extinctions over the past 500 million years caused by extremes of climate change. Increasing evidence suggests that we may now be entering the sixth, aided by our own ingenuity and cavalier dominance.

In this *Age of Man* we are again losing species at a rapid rate. Without a course correction and a change in our behavior, *Homo sapiens* may soon be facing the same fate. If we continue to pursue maximization of material growth as a global economic strategy, with little regard for human well-being and the health of our planet, then potentially we are flirting with our own extinction. We are building our own doomsday machine, one that is slower in its impact than acute nuclear disaster but that is of similar epic proportions over the long term. The coming crisis—given our growing knowledge—presents a moral issue only if we choose to ignore it.

AS OGDEN NASH, the American humorist and poet, prophetically observed before his death in 1971, "Progress might have been all right once, but it has gone on too long." I find myself imagining the fate of the urban finches that shared my breakfast table during my visit to the Galápagos, should they be faced once more with seed foraging after decades of feeding on scrambled eggs. Deprived of their ease, the adaptive retuning of their behavior to the realities of the natural world would be no simple task.

Nor will it be a simple task for us, but fortunately we are not finches. As individuals we have the knowledge to imagine adaptive strategy beyond exponential growth. But do we have the collective will to change our habits? Do we have the determination to retune the way we think? If human progress is to be made rational and sustainable, the complex interaction between our instinctual drives and our cultural choices must be tempered and brought into balance. To achieve success, this will be necessary for each of us. In resonance with my metaphor of Bach's *Well-Tempered Clavier* (which you will recall from the introduction), our efforts at cultural standardization—as in tuning the today's family piano to equal temperament—will get us only so far. Tuning our habits to accept the uniformity of consumerism squeezes out flexibility and ingenuity. Bach's "customized" approach, as in tuning his clavier, is what we need.

Human beings are so good at simply copying the behaviors of others that, when the drumbeat is demand-driven and attention-grabbing, we stop thinking for ourselves and forget the future: in the consumer society we become imprinted on immediate reward. Such ingrained habits—embedded in our culture, politics, and business practices— are dangerously soporific when it comes to changing anything. The social engineering of 1950s communism, which so preoccupied Hayek, and the oligarchies of crony capitalism that are prevalent today do not work. The order they create is brittle and snaps under duress. That social balance can be achieved through top-down intervention is a "fatal conceit," to borrow Hayek's phrase. Nor will that balance be fostered by excessive social standardization and legal oversight, as Philip K. Howard, the American lawyer and social critic, has argued in his book *The Rule of Nobody: Saving America from Dead Laws and Broken Government.*

No, rather it is the creativity of resilient, knowledgeable, and innovative individuals working together that we need. It is through self-awareness—the wisdom acquired over a lifetime of self-tuning— that we will progressively take ownership of our behavior. To shape a sustainable future, we must each challenge the preconscious, personal narrative of habit. Through this conscious process, harnessing the extraordinary powers of human reason—of perception, analysis, imagination, and choice—the dynamics of biology, ecology, and cultural change can be thoughtfully aligned and brought into closer harmony. Insights from neuroscience and evolutionary theory will help us navigate the social transformation. We also need to take on the responsibility for rational problem solving and active participation in crafting and strengthening the social institutions that enhance education, independent choice, the development of character, and social fellowship. In reality, the future we create will be determined by the individual choices we make. We must again, consciously, respect and embrace our place in the natural world.

THE GOOD NEWS IS that we do not start from scratch when it comes to seeking the change that we need. Throughout the United States and across the world there are many individuals who are thinking and working "outside the box" of consumerism. I have had the privilege of profiling a tiny sample of such individuals in these pages. A stirring of public sentiment for change is apparent and widespread. Social inequality is of growing concern in America and Britain and is on the political agenda. Since the recession that began in 2008, many Americans have become savers again, in part by necessity. In what may be just a Panglossian moment, the addictive appetite for material goods appears to be waning, especially in young people. Similarly, as weather patterns become extreme and the unusual becomes the routine, the idea that global warming may have human consequences has begun its move to center stage. Things are changing, but slowly.

Industry, again by necessity, has begun to pay attention. Businesses, especially those with global reach, are awakening to the threats that resource limitation, climate change, and extreme weather events pose to their profits and their traditional practices. As one example, the global giant Coca-Cola, was chastened in 2004 by the loss of its license to operate India's largest bottling plant in Plachimada, Kerala, where the company was drawing nearly one million liters of water each day from underground aquifers, destroying the local agricultural economy in the process. Similarly Nike, the manufacturer of athletic shoes, with seven hundred factories in forty-nine countries, many in Asia, has felt the impact of extreme weather. In Thailand in 2008 floods shut down four factories, and sporadic drought threatens the company's supply of cotton.

Responding to these economic concerns and to spreading anxiety, in 2014 the challenges of a changing environment featured prominently on the agenda of the World Economic Forum—the pantheon of the world's business and political leaders—that is held each winter in Davos, Switzerland. That year no fewer than thirty-five sessions were devoted to climate change, green investment, and the potential for a sustainable, "circular" economy. The latter, a concept first proposed in the 1970s by the Swiss architect Walter Stahel, is seen as a substitute for the existing linear industrial model of progressive, resource-depleting growth. Pertinent to my discussion here is that the model of "circularity" takes inspiration from the regenerative dynamics of biological systems.

Essentially, it is argued, the industrial economy favored today harvests raw materials—both those grown through photosynthesis and those from the earth's natural resources—to manufacture a product, which is then discarded as waste at the end of its useful life. A circular economy, on the other hand is designed to be regenerative from the beginning: foodstuffs and other organic products return to the soil; source materials from the earth's supply, including petroleum derivatives such as plastics, are cycled for remanufacture. Durable goods are designed for disassembly such that they may be upgraded at minimal cost. Everybody wins—the consumer, the manufacturer, and the planet.

Dame Ellen MacArthur—the British yachtswoman, who in 2005 at the age of twenty-eight was knighted after achieving what was then the fastest single-handed circumnavigation of the globe—brought the circular economy to popular attention in 2010, when she founded a charity explicitly for the purpose. MacArthur proved to be an articulate spokeswoman, and the program rapidly garnered wide interest, with significant international companies—including McKinsey, Philips, Cisco, Kingfisher, and Renault, among others—providing partnership and financial support.

For MacArthur, primed by her professional experience in yacht racing, the conservation and reuse of resources through commitment to a circular economy makes both environmental and business sense. "When you set off around the world, you take with you everything that you need for your survival," she explained in a 2014 interview. "For three and a half months you are on a boat with everything that you have . . . only so much food, only so much diesel. As you watch those resources go down, you realize just what 'finite' means, because in the Southern Ocean you're 2500 miles away from the nearest town. I realized that our global economy is no different. It's powered on resources that are ultimately finite."

THERE IS SOMETHING POETIC about a charismatic and accomplished woman, one who understands and knows the seas, championing the call for an ecologically sensitive economy. Staring at the Pacific Ocean roiling against the rugged volcanic shore—as I did sitting on Darwin's beach one afternoon during my Galápagos visit—it is difficult to imagine that a presence so vast and powerful could be vulnerable. But sadly it is so. The oceans cover approximately 70 percent of the earth's surface, and yet through our exploitation and inattention they have become dangerously degraded. The story offers a cautionary tale, but one not without hope that sustainable practices can be achieved.

Coastal pollution from industrial agriculture, warming temperatures, acidification, and the destruction of habitat—each of these has taken its toll on marine life. But most destructive of the ocean's finite resources has been their depletion by industrialized fishing. We have allowed our myopic propensity for short-term reward to cripple many fishing grounds. Britain's Dogger Bank fishery, once a fine source of herring, collapsed in the 1960s, and the Newfoundland cod-fishing grounds followed in the 1990s. Overall it is estimated that the global fishing catch rose from 35 million tons a year in 1950, to 150 million tons in 2009—well above what the oceans can sustain. Some of the most preferred commercial fish—cod, tuna, haddock, and flounder— are so depleted that they face extinction by 2050. The French-born Marine biologist Daniel Pauly, a professor of zoology who runs the Sea Around Us Project at the University of British Columbia in Vancouver, estimates that the biomass of big fish in the sea has decreased by more than 95 percent over the past century. We are heading rapidly toward the creation of marine deserts.

In efforts to manage this looming, man-made disaster of ecosystem decline, the development of marine reserves has been popular with government authorities. One such reserve was first established in the Galápagos islands in 1974 and was extended to protect a radius of forty nautical miles around the archipelago in 1998. As in all coastal regions, but as is particularly evident in the Galápagos, the marine ecology and that of the landmass are intertwined. Many birds, including the unique flightless cormorant, are entirely dependent on the sea for their food supply. And so too do the local *human* fishers depend on the marine reserve for their economic livelihood, in supplying fish to the island population and to those visiting Galápagos National Park. Thus wisdom is called for in balancing these human needs, while at the same time sustaining the entire ecosystem of the archipelago. Zoning is essential to constrain human activity, but it must also be sensitive to changing environmental circumstance and the varying profitability of the fisheries.

Evidence from a variety of studies across the world emphasizes that an understanding of human behavior is essential in managing marine resources or any other ecological system. As contrived carve-outs of the natural world, these complex, dynamic systems will find their own extended order if protected from predatory practices. But they also represent an economy that is a vital source of human sustenance.

Around the world approximately 1 billion people depend on the ocean for their nutrition and livelihood. As a microcosm of the larger challenge, such systems therefore offer valuable insights into how sustainability can be achieved.

One thing that clearly does not work in shaping human behavior is to appeal to moral virtue without regard to self-interest. Reason, as David Hume understood, is the slave of the passions. This edict holds true in fishing. In changing behavior incentive-based systems are essential. Hence in commercial fisheries, just declaring a region to be a marine preserve and imposing catch limits usually backfires. Such regulation increases short-term, myopic behavior, leading to competitive large-scale "race to fish" practices where less valuable species are dumped from the reported catch. The trick is to turn personal short-term interest into a genuine sense of shared, long-term responsibility.

A proven way of achieving this shift is to provide fishermen with individual fishing rights to a specific territory that are long term and secure. Such strategies work especially well if those involved are bound together in a collective enterprise of mutual advantage. Then, as the vitality of the ecosystem's extended order returns through greater knowledge, good husbandry, and fair practice, the catch improves in quality and everyone wins, including the fish and other marine life. As you may have realized, what I am describing is a fisherman's version of Mischel's famous marshmallow test, which you will recall from Chapter 7. As it is in childhood, so it is in fishing: delayed gratification pays off.

Indeed, using such a paradigm in her research, Ayana Elizabeth Johnson, a marine biologist with the Wiatt Institute, in Washington, D.C., who has a passionate interest in the sustainable use of ocean resources, has explored the role of behavior and social factors in shaping conservation success. In a clever study, originally conceived for her Ph.D. thesis at San Diego's Scripps Institution of Oceanography, Johnson studied the time preferences and resource management approaches of 350 fishermen and scuba divers in Curaçao and Bonaire, of the Netherlands Antilles, in the Caribbean. In a design similar to that used by

Mischel, Johnson offered the participants enrolled in the conservation study $50 at a future date or a smaller amount immediately and logged their preferences. The cut-off that emerged as an acceptable immediate reward was around $35: below that number—which was about the cost of a case of the most popular local beer at the time—most individuals were prepared to wait for the larger sum.

But the details are interesting. Not surprisingly, being hard up financially played a major role in the decision making. That was particularly true for the local fishermen who frequently had families to support: the scuba divers, often young people from Holland, tended to be wealthier. This difference also played out in the attitude of the two groups toward conservation: the fisher's income depended on taking fish *out* of the ocean, while the scuba divers—dependent on the tourist trade for their living—benefited from keeping fish *in* their habitat. The implications of Johnson's studies are clear: if sustainable fishing practices are the goal, then behavioral preferences and the socioeconomic issues that shape those preferences must be taken into consideration. Behavior matters.

If sustainable ecosystem practices are to succeed, the importance of understanding human behavior must be placed front and center. Without systems of balanced incentive, individuals acting in their own interest will deplete any common resource, to the detriment of the greater good. The American ecologist Garrett Hardin famously described this dilemma in his 1968 paper published in *Science* magazine, provocatively titled "The Tragedy of the Commons." Hardin, being an expert on population growth, expressed a certain Malthusian misanthropy in his writings. But he was also a systems thinker and a great believer in the destructive consequences of selfishness—including death and starvation as the feedback mechanism through which the extended order would eventually return to equilibrium. Ideally, some less drastic method of self-correction is to be fostered.

The political economist Elinor Ostrom, who won the Nobel Prize for economics in 2009, and who studied common resource management across the world—from lobster fisheries in Maine to irrigation systems in Nepal—felt more sanguine about human nature. In her research she found that communities with investment in the long-term viability of a local resource frequently developed successful and sophisticated systems of governance. The critical factors are the size of the community involved and the relationships among the principal players invested in the shared resource. And yes, of course, we are back to Adam Smith: small communities, with the interlocking interests of the participating members, do find their own extended order.

Hayek was right. The understanding that promotes social order and human progress is widely distributed among us: it is a function of the personal relationships we build and cannot be duplicated by top-down planning. But as Ostrom's studies demonstrate, such relationships are weakened and tend to be replaced by self-interest as communities grow in size and drift toward anonymity. Our challenge today, in the shadow of extraordinary material achievement, is to reverse that process of social erosion. I share Ostrom's sanguinity: I'm optimistic that collectively we can acquire the wisdom to sustain a vibrant and balanced society. As I have outlined in these pages, the challenge is one of assuming personal responsibility for the health of our families, our schools, and our communities, and for the ecology that feeds us. In our educational practice, in the workplace, and around the table, it is through the rewards of mutual attachment that collective change becomes possible. Throughout the adventure that is human history, cooperation has repeatedly proven to be more interesting and more profitable than unbridled self-interest. I believe that cultural sentiment, deep down, has not changed.

AS I WRITE THIS, spring has come to England after a long cold winter. The daffodils know that, the geese on the lake know it too, and in our bodies so do we. It is part of the seasonal cycle of being. Each living creature is embedded in the natural world; human beings do not stand independent of it. Each of us, as a self, is a pattern of interaction: take away the interaction, and you take away the person. This is the ecological vision. *Ecology* is a word that in Greek means "household." And as in the case of a household it is not the disagreements and the competition among the members of the family that determine its health but their compassion and collaboration. The ecology of the family is a multitude of sympathetic, synergistic, and symbiotic interactions. Personal freedom and individual responsibility are forged, honed, and expressed within this ecology.

Our science, in its inquiry, first takes this ecology of nature and reduces it to a series of elements. The human mind, in awe at the complexity of it all, finds it easier to think that way—in a linear fashion. We have made great progress with this method in understanding the pieces of the jigsaw puzzle and in moving forward with our social enterprise. And there is more to learn. It is exciting and seductive to believe that, in teasing biology apart, we may find a path and an efficiency that will serve our immediate and greater purpose.

But if we are serious about understanding our future on this planet, then science, broadly defined, must also be committed to integration—to understanding and respecting the complexity of the ecological paradigm. How, we must ask, with our new-found knowledge, can we better imagine ourselves in the natural order of things? How may we better assume the responsibilities that will secure for future generations a sustainable human experience? How may we better tune the human brain for the complexities and challenges ahead? Seated now at the keyboard, in this *Age of Man*, how may the musician find greater harmony? It's a metaphor, of course. But it was through metaphor that we first sought to understand our world.

Acknowledgments

I HAVE HAD MUCH HELP in putting this book together. First, I have been blessed in my own education and in my professional development with fine teachers, colleagues, students, and friends who have taught me much, not only about ideas and about thinking but also about life and about myself. That education is ongoing. Some mentors are referenced here in these pages, others are not—but to each I give thanks.

I am particularly indebted to Morten Kringelbach, to Joaquín Fuster, and to David Gregory for helping frame the arguments that I have set forth, and for many of the discussions that have refined them. Each gave generously of his time and offered sage advice. In addition, both Joaquín and David carefully critiqued the full manuscript, as did my partner, Nancy Main. In each instance I benefited greatly from their comments. Similarly Hans Wirz helped improve my understanding of the practical challenges facing today's architects and town planners, as David McGough sharpened my knowledge of the complex debates that confound policy making in public education. Deepak Lal, through his lucid writings and illuminating debate, sharpened my respect for economics. A special thanks is also owed to those who permitted the inclusion of their personal stories. All, in offering their insights and experience, have immeasurably enriched the narrative.

I owe particular thanks to Zoe Pagnamenta, my literary agent and longtime friend, for her unflagging support. Without Zoe's consistent, caring, perceptive vision and wise counsel, I would have been lost long ago. In the early stages of structuring the book, as with past writings, Helen Whybrow provided insightful editorial guidance. At Norton, from the beginning, Angela von der Lippe championed my efforts to meld science and social commentary. Amy Cherry, now my editor at Norton, enthusiastically continued that endorsement and, to my great benefit, employed her many talents both to refine the manuscript and to shepherd it through the process of publication. Finally, on the production side, I am deeply grateful to Betsy McNeely, who miraculously, and quickly, through her artistry transformed my clunky PowerPoint slides and rough scribbles into the clear grayscale drawings that illustrate the text.

At UCLA, on the academic front, I particularly thank Fawzy Fawzy, my trusted colleague and friend, and the many colleagues who, in our discussions, have been willing to cross the usual boundaries of science to share their ideas. Particularly at the Semel Institute, thanks to the personal interest and generous support of Jane and Terry Semel, we are blessed with such cross-disciplinary opportunities. This eclecticism greatly facilitated my early research, as did a period of sabbatical spent at Oxford University, made possible through the generosity of Guy Goodwin, George Bowen, and Paul Madden, the provost of Queen's College. Special thanks also to Matthew Neilson, of the Blenheim Estate, whose efficiency and kindness helped secure a quiet haven for thinking and writing, one to which I have consistently returned. And finally, sincere thanks to my staff; to Tracey Alberi for all her support, and to Sharon Chavez, without whose humor and unwavering good judgment nothing would have gone smoothly, my greatest gratitude. Once again, together with Fawzy Fawzy, it was Sharon who gave me time.

Notes

Introduction: IN THE AGE OF MAN

1   **". . . progress, man's distinctive mark":** "A Death in the Desert" is one of several dramatic monologues by the English poet Robert Browning (1812–69), published in 1864. Here Browning attempts to define the place of humankind as being between God and the beasts, and progress as the mark of our intellectual distinction.

1   **explosive economic growth:** Angus Maddison, *Contours of the World Economy 1–2030 AD: Essays in Macro-Economic History* (New York: Oxford University Press, 2007).

2   **the power of fossil fuels:** E. A. Wrigley, *Energy and the English Industrial Revolution* (Cambridge, UK: Cambridge University Press, 2010).

2   **economic growth continues to quicken:** "Global Poverty: A Fall to Cheer," *Economist*, March 3, 2012.

2   **the emerging world:** "Mammon's New Monarchs: The Emerging-World Consumer Is King," *Economist*, January 5, 2013; John Stutz, "The Three-Front War: Pursuing Sustainability in a World Shaped by Explosive Growth," *Sustainability: Science, Practice and Policy* 6 (2010): 49–59.

2   **the disappearing Aral Sea . . . Athabasca tar sands:** Robert Kunzig, "Scraping Bottom: Once Considered Too Expensive, as Well as Too Damaging to the Land, Exploitation of Alberta's Oil Sands Is Now a Gamble Worth Billions," *National Geographic Magazine* (March 2009); Philip Micklin and Nikolay V. Aladin, "Reclaiming the Aral Sea," *Scientific American*, March 17, 2008.

3   **human appetites play a significant role in climate change:** Katherine Leitzell, "Greenland's Glaciers and the Arctic Climate," National Snow and Ice Data Center, September 21, 2011, Nsidc.org; "The Melting North, Special Report: The Arctic," *Economist*, June 16, 2012; Justin Gillis, "Satellites Show Sea Ice in Arctic Is at Record Low," *New York Times*, August 28, 2012; "Climate Change: The Heat is On," *Economist*, October 22, 2011; Thomas Kaplan, "Most New Yorkers Think Climate Change Caused Hurricane, Poll Finds," *New York Times*, December 3, 2012; Intergovernmental Panel on Climate Change, *Climate Change 2013: The Physical Science Basis*, www.climatechange2013.org.

3   **a new planet "Eaarth":** Bill McKibben, *Eaarth: Making a Life on a Tough New Planet* (New York: St. Martin's Press, 2011).

3   **The distinguished biologist E. O. Wilson:** Elizabeth Kolbert, "Enter the Anthropocene—Age of Man," *National Geographic*, March 2011.

3   **The *Age of Man*:** Jan Zalasiewic et al., "The New World of the Anthropocene," *Environmental Science and Technology* 44 (2010): 2228–31; "A Man-made World: Science Is Recognizing Humans as a Geological Force to Be Reckoned With," *Economist*, May 28, 2011.

4   **the indiscretions of others:** Daniel Henniger, "The Age of Indiscretion," *Wall Street Journal*, April 21, 2012.

6   **difficult to change our ways:** William Rees, "What's Blocking Sustainability? Human Nature, Cognition and Denial," in *Sustainability: Science, Practice and Policy* 6 (2010): 1–13.

9   **"Happiness . . . consists in tranquillity and enjoyment":** Adam Smith, *The Theory of Moral Sentiments* (1759; reprint edition Indianapolis: Liberty Classics, 1976), bk. 3, chap. 3.

9   **the American Dream:** Jon Meacham, "Making of America: Keeping the Dream Alive," *Time*, June 21, 2012; Gus Speth, "What Is the American Dream? Dueling Dualities in the American Tradition," *Grist*, June 25, 2011, Grist.org.

9   **the myth of material happiness:** Michael Foley, *The Age of Absurdity: Why Modern Life Makes It Hard to Be Happy* (New York: Simon & Schuster, 2010); and Hilke Brockmann and Jan Delhey, eds., *Human Happiness and the Pursuit of Maximization: Is More Always Better?* (New York: Springer, 2013).

13   **sustaining a human-friendly planet ecology:** Tim Jackson, *Prosperity Without Growth? The Transition to a Sustainable Economy* (UK: Sustainable Development Commission, 2009).

14   **The *Well-Tempered Clavier*:** For a concise discussion of tuning and temperament, see Percy A. Scholes, *The Oxford Companion to Music*, ed. John Owen Ward, 10th ed. (New York: Oxford University Press, 1970), pp. 1012ff. Also see Bradley Lehman, "Bach's Extraordinary Temperament: Our Rosetta Stone," *Early Music* 33, no. 1 (2005): 3–23, and *Early Music* 33, no. 2 (2005) 211–32. Lehman believes that what appear to be mere decorative hieroglyphics on the face page of Bach's workbook are, in fact, the key to his tuning method. Rather than random doodles, the looping illustration at the top of the frontispiece is a specific diagrammatic guide to the tuning method Bach used. See John Marks, "Better than the Da Vinci Code," *Stereophile* (February 2007): 47–53. For those interested in a comprehensive history of this debate and Bach's tuning method, see Ross Duffin, *How Equal Temperament Ruined Harmony (and Why You Should Care)* (New York: Norton, 2007). Duffin, a distinguished professor at Case Western Reserve University, believes that Lehman is correct in his interpretation of Bach's tuning methods.

Chapter 1: OFF BALANCE

19   **"Man with all his noble qualities . . .":** Charles Darwin, *The Descent of Man* (1871; 2nd edition London: John Murray, 1890), p. 619: "We must, however, acknowledge, as it seems to me, that man with all his noble qualities, with sympathy which feels for the most debased, with benevolence that extends not only to other men but to the humblest living creature, with his god-like intellect which has penetrated into the movements and constitution of the solar system—with all these exalted powers—Man still bears in his bodily frame the indelible stamp of his lowly origin."

22   **Affluence—defined as an abundance of choice:** Avner Offer, *The Challenge of Affluence: Self-Control and Well-Being in the United States and Britain Since 1950* (Oxford: Oxford University Press, 2006).

23   **a body-mass index above 30:** The BMI is derived by dividing a person's body weight by the square of their height. Normal range of the index is considered to be between 18.5 and 24.9. An index of 25 is overweight: this translates for a man 5 feet 9 inches in height into a weight of 170 pounds. An index of 30 or over is obese.

23   **U.S. statistics for obesity:** Sixty-eight percent of the U.S. population is overweight and of that group some 33 percent are considered to be obese. The most up-to-date data sets, from which these figures were taken, and maps of the spread of the epidemic over the past two decades, state by state, are to be found on the Centers for Disease Control and Prevention website at www.cdc.gov. The data reflecting obesity around the world date to 2009 and are gathered from the Organization for Economic Cooperation and Development and reported in Trenton G. Smith, "Behavioural Biology and Obesity," in Avner Offer, Rachel Pechey, and Stanley Ulijaszek, eds., *Insecurity, Inequality and Obesity in Affluent Societies* (Oxford: Oxford University Press, 2012).

23   **Americans have been slowly gaining weight:** John Komlos and Marek Brabec, "The Trend of Mean BMI Values of U.S. Adults, Birth Cohorts 1882–86, Indicates That the Obesity Epidemic Began Earlier than Hitherto Thought," Working Paper no. 15862, National Bureau of Economic Research, April 2010.

23   **shift in our dietary habits:** A. Drewnowski and N. Darmon, "Food Choices and Diet Costs: An Economic Analysis," *Journal of Nutrition* 135 (2005): 900–4.

24   **Multiple genes are involved:** S. O'Rahilly, "Human Genetics Illuminates the Paths to Metabolic Disease," *Nature* 462 (2009): 307–14; Yung Seng Lee, "The Role of Genes in the Current Obesity Epidemic," *Annals of the Academy of Medicine Singapore* 38 (2009): 45–47.

25   **Pima Indians of Arizona:** P. H. Bennett, "Type 2 Diabetes Among the Pima Indians of Arizona: An Epidemic Attributable to Environmental Change?" *Nutritional Reviews* 57 (1999): S51–S54; and Eric Ravussin et al., "Effects of Traditional Lifestyle on Obesity in Pima Indians," *Diabetes Care* 17 (1994): 1067–74.

26   **a jerry-rigged organ of expedience:** Paul D. MacLean, *The Triune Brain in Evolution* (New York: Plenum Press, 1990); Peter C. Whybrow, "Dangerously Addictive: Why We Are Biologically Ill-Suited to the Riches of Modern America," *Chronicle Review: The Chronicle of Higher Education*, March 13, 2009.

28   **a common cultural driver [in obesity]:** K. M. Flegal et al., "Prevalence of Obesity and Trends in the Distribution of Body Mass Index Among U.S. Adults, 1999–2010," *Journal of the American Medical Association* 307 (2012): 491–97.

29   **the price of a McDonald's Big Mac:** See "Big Mac Index," *Economist*, January 14, 2012.

29   **pervasive *metabolic stress*:** Avner Offer, Rachel Pechey, and Stanley Ulijaszek, "Obesity Under Affluence Varies by Welfare Regimes: The Effect of Fast Food, Insecurity, and Inequality," *Economics and Human Biology* 8 (2010): 297–315; Avner Offer, Rachel Pechey, and Stanley Ulijaszek, eds., *Insecurity, Inequality and Obesity in Affluent Societies* (Oxford: Oxford University Press, 2012); and Trenton G. Smith, "Behavioural Biology and Obesity," ibid., pp. 69–81.

30   **a demand-driven "fast new world" that never rests:** Peter C. Whybrow, *American Mania: When More Is Not Enough* (New York: Norton, 2006).

30   **A *subjective sense of control*:** Peter C. Whybrow, *A Mood Apart; The Thinker's Guide to Emotion and Its Disorders* (New York: HarperPerennial, 1998), pp. 169–94.

31   **When cytokines are produced in excess:** J. G. Cannon, "Inflammatory Cytokines in Non-pathological States," *News in Physiological Science* 15 (2000): 298–303; S. W. Coppack, "Pro-inflammatory Cytokines and Adipose Tissue," *Proceedings of the Nutrition Society* 60 (2001): 349–56; and K. P. Karalis et al., "Mechanisms of Obesity and Related Pathology: Linking Immune Responses to Metabolic Stress," *Federation of European Biochemical Societies Journal* 276 (2009): 5747–54.

31   **chronic work stress in America:** Peter Gosselin, "If America Is Richer, Why Are Its Families So Much Less Secure?" *Los Angeles Times*, October 10, 2004.

32   **Social inequality:** Joseph Stiglitz, *The Price of Inequality: How Today's Divided Society Endangers Our Future* (New York: Norton, 2012); Charles Murray, "The New American Divide," *Wall Street Journal*, January 21, 2012; and Andrew Hacker, "We're More Unequal than You Think," *New York Review of Books*, February 23, 2012. Despite lengthening work hours and fewer vacations (in 2007 Americans labored nine weeks longer per year than Germans and four more than British), by 2007 the median wage in the United States had been stagnant for two decades, with growing disparity between rich and poor: See *Trends in the Distribution of Household Income Between 1979 and 2007* (Congressional Budget Office, October 2011). In this growing inequality America is not alone: a similar trend is occurring in Britain. See review by Nick Cohen, "The Haves and the Have-Some-Mores," *Literary Review*, May 2012.

32   **lack of sleep:** D. F. Kripke et al., "Mortality Associated with Sleep Duration and Insomnia," *Archives of General Psychiatry* 59 (2002): 131–36; Peter C. Whybrow, "Time Urgency, Sleep Loss and Obesity," in Avner Offer, Rachel Pechey, and Stanley Ulijaszek, eds., *Insecurity, Inequality and Obesity in Affluent Societies* (Oxford: Oxford University Press, 2012).

32   **sleep loss further feeds the body's pro-inflammatory cytokine response:** S. J. Motivala and M. R. Irwin, "Sleep and Immunity: Cytokine Pathways Linking Sleep and Health Outcomes," *Current Directions in Psychological Science* 16 (2007): 21–25; and K. Spiegel, R. Leproult, and E. Van Cauter, "Impact of Sleep Debt on Metabolic and Endocrine Function," *Lancet* 354 (1999): 1435–39.

33   **the appetite-controlling hormones *leptin* and *ghrelin*:** K. Spiegel et al., "Brief Communication: Sleep Curtailment in Healthy Young Man Is Associated with Decreased Leptin Levels, Elevated Ghrelin Levels and Increased Hunger and Appetite," *Annals of Internal Medicine* 14 (2004): 846–50; V. D. Dixit et al., "Ghrelin Inhibits Leptin and Activation Induced Pro-inflamatory Cytokine Expression by Human Monocytes and T Cells," *Journal of Clinical Investigation* 114 (2004): 57–66; and S. J. Motival et al., "Nocturnal Levels of Ghrelin and Leptin and Sleep in Chronic Insomnia," *Journal of Psychoneuroendocrinology* 34 (2009): 540–45.

34   **health problems . . . driven by the choices we make:** "Americans Have Worse Health than People in Other High-income Countries," *News from the National Academies*, January 9, 2013, NationalAcademies.org.

35   **a culture of excess:** Jeanne Arnold, Anthony Graesch, Elinor Ochs, and Enzo Ragazzini, *Life at Home in the Twenty-first Century: 32 Families Open their Doors* (Los Angeles: Cotsen Institute of Archaeology, 2012); and Judith Warner, "The Way We Live Now: Dysregulation Nation," *New York Times Magazine*, June 14, 2010.

36   **Delphic maxim "know thyself":** This ancient Greek aphorism, used extensively by Plato in his dialogues, is purported to have been inscribed in the forecourt of the Temple of Apollo at Delphi. See Timothy D. Wilson, "Know Thyself," *Perspectives on Psychological Science* 4 (July 2009): 384–89.

36   **morbid obesity is now a global challenge:** See "Obesity: Preventing and Managing the Global Epidemic," *WHO Obesity Technical Report Series* (Geneva: World Health Organization, 2000), p. 894; "Growing Pains: Chronic Diseases in Developing Countries," *Economist*, September 24, 2011; "The Big Picture," *Economist*, December 12, 2012; and "A Sense of Crisis as China Confronts Ailments of Affluence," *Science* 328 (2010): 422–24.

37   **exponential growth of obesity was leveling off:** Cynthia L. Ogden, Margaret D. Carroll, Brian K. Kit, and Katherine M. Flegal, "Prevalence of Obesity in the United States, 2009–2010," NHCS Data Brief no. 82, January 2012, www.cdc.gov. For a detailed report regarding California, see *A Patchwork of Progress: Changes in Overweight and Obesity Among California 5th, 7th, and 9th Graders, 2005–2010* (Los Angeles: UCLA Center for Health Policy Research and the California Center for Public Health Advocacy, 2011). For the decline in childhood obesity reported in 2014, see "Obesity Rate for Young Children Plummets 43% in a Decade," *International New York Times*, February 25, 2014; and Cynthia Ogden et al., "Prevalence of Childhood and Adult Obesity in the United States, 2011–2012," *Journal of the American Medical Association* 311 (2014): 806–14.

37   **Potential remedies:** Joy Pullmann, "Michelle Obama's School Lunch Program Leaves Children Hungry," *Washington Times,* October 2, 2012; "Lexington: Stick or Carrot?" *Economist*, June 9, 2012; and James Surowiecki, "The Financial Page: Downsizing Supersize," *New Yorker*, August 13–20, 2012.

37   **health-monitoring applications:** "The Quantified Self: Counting Every Moment," *Economist Technology Quarterly*, March 3, 2012. Free smartphone applications were also proliferating rapidly. One popular weight-loss and calorie-counting program, MyFitnessPal, had gained wide use by 2012 but had not

been objectively evaluated. Unfortunately this was true of many of the electronic devices purported to enhance self-regulation.

38   **interventions designed to help adolescent children:** David R. Lubans et al., "Preventing Obesity Among Adolescent Girls: One-Year Outcomes of the Nutrition and Enjoyable Activity for Teen Girls (NEAT Girls) Cluster: Randomized Controlled Trial," *Archives of Pediatric Adolescent Medicine* 41 (2012): 1–7.

39   **we are creatures of habit:** "Economics Focus: The Marmite Effect," *Economist*, September 25, 2010; Mark Bittman, "Selling Junk to Kids Department," *New York Times*, November 7, 2011, Bittman.blogs.nytimes.com; and Teresa Watanabe, "Los Angeles Schools' Healthful Meal Program Panned by Students," *Los Angeles Times*, December 17, 2011.

39   **in shaping eating preferences it's essential to start early:** Wendy Slusser et al., "Pediatric Overweight Prevention Through a Parent Training Program for 2–4 Year Old Latino Children," *Childhood Obesity* 8 (2012): 52–59.

40   **obesity spreads among friends:** Nicholas A. Christakis and James H. Fowler, "The Spread of Obesity in a Large Social Network over 32 Years," *New England Journal of Medicine* 357 (2007): 370–79; Alison L. Hill et al., "Infectious Disease Modeling of Social Contagion in Networks," *PLoS Computational Biology*, November 4, 2010, doi: 10.1371/journal.pcbi.1000968.

42   **subtle environmental triggers further promote:** Brian Wansink, *Mindless Eating: Why We Eat More Than We Think* (New York: Bantam Dell, 2006).

Chapter 2: HABIT AND INTUITION

45   **"The mind of man is more intuitive":** Luc de Clapiers (1715–47), the marquis of Vauvenargues, was an impoverished French nobleman and friend of Voltaire. See *The Reflections and Maxims of Luc de Clapiers, Marquis of Vauvenargues*, ed. F. G. Stevens (London: Humphrey Milford Press, 1940).

45   **"Watch your habits":** Abi Morgan is a British screenwriter. This quotation is taken from Morgan's film script *The Iron Lady*. The 2011 film explores Margaret Thatcher's career as a politician told in flashbacks during the struggles with memory loss and dementia that developed in her later years. The full quotation is within the context of a scene (page 55) when her doctor asks, "Margaret, What are you thinking?" Margaret answers, "Watch your thoughts, for they become words. Watch your words, for they become actions. Watch your actions, for they become habits. Watch your habits, for they become your character. And watch your character, for it becomes your destiny. What we think, we become. My father always said that."

46   **The human brain . . . unique evolutionary history:** See Paul MacLean, *The Triune Brain in Evolution* (New York: Plenum Press, 1990). MacLean, a neuroscientist working at the National Institutes of Health in Bethesda, was the first to propose the concept of a "triune" brain as an aid to understanding the mix of primitive and evolved behaviors characteristic of human beings. MacLean's research, spanning thirty years, led to the general acceptance of the limbic system as the anatomical home of emotion. For those interested in the evolution of

the human behavior, it is a text worth exploring, being full of anatomical and research details while adding a philosophical, sometimes whimsical, view of the complexity of human development. For a brief essay by Paul MacLean on his basic concepts and ideas, see *Human Evolution: Biosocial Perspectives*, ed. S. L. Washburn and E. R. McCown (Menlo Park, CA: Benjamin Cummings Publishing Co., 1978), pp. 33–57.

46   the frontal regions of the cortex: Joaquín M. Fuster, *The Prefrontal Cortex* (New York: Academic Press, 2008).

50   Sigmund Freud, more than any other: See Ernest Jones, *The Life and Work of Sigmund Freud*, abridged ed. (New York: Basic Books, 1961). In his writings Freud drew upon a long history of thought on the subject of the subconscious. In the fourth century B.C. Plato had embraced dreams and the imagination as evidence of preconscious knowledge. Schopenhauer and Nietzsche, pillars of the German philosophical tradition, set the stage for Freud's dynamic theory of mind, which argued that instinctual strivings, early experience, and memories beyond conscious awareness helped shape our everyday behavior. But perhaps most immediately Freud's investigation had roots in the psychological writings of Johann Friedrich Herbart (1776–1841), who had a significant impact on German education in the nineteenth century and formulated his own dynamic theory of the unconscious mind, complete with the concept of repression, thus greatly influencing Freud and Josef Breuer in their early studies of hysteria. For further discussion, see Peter C. Whybrow, "The Meaning of Loss: Psychoanalytic Explorations," in Peter C. Whybrow, Hagop S. Akiskal, and William T. McKinney, eds., *Mood Disorders: Toward a New Psychobiology* (New York: Plenum Press, 1984), pp. 81–93.

50   a reaction to the Enlightenment ideal: Eric R. Kandel, *The Age of Insight* (New York: Random House, 2012).

51   modern brain-imaging technology: Michael I. Posner and Marcus E. Raichle, *Images of Mind* (New York: Scientific American Library, 1994) provides a concise and useful history of the mapping of the brain. Over decades wiring diagrams of the motor and sensory systems in the brain were slowly drawn from the study of those who suffered stroke and other neurological disorders or needed surgery for uncontrollable epilepsy. This progress was accelerated by electrode studies in living animals, including nonhuman primates. But the secrets of the mind—those complex activities of brain that conjure the living self—remained mysterious. It wasn't until the last decades of the twentieth century that advancing computer technology coupled with applied biophysics made it possible to begin mapping the processes underpinning human thought and emotion. Magnetic resonance imaging technology (MRI) has been the linchpin in our advance. The physics of this opportunity lies in a discovery made by Linus Pauling in 1935, when he found that the amount of oxygen carried by hemoglobin—which gives blood its red color—changes the magnetic properties of the hemoglobin molecule, making it possible to differentiate between arterial and venous blood. As neurons become active in a brain region, blood flow increases, with oxygen-rich hemoglobin displacing that which is depleted. Technically the gradient of this change is detectable by measurement of the shifting magnetic properties of the hemoglobin at the site of metabolic action, giving a quantifiable measure of brain activity.

52 **social cognitive neuroscience:** Matthew D. Lieberman, "A Geographical History of Social Cognitive Neuroscience," *Neuroimage* 61 (2012): 432–36; and Matthew D. Lieberman, "Social Cognitive Neuroscience: A Review of Core Processes," *Annual Review of Psychology* 58 (2007): 259–89.

54 **the renowned psychologist Daniel Gilbert:** Daniel Gilbert, *Stumbling on Happiness* (New York: Knopf, 2006).

54 **intuitive thinking, rather than being mysterious:** Matthew D. Lieberman, "Intuition: A Social Cognitive Neuroscience Approach," *Psychological Bulletin* 126 (2000): 109–37.

55 **brain can initiate . . . routine motor behaviors:** Scott B. Kaufman et al., "Implicit Learning as an Ability," *Cognition* 116 (2010): 321–40.

55 **reflective . . . and *reflexive* . . . self-knowledge:** Matthew D. Lieberman, Johanna M. Jarcho, and Ajay B. Satpute, "Evidence-based and Intuition-based Self-knowledge: An fMRI Study," *Journal of Personality and Social Psychology* 87 (2004): 421–35. As an aid to communication Lieberman has labeled the neural centers activated in the *conscious* processing of evidence-based information about the self, a process that draws heavily upon memory and the retrieval of personal information, as the C system (C for reflective). The *intuitive,* preconscious neural network, which has the capacity for self-judgment based upon accumulated evidence without resort to explicit conscious retrieval, he has dubbed the X system (X for reflexive).

57 **two separate but parallel brain processes:** William Schneider and Richard M. Shriffrin, "Controlled and Automatic Human Information Processing I. Detection, Search and Attention," *Psychological Review* 84 (1977): 1–66.

58 **the concept of dual process thinking:** Daniel Kahneman, *Thinking Fast and Slow* (New York: Farrar, Straus & Giroux, 2011).

59 **as in Parkinson's disease:** In Parkinson's disease before treatment with L-dopa, individuals are less capable of learning from positive feedback. See Michael Frank, Lauren Seeberger, and Randall O'Reilly, "By Carrot or by Stick: Cognitive Reinforcement Learning in Parkinsonism," *Science* 306 (2004): 1940–43. Similar underlying mechanisms seem to operate in other brain disorders such as attention deficit disorder and in the compulsive repetition of movements and thoughts. Similarly dopamine activity is excessive in drug addiction and other addictive states such as habitual risk-taking that are also examples of habit behaviors that are difficult to overcome. Just as chocolate cake makes us feel good and want to eat it again, so can myriad social behaviors make us feel rewarded.

60 **across mammalian species:** Ann M. Graybiel, "The Basal Ganglia: Learning New Tricks and Loving It," *Current Opinion in Neurobiology* 15 (2005): 638–44; Terra Barnes et al., "Activity of Striatal Neurons Reflects Dynamic Encoding and Recoding of Procedural Memories," *Science* 437 (2005): 1159–61; Kaytl Sukel, "Basal Ganglia Contribute to Learning but Also Certain Disorders," *Brain Work* (New York: Dana Foundation, 2007); and Ann Graybiel, "The Basal Ganglia: Moving Beyond Movement," *Advances in Brain Research* (New York: Dana Foundation, 2007).

61 **the brain makes autonomous and preconscious judgments:** See Joseph E. Ledoux, "Rethinking the Emotional Brain," *Neuron* 73 (2012): 653–76; and Ledoux's earlier book on the same subject, *The Emotional Brain: The Mysterious Underpinnings of Emotional Life* (New York: Simon & Schuster, 1996).

62 **an intensely social species:** Susanne Schultz and Robin Dunbar, "Encephalization Is Not a Universal Macroevolutionary Phenomenon in Mammals But Is Associated with Sociality," *Proceedings of the National Academy of Science* 107, no. 50 (2010): 21582–86.

63 **mental "heuristics"—innate rules:** Leda Cosmides and John Tooby, *The Adapted Mind: Evolutionary Psychology and the Generation of Culture* (Oxford: Oxford University Press, 1992).

64 **how morality varies across cultures:** See Jonathan Haidt and Selin Kesebir, "Morality," in S. Fiske, D. Gilbert, and G. Lindzey, eds., *Handbook of Social Psychology*, 5th ed. (Hoboken, NJ: John Wiley & Sons, 2010), vol. 1. Increasingly Haidt has turned his attention to the moral foundations of politics and how to transcend the "culture wars" of political partisanship using the findings of moral psychology. See J. Haidt, J. Graham, and C. Joseph, "Above and Below Left-Right: Ideological Narratives and Moral Foundations," *Psychological Inquiry* 20 (2009): 110–19. For a report in the popular press on the same subject, see Clive Crook, "US Fiscal Crisis Is a Morality Play," *Financial Times*, July 4, 2011.

65 **intuition is unreliable:** Daniel Kahneman and Gary Klein, "Conditions for Intuitive Expertise: A Failure to Disagree," *American Psychologist* 64 (2009): 515–26.

65 **"strangers to ourselves":** Timothy D. Wilson, *Strangers to Ourselves: Discovering the Adaptive Unconscious* (Cambridge, MA: Harvard University Press, 2002).

67 **"Yes, in modern times the concept of the self":** See also Matthew Lieberman and Naomi Eisenberger, "Conflict and Habit: A Social Cognitive Neuroscience Approach to the Self," in A. Tesser, J. V. Wood, and D. A. Stapel, eds., *On Building, Defending and Regulating the Self: A Psychological Perspective* (New York: Psychology Press, 2004), pp. 77–102.

68 **personal identity today is . . . self-determined and choice-driven:** Roy F. Baumeister; "How the Self Became a Problem: A Psychological Review of Historical Research," *Journal of Personality and Social Research* 52 (1987): 163–76.

Chapter 3: ENLIGHTENED EXPERIMENTS

69 **"Money begats trade":** Thomas Mun, "England's Treasure by Forraign Trade," in John Ramsay McCulloch, ed., *A Select Collection of Early English Tracts on Commerce* (London: Political Economy Club, 1856). Little is known about Thomas Mun save that he was an eminent merchant of London in the mid-seventeenth century and a director of the East India Company.

69 **"And who are you? said he":** Laurence Sterne, *The Life and Opinions of Tristram Shandy, Gentleman* (London: Folio Society, 1970), bk. 7, chap. 33, p. 399. Sterne (1713–68) was an English parson and humorist who rocketed to fame at forty-six after the publication of the first two volumes of *Tristram Shandy*.

69   **the Domesday Survey:** Commissioned by William the Conqueror in 1085, the survey reviewed more than thirteen thousand hamlets and towns in England and Wales and was completed in one year. See www.domesdaybook.co.uk/oxford shire1.html.

70   **Combe Mill was retired:** The historical details regarding the mill are taken from *Guide to Combe Mill* (Combe Mill Society, 2009). Further information may be found at www.combemill.org.

70   **steam engines . . . initiated our dependence on fossil fuel:** E. A. Wrigley, *Energy and the English Industrial Revolution* (Cambridge, UK: Cambridge University Press, 2010).

70   **the Lunar Society of Birmingham:** Robert Schofield, *The Lunar Society of Birmingham* (Oxford: Oxford University Press, 1963); and Jenny Unglow, *The Lunar Men: Five Friends Whose Curiosity Changed the World* (New York: Farrar, Straus & Giroux, 2002).

71   **"a little philosophical laughing":** Erasmus Darwin to Matthew Boulton, March 11, 1766, quoted in Unglow, *Lunar Men*, p. xv.

72   **Charles needed money:** See Jenny Unglow, *A Gambling Man: Charles II's Restoration Game* (New York: Farrar, Straus & Giroux, 2002), particularly pp. 289–304.

73   **William of Orange gave political stability to England:** J. R. Jones, *Country and Court: England 1658-1714* (Cambridge, MA: Harvard University Press, 1978).

73   **the battle of Blenheim:** Charles Spencer, *Blenheim: Battle for Europe* (London: Weidenfeld & Nicolson, 2004).

74   **"nervous" and "of the sensorium":** Erasmus Darwin's *Zoonomia: The Laws of Organic Life* (1794) is essentially a medical text that explores the functioning of the body, including anatomy, psychology, and pathology. Darwin had studied medicine at Cambridge, receiving his degree in 1755, and he maintained a busy practice for most of his life.

75   **felt they held the future in their own hands:** See William Hutton, *An History of Birmingham* (1783), online at www.gutenberg.org/ebooks/13926. "Every man has his fortune in his own hands," wrote Hutton (1723–1815), a printer and local historian.

75   **"that conscious thinking thing":** John Locke (1632–1704) was the son of a country lawyer who had served with Cromwell; partly through those connections Locke attended the Westminster School and went on to Christ Church, Oxford. There he was exposed to some of the best scientific minds, men who were breaking with the Aristotelian tradition and moving toward systematic observation as the bedrock of science and medicine. In 1666 he met Lord Ashley, later the Earl of Shaftesbury and one of the richest men in England, becoming his personal physician, secretary, and political operative. Living with Ashley in London, Locke found himself at the center of English political life during the turbulent reign of Charles II. Ashley believed that England would prosper through trade and persuaded the king to develop the Board of Trade, the legal body that administered the American Colonies before the revolution. Locke became its secretary, including drafting the constitution of the Carolinas in America. Throughout, Locke remained a philosopher in his thinking. His *An Essay Concerning Human Understanding*, with his reflections upon the nature of the self, first appeared in 1688; he made several revisions before his death in 1704.

75   **self-scrutiny was a rare activity:** Roy Baumeister, "How the Self Became a Problem: A Psychological Review of Historical Research," *Journal of Personality and Social Psychology* 52 (1987): 163–76.

75   **Michel de Montaigne:** Sarah Bakewell, *How to Live, or A Life of Montaigne in One Question and Twenty Attempts at an Answer* (UK: Other Press, 2010).

76   **human judgment is unreliable:** Thomas Hobbes (1588–1679) was a pessimist, although perhaps he may be excused given what he experienced. Born in the time of Elizabeth I, he endured the cruelty and chaos of the English Civil War, including the beheading of Charles I. Hobbes's greatest fear over his long life was the threat of social and political chaos. Only science, he asserted, and "the knowledge of consequences" offered hope in overcoming human frailty. Hobbes was committed to the emerging scientific method; indeed, the mechanistic reasoning that he employed was in some ways a personal means of avoiding the messy emotional and political time in which he lived. He saw the body and its control by the head—the brain—as comparable to the need for the body politic to have a head that would decide what should be done. His thinking, however, was constrained by this mechanistic viewpoint when it came to describing human nature. A medievalist at heart, in the political realm his vision was darker still: in the face of declining religious influence, he asserted, only sovereign autocracy was capable of sustaining a stable social order.

76   **greed and a love of luxury were the engines:** Bernard de Mandeville, *The Fable of the Bees, or Private Vices, Public Benefits* (1732; reprinted Oxford University Press/Sandpiper Books, 2001).

76   **with profit for both the individual and society:** See Peter Gay, *The Enlightenment: An Interpretation: The Science of Freedom* (New York: Norton, 1969).

77   **"psychology of action":** David Hume, *A Treatise of Human Nature* (1738; reprint edition London: Everyman's Library, 1939).

79   **the patron saint of capitalism:** Of the numerous books written about Adam Smith, one that best balances the philosopher and the economist is Nicholas Phillipson's *Adam Smith: An Enlightened Life* (New Haven, CT: Yale University Press, 2010). Another is James Buchan, *The Authentic Adam Smith: His Life and Ideas* (New York: Norton, 2006).

80   **"by which we perceive virtue or vice":** For a concise discussion of Francis Hutcheson's contribution to Enlightenment philosophy and his influence on Smith's thinking and writing, see Phillipson, *Smith: Enlightened Life*, pp. 24–55.

81   **"on which all forms of human communication":** Ibid., p. 148.

81   **"Though our brother is upon the rack":** Adam Smith, *The Theory of Moral Sentiments* (1759; reprint edition Indianapolis: Liberty Fund, 1976), sec. 1, chap. 1, p. 48.

82   **in the pursuit of mutual sympathy:** James R. Otteson, *Adam Smith's Marketplace of Life* (Cambridge, UK: Cambridge University Press, 2002).

82   **"It is not from the benevolence of the butcher":** Adam Smith, *The Wealth of Nations* (1776; reprint edition New York: Random House, 1994), bk. 1, chap. 2, p. 15.

83   **"it is the most insistent":** Adam Gopnik, "Market Man: What Did Adam Smith Really Believe?" *New Yorker*, October 18, 2010.

86   **the transition from community to society:** Ferdinand Tönnies, *Community*

and Society, trans. Charles P. Loomis (New York: Dover, 2002). Tönnies first published *Gemeinschaft und Gesellschaft* in 1887.

87   **"maximize economic return":** E. A. Wrigley, *Energy and the English Industrial Revolution* (Cambridge, UK: Cambridge University Press, 2010), chap. 8.

88   **preoccupations with Newtonian science and moral philosophy:** Garry Wills, *Inventing America: Jefferson's Declaration of Independence* (New York: Doubleday, 1978).

89   **happiness is similar to the concept of price:** Jason Potts, "The Use of Happiness in Society: An Evolutionary/Hayekian Approach to Happiness Economics," *Proceedings of the Mont Perelin Society*, Annual Meeting, 2010.

90   **the Tea Party movement:** "Lexington: The Perils of Constitution-worship," *Economist*, September 25, 2010.

Chapter 4: CHOICE

91   **"Give me the liberty to know":** John Milton, *Areopagitica, in Defense of the Right to Publish Without License*, November 23, 1644. The speech was given before Parliament and published simultaneously as a pamphlet.

92   **Joaquín Fuster:** For Fuster's autobiography, see Joaquín M. Fuster, *The History of Neuroscience in Autobiography*, ed. Larry R. Squire (Oxford: Oxford University Press, 2011), pp. 7:58–97.

92   **the Orient Express:** Jonathan Bastable, "Orient Express, 1982," *Condé Nast Traveller*, April 2009.

93   **Human "Connectome" Project:** Francis Collins, "The Symphony Inside Your Brain," NIH Director's Blog, November 5, 2012, http://directorsblog.nih.gov/the-symphony-inside-your-head. See also A. Paul Alvisatos et al., "The Brain Activity Map," *Science* 339 (March 7, 2013).

94   **the hippocampus:** That the hippocampus is essential to memory formation is dramatically and tragically demonstrated by the case of Henry Molaison, known during his lifetime as HM. Henry, born in 1926, developed epilepsy in his teens and by the age of twenty-seven it had become intractable with as many as eleven severe seizures each week. The seizure activity was localized to the temporal lobes of the brain, which contain the hippocampus and the amygdala; both of these structures were removed in an effort to control the seizures. The control of epilepsy was achieved but with the startling and immediate result of his complete loss of the capacity for recent memory, although distant memories, acquired before the surgery, remained intact. Henry lived until 2008, but his incapacity to remember recent events persisted throughout his lifetime. He became the object of considerable neuropsychological study; the tragedy of his disability has contributed enormously to our understanding of the role of the hippocampus in memory acquisition and retrieval. For the original article published by the surgeon who performed the operation, see William Beecher Scoville and Brenda Milner, "Loss of Recent Memory After Bilateral Hippocampal Lesions," *Journal of Neurology Neurosurgery and Psychiatry* 20 (1957): 11–21; it was reprinted in *Journal of Neuropsychiatry and Clinical Neuroscience* 12 (2000):1ff. For a popular review at the time of HM's death, see "Obituary: HM," *Economist*, December 20, 2008.

94 **the frontal lobes:** Joaquín M. Fuster, *The Prefrontal Cortex*, 4th ed. (London: Elsevier Press, 2008); and Fuster, *The Neuroscience of Freedom and Creativity* (Cambridge, UK: Cambridge University Press, 2013).

95 **a tapestry of personal knowledge:** Joaquín M. Fuster, *Cortex and Mind: Unifying Cognition* (Oxford: Oxford University Press, 2003).

96 **to remember the past . . . enables us to imagine the future:** Daniel L. Schachter and Donna Rose Addis, "Constructive Memory: The Ghosts of Past and Future," *Nature* 445 (2007): 27.

96 **the fundamentals of neuronal action have been conserved:** Eric R. Kandel, "The Molecular Biology of Memory Storage: A Dialog Between Genes and Synapses," Nobel lecture, December 8, 2000; in *Bioscience Reports* 24 (2004): 477–522.

97 **clusters of neurons can be . . . consistently excited:** For an elegant and concise summary of the work of Itzhak Fried and his colleagues, see Rodrigo Quiroga, Itzhak Fried, and Christof Koch, "Brain Cells for Grandmother," *Scientific American* 308 (2013): 30–35.

100 **the fatty insulation called myelin:** George Bartzokis et al., "Lifespan Trajectory of Myelin Integrity and Maximum Motor Speed," *Neurobiology of Aging* 31 (2010): 1554–62.

101 **"there was likely much more to brain function":** Marcus Raichle and Abraham Snyder, "A Default Mode of Brain Function: A Brief History of an Evolving Idea," *NeuroImage* 37 (2007): 1083–90.

102 **the brain's functional networks change with age:** Damien Fair et al., "Functional Brain Networks Develop from a 'Local to Distributed' Organization," *PLoS Computational Biology* 5 (May 2009); and Jonathan Power et al., "The Development of Functional Brain Networks," *Neuron* 67 (2010): 735–48.

105 **the tragedy of Phineas Gage:** John Van Horn et al., "Mapping Connectivity Damage in the Case of Phineas Gage," *PLoS One* 7 (May 2012), doi:10.1371/journal.pone/0037454.

110 **the central role of pleasure in driving human behavior:** Morten L. Kringelbach, "The Human Orbitalfrontal Cortex; Linking reward to Hedonic Experience," *Nature Reviews: Neuroscience* 6 (2005): 691–702; and Kringelbach, *The Pleasure Center: Trust Your Animal Instincts* (Oxford: Oxford University Press, 2009).

110 **a brain area . . . particularly active . . . in "resting" blood flow studies:** The ventromedial prefrontal cortex is consistently active in fMRI and PET studies of the brain's default networks. It appears to be one anchor in the cross-talk among the several centers of the "executive" brain. The other is the posterior cingulated cortex, which is part of the first layer of the "new" cortex that wraps itself around the older limbic brain structures. For a summary see Tina Hesman Saey, "You Are Who You Are by Default," *Science News*, July 18, 2009.

110 **The ventrolateral prefrontal cortex . . . braking system:** Jessica Cohen and Matthew Lieberman, "The Common Neural Basis of Exerting Self-Control in Multiple Domains," in Y. Trope, R. Hassin, and K. N. Ochsner, eds., *Self Control* (Oxford: Oxford University Press, 2010), pp. 141–60.

112 **"inter-temporal or delayed discounting":** George Ainslie, "Précis of Breakdown of Will," *Behavioral and Brain Sciences* 28 (2005): 635–73.

113 **separate brain systems ... immediate and delayed rewards:** S. M.
McClure et al., "Separate Neuronal Systems Value Immediate and Delayed
Monetary Awards," *Science* 306 (2004): 503–7. For a commentary, see George
Ainslie and John Monterosso, "A Marketplace in the Brain?" *Science* 306 (2004):
421–23. The timing of a reward is also important, with immediate reward dominating long-term decision making. See S. M. McClure et al., "Time Discounting
for Primary Rewards," *Journal of Neuroscience* 27 (2007): 5796–804; and Lucy
Gregorios-Pippas, Philippe N. Tobler, and Wolfram Schultz, "Short-term Temporal Discounting of Reward Value in Human Temporal Striatum," *Journal of Neuro-
physiology* 101 (2009): 1507–23.

114 **the brain's two systems of choosing:** Bernard Balleine and John O'Doherty,
"Human and Rodent Homologies in Action Control: Corticostriatal Determinants
of Goal-Directed and Habitual Action," *Neuropharmacology* 35 (2009): 48–69.

115 **"we *learn* to be thoughtless":** Joshua M. Epstein, "Learning to Be Thoughtless: Social Norms and Individual Computation," *Computational Economics*
18 (2001): 9–24. A variation of this phenomenon is the "Einstellung effect,"
where in solving problems we persist in approaching tasks with a biased mindset
that has been developed from previous experience. See Merim Bilalic, Peter
McLeod, and Fernand Gobet, "The Mechanism of the Einstellung (Set) Effect:
A Pervasive Source of Cognitive Bias," *Current Directions in Psychological Science* 19 (2010): 111–15.

Chapter 5: MARKET MAYHEM

117 **"This division of labour":** One of Smith's most famous quotations from *The
Wealth of Nations* focuses upon exchange as the core activity of the social relationships from which the various institutional arrangements we call the "free"
market then develop. See Adam Smith, *An Inquiry into the Nature and Causes of
the Wealth of Nations* (1776; reprint edition New York: Modern Library, 1994), bk.
1, chap. 2, p. 14.

117 **Beyond *Babylon*:** Joan Aruz, Kim Benzel, and Jean Evans, eds., *Beyond Babylon:
Art, Trade, and Diplomacy in the Second Millennium B.C.* (New York: Metropolitan Museum of Art, 2008).

118 **destined to change American capitalism:** "The Week that Changed American Capitalism," *Wall Street Journal*, September 20, 2008.

118 **"the simple and obvious system of natural liberty":** Smith, *Wealth of
Nations*, bk. 4, chap. 9, p. 745.

119 **Barter and exchange are older than the practice of agriculture:** Smith
employed a four-stage theory of economic history—hunters, herding, agriculture,
and commercial society—based upon the taxonomy laid down by Henry Home,
later Lord Kames, in *Sketches on the History of Man* (1734). In the hunter-gatherer
society, competition for resources was resolved by seeking new territory; herding provided opportunities for larger groups to be sustained, but few laws were
required because social control was provided by the family unit; settlement and
agriculture were a social order of greater complexity requiring agreements and obli-

gations. Finally in commercial society clear regulatory practices were required to protect property and to distribute responsibility across individuals and the social group. Honesty in practice is fundamental, both in respecting of the property of others and in establishing the fair price of the goods to be exchanged. Most important, those involved in the exchange must demonstrate integrity, without which trust erodes and the market culture's delicate web of social interaction is rapidly destroyed.

119   **In the late Bronze Age the Mediterranean was a trading hub:** Karl Polanyi, Conrad Arensberg, and Harry Pearson, eds., *Trade and Market in the Early Empires* (Chicago: Henry Regnery Co., 1971); and S. C. Humphreys, "History, Economics, and Anthropology: The Work of Karl Polanyi," *History and Theory* 8 (1969): 165–212.

119   **a Bronze Age trading vessel:** The Uluburun was salvaged by George Bass, considered by many to be the father of underwater archaeology. Bass founded the Institute of Nautical Archaeology, which has a major research center in Bodrum, Turkey, where many of the Uluburun artifacts are on display. See Dale Keiger, "The Underwater World of George Bass," *Johns Hopkins Magazine*, April 1997.

120   **Commerce flourished among these ruling elites:** "The First Civilizations of Europe: 3000–600 BC," *Hammond Concise Atlas of World History* (HarperCollins, 1998).

123   **palace economies:** M. I. Finley, *The World of Odysseus* (1954; reprint edition New York: NYRB Classics, 2002).

123   **The value of most commodities was determined by weight:** The weight of the volume of water filling an amphora was called a *talent*, in ancient Greek meaning "scale" or "balance." Talent, as a unit of mass, was also the name given to a unit of precious metal of equivalent mass. This represented the first stage of currency development, where valuable metals including copper ingots were held as the receipt of purchase for stored grain or other commodities. The concept of gold and silver as money grew only later as trade became organized. It was to be many centuries, however, before Alyattes, the father of Croesus, had the bright idea, around 600 B.C. in Anatolia, of guaranteeing the weight and purity of the precious metals circulating in his dominion, thus greatly simplifying trading.

125   **the economies of the eastern Mediterranean feudal states collapsed:** Robert Drews, *The End of the Bronze Age* (Princeton: Princeton University Press, 1995); and Eric H. Cline, *1177 B.C.: The Year Civilization Collapsed* (Princeton: Princeton University Press, 2014).

126   **the equilibrium of political and military power:** Eberhard Zangger, "Who Were the Sea People?" *Saudi Aramco World*, May–June 1995.

126   **the siege of Troy to which Homer:** Joachim Latacz, *Troy and Homer: Towards a Solution of an Old Mystery* (Oxford: Oxford University Press, 2005); and Caroline Alexander, *The War That Killed Achilles: The True Story of the Iliad* (New York: Viking Penguin, 2009).

127   **bands of hungry seagoing predators:** Mark Schwartz, "Darkness Descends," *Ancient Warfare* 4 (August–September 2010): 4.

128   **the great slab of memory that is human history:** Madeline Bunting, "The Memory of Humankind Preserves Our Global Sanity," *Guardian*, March 15, 2007.

129   **interactive equilibrium with their surroundings:** Ludwig von Bertalanffy, *General Systems Theory* (New York: George Braziller, 1969).

129   **the brain as a self-organizing and goal-directed system:** F. A. Hayek, *The Sensory Order: An Inquiry into the Foundations of Theoretical Psychology* (Chicago: University of Chicago Press, 1976).

129   **Markets . . . a natural product of human social interaction:** F. A. Hayek, *The Fatal Conceit: The Errors of Socialism* (Chicago: University of Chicago Press, 1988).

130   **"invisible hand":** While the metaphor of the "invisible hand" is much quoted, in fact Smith used it sparingly. In *The Wealth of Nations,* for example, it appears in relation to foreign trade as follows: "By preferring the support of domestic to that of foreign industry, he intends only his own security; and by directing that industry in such a manner as its produce may be of the greatest value, he intends only his own gain, and he is in this, as in many other cases, led by an *invisible hand* to promote an end which was no part of his intention" (book 4, chapter 2). Today classical economists extend the meaning of the phrase to infer cooperation without coercion.

132   **"we are no longer living in Adam Smith's village economy":** John Komlos, "A Critique of Pure Economics," *Challenge: The Magazine of Economic Affairs* 55 (2012): 21–57.

133   **"The moment that barter is replaced":** Hayek, *Fatal Conceit,* p. 101.

134   **the fable of King Midas:** Richard Seaford, "World Without Limits: The Greek Discovery That Man Could Never Be Too Rich," *Times Literary Supplement,* June 19, 2009. In mythology the story of King Midas offers a cautionary note. Midas, the king of Phrygia, "was a wise and pious king." One day he was offered a wish by the god Dionysus. "Midas asked that everything he touched should be turned to gold. He soon regretted his indiscretion, for even the food he ate immediately turned to gold. Dionysus took pity on him and sent him to purify himself in the river Pactolus, which thenceforth flowed with gold dust." *New Larousse Encyclopedia of Mythology* (New York: Crescent Books, 1989), p. 150.

134   **entrepreneurs at JPMorgan Chase dreamed up:** Gillian Tett, *Fool's Gold: The Inside Story of J.P. Morgan and How Wall Street Greed Corrupted Its Bold Dream and Created a Financial Crisis* (New York: Free Press, 2010). Finance began as a service industry in support of commerce and development. Acting as a "market-maker"—buying and selling stocks, commodities and other financial instruments—the goal was to make profit from the price differentials between the bid and the sale, thus providing liquidity in the market and facilitating trade. See also Gillian Tett, "Genesis of the Debt Crisis," *Financial Times,* May 1, 2009.

135   **"high latent demand" zip codes:** "Chain of Fools: Hard Evidence That Securitization Encouraged Lax Mortgage Lending in America," *Economist,* February 9, 2008.

136   **"debt economy," based on an assumption of continuous growth:** James Surowiecki, "The Debt Economy," *New Yorker,* November 23, 2009.

136   **making debt acceptable:** Richard Duncan, *The New Depression: The Breakdown of the Paper Money Economy* (Hoboken, NJ: John Wiley & Sons, 2012).

136 **The explosion of credit . . . changed our habits:** "Buttonwood: Duncan Dough Notes, A Thought Provoking Analysis of the Debt Crisis," *Economist*, July 7, 2012. Private indebtedness in the United States grew from 120 percent of GDP in 1980 to 300 percent in 2009, which was proportionally higher than in 1929 at the start of the Great Depression. As part of this increase, the household debt that fueled the mortgage bubble, which first began leaking in 2007, rose from $6.5 trillion in 2000 to almost $15 trillion by 2008. Michael Clark, "It's Private Debt, Not Public Debt That Got Us into This Mess," Seekingalpha.com, May 7, 2012.

138 **the finance industry's changing share:** Deepak Lal, "The Great Crash of 2008: Causes and Consequences," *Cato Journal* 30 (2010): 265–77. Goldman Sachs as the leader of the banking oligarchy had helped facilitate the growth of the credit economy by promoting liberalization of capital requirements. Two treasury secretaries and innumerable government advisers had been recruited from the firm. In parallel to the nation's growing indebtedness the finance industry had been lobbying Washington to diminish its financial oversight of its activities. Most of this effort had been focused upon dismantling the controls—notably the Glass-Steagall Act—that had been put in place after the Great Depression in an effort to curb financial speculation. In this legislation retail banks—those traditionally dealing directly with the customer in evaluating loans and managing deposits, which were covered by federal insurance to a specified limit—were distinguished from investment banks, which were free to gamble in the open market. The principal argument mounted against this "firewall" legislation was that it stifled healthy competition. After years of slow erosion the act was finally repealed in 1999 under President Clinton. In a similar move toward deregulation, the City of London had opened its financial markets to global competition and electronic trading in the 1980s.

138 **"if discretionary distributions":** Patrick Hosking, "Bank Says Crisis Could Have Been Avoided If Bonuses Had Been 20 Percent Less," *Times* (London), December 18, 2009.

138 **With hindsight the facts are simple:** Martin Wolf, "The World after the Financial Crisis," in Nick Kuenssberg, ed., *Argument Amongst Friends: Twenty-five Years of Sceptical Inquiry* (Edinburgh: David Hume Institute, 2010).

139 **"too big to fail":** Andrew Ross Sorkin, "Realities Behind Prosecuting Big Banks," *New York Times*, March 12, 2013; Anat Admati and Martin Hellwig, *The Banker's New Clothes: What's Wrong with Banking and What to Do About It* (Princeton: Princeton University Press, 2013); and "Prosecuting Bankers: Blind Justice, Why Have So Few Bankers Gone to Jail For Their Part in the Crisis?" *Economist*, May 4, 2013.

139 **the oligarchy . . . came away essentially unharmed:** U.S. Senate Permanent Subcommittee on Investigations, *Wall Street and the Financial Crisis: Anatomy of a Financial Collapse*, April 13, 2011. In this bipartisan report on the collapse of the global financial system the Senate Subcommittee on Investigations concluded that "the crisis was not a natural disaster, but the result of high risk, complex financial products, undisclosed conflicts of interest; and the failure of regulators, the credit rating agencies and the market itself to rein in the excesses of Wall

Street" (pt. 1, p. 9). See also Gretchen Morgenson and Louise Story, "Naming Culprits in the Financial Crisis," *New York Times*, April 13, 2011.

139 **social inequality . . . instability of America's financial system:** Chrystia Freeland, "The New Global Super-Rich No Longer Look So Benign," *Financial Times*, January 2, 2010; Robert B. Reich, "The Limping Middle Class," *New York Times*, September 4, 2011; "Free Exchange: Body of Evidence; Is a Concentration of Wealth at the Top to Blame For Financial Crises?" *Economist*, March 17, 2012.

140 **combination of social inequality and the easing:** Raghuram Rajan, *Fault Lines: How Hidden Fractures Still Threaten the World Economy* (Princeton: Princeton University Press, 2011).

140 **"We have met the enemy":** The American cartoonist Walt Kelly (1913–73) first used the quote "We have met the enemy and he is us" on a poster for Earth Day in 1970, http://www.igopogo.com/we_have_met.htm.

140 **the American economy was in recession only 5 percent of the time:** "US Business Cycle Expansions and Contractions," National Bureau of Economic Research, www.nber.org/cycles.html.

141 **the sin of extrapolation:** Probably the first individual to describe the phenomenon was the economist Hyman Minsky, who in the mid-twentieth century drew attention to the role that the finance industry played in exaggerating economic cycles. See "Buttonwood: Minsky's Moment," *Economist*, April 4, 2009.

141 **economic growth had been built on debt:** David Manuel, "Savings Rates in the United States Have Collapsed Since Mid-'80s," Davemanuel.com, January 1, 2010, http://bit.ly/1sC111t.

142 **"of self-denial, of self-government . . .":** Adam Smith, *The Theory of Moral Sentiments* (1759; reprint edition Liberty Fund Classics, 1976), pt. 1, sec. 1, chap. 5.

142 **Character is built, not born:** Richard Reeves, "A Question of Character," *Prospect*, August 2008.

143 **As trust declines, the social glue erodes:** CESifo Group Munich, *EEAG Report on the European Economy 2010*, http://bit.ly/Vj4Biq; Veronica Hope-Hailey, "Trust Is in Short Supply—If We Want Our Economy to Grow, We Need It," *Guardian*, January 23, 2012; Ron Fournier and Sophie Quinton, "How Americans Lost Trust in Our Greatest Institutions," *Atlantic*, April 20, 2012.

143 **a seemingly endless list of improprieties:** "MPs' Expenses Scandal: The Timeline," *Independent*, February 2010; Francesco Guerrera, Henry Sender, and Justin Baer, "Goldman Sachs Settles with SEC," *Financial Times*, July 16, 2010; "Banks Shares Suffer As J.P. Morgan's $2 Billion Loss Raises Heat over Risk-Taking," *Financial Times Weekend*, May 12–13, 2012; "Dimon and His Lieutenants Caught in the Spotlight Over Risk Management," *Financial Times Weekend*, March 16–17, 2013; "The LIBOR Scandal: The Rotten Heart of Finance," *Economist*, July 7, 2012; and "Retirement Benefits: Who Pays the Bill?" *Economist*, July 27, 2013.

143 **greed and fraud in high places:** Chrystia Freeland, "Is Capitalism in Trouble? CEOs Are Growing Nervous. Can They Help Save Our System From Its Worst Excesses?" *Atlantic*, December 2013.

Chapter 6: LOVE

147 **"Mary had a little lamb":** The nursery rhyme was published in 1830 by Sarah Josepha Hale, an American self-educated writer and novelist. It is now generally accepted, although it was denied by Mistress Hale just before her death, that the poem was built upon three stanzas written by a young man named John Roulstone. Roulstone is purported to have witnessed firsthand Mary Sawyer's pet lamb following her to school in Sudbury, Massachusetts. *The Oxford Dictionary of Nursery Rhymes* (Oxford: Oxford University Press), p. 354.

147 **"How selfish soever man may be supposed":** Adam Smith, *The Theory of Moral Sentiments* (1759; reprint edition Indianapolis: Liberty Classics, 1976), sec. 1, chap. 1. Just as Smith built his theory of commerce upon the human propensity for barter and exchange and the efficiency of the division of labor, so did he argue that those sentiments in man's nature that *"interest him in the fortunes of others"* are the foundation of organized society.

148 **Helen started her flock:** Helen Whybrow, "Lambing Time," *Vermont's Local Banquet*, no. 16, (Spring 2011). Wren, the youngest of her family, lives with her sister, Willow, and her parents, Helen Whybrow and Peter Forbes, at Knoll Farm in Fayston, Vermont.

150 **the Brothers Grimm:** Wilhelm and Jacob Grimm were German literary scholars born just eighteen months apart in the latter part of the eighteenth century. Their collection of German folk tales, first published in 1812, contained several stories of wolves and their escapades, perhaps the most famous of which is Little Red Cap (Rotkäppchen), now known as Little Red Riding Hood. For an excellent translation, see *Grimm's Complete Fairy Tales*, trans. Margaret Hunt (San Diego, CA: Canterbury Classics, 2011).

152 **the faithful prairie vole has many more receptors for oxytocin and vasopressin:** For original studies, see Thomas R. Insel and Lawrence Shapiro, "Oxytocin Receptor Distribution Reflects Social Organization in Monogamous and Polygamist Voles," *Proceedings National Academy of Sciences* 89 (1992): 5981–85; Larry J. Young and Zuoxin Wang, "The Neurobiology of Pair Bonding," *Nature Neuroscience* 7 (2004): 1048–54; and Larry J. Young, Anne Z. Murphy Young, and Elizabeth A. D. Hammock, "Anatomy and Neurochemistry of the Pair Bond," *Journal of Comparative Neurology* 493 (2005): 51–57. For an easily accessible summary, see "The Science of Love: I Get a Kick Out of You," *Economist*, February 14, 2004.

153 **smell and close attachment are intimately intertwined in human bonding:** R. H. Porter, J. M. Cernoch, and F. J. McLaughlin, "Maternal Recognition of Neonates Through Olfactory Cues," *Physiology And Behavior* 30 (1983): 151–54; and "Paternity and Parental Investment: Like Father, like Son," *Economist*, June 18, 2009.

153 **human infants . . . will show concern for others:** Felix Warneken and Michael Tomasello, "Altruistic Helping in Human Infants and Young Chimpanzees," *Science* 311 (2006): 1301–3.

153 **the smiles and babbling of young children:** Charles Darwin, *The Expres-*

sion of the Emotions in Man and Animals was first published in 1872, thirteen years after *The Origin of Species*. It had been long in genesis, however, for there is evidence that Darwin began keeping notebooks about the possible interaction of inherited traits and emotion back in 1838. In Victorian times emotion was a tricky subject, tied in the public mind to spirituality, good and evil. A scientific understanding of human behavior was thus likely to receive public and church opposition. Hence Darwin in his book focused on the expression of human emotion in animals rather than the other way around.

153 **babies . . . change the behavior of those around them:** Morten Kringelbach et al., "A Specific and Rapid Neural Signature for Parental Instinct," *PLoS* 3 (2008): 1–7, doi: 10.137/journal.pone.0001664. In a study using magnetoencephalography (MEG) the investigators provided evidence that within milliseconds the adult brain responds to unfamiliar infant faces but not to the faces of unfamiliar adults.

154 **"cooperative breeding":** Sarah Blaffer Hrdy, *Mothers and Others: The Evolutionary Origins of Mutual Understanding* (Cambridge, MA: Harvard University Press, 2009). Hrdy presents a powerful argument for the unique nature of human cooperation. What other primate species, she asks at the beginning of her book, is willing to spend several hours locked up together in a metal tube (an airliner) and emerge at the other end with all limbs intact and no combat deaths? No other ape has such a capacity for tolerance and mutual understanding—behaviors that Hrdy believes evolved from collaborative childrearing practices.

155 **Kalahari Bushmen:** Polly Wiessner, "Taking the Risk Out of Risky Transactions: A Forager's Dilemma," in F. Salter, ed., *Risky Transactions: Trust, Kinship and Ethnicity* (New York: Berghahn Books, 2002), pp. 21–43. See also "Where Gifts and Stories Are Crucial to Survival: A Conversation with Pauline Wiessner," *New York Times*, May 25, 2009. For a rich first-hand account of the nomadic life of the Kalahari Bushmen before and after the encroachments of industrialized culture, which has annexed some 95 percent of their habitat, see Elizabeth Marshall Thomas, *The Harmless People* (New York: Vintage, 1959). Thomas, an anthropologist, lived with the Bushmen from the 1950s to the 1980s. See also Spencer Wells, *The Journey of Man: A Genetic Odyssey* (New York: Random House, 2004).

156 **in moments of disaster:** Shankar Vedantam, "The Key to Disaster Survival? Friends and Neighbors," National Public Radio, July 4, 2011. Stories of group support are consistently present in the news reports that follow natural disasters. See as another example a press story following the Rancho Bernardo fire in southern California, which destroyed seventeen hundred homes: Molly Hennessy-Friske, "Amid Ashes, Neighbors Rally and Life Stirs Anew; They Lost So Much, but They May Have Regained a Sense of Community," *Los Angeles Times*, November 3, 2007.

156 **the Ultimatum Game:** Werner Güth, Rolf Schmittberger, and Bernd Schwarze, "An Experimental Analysis of Ultimatum Bargaining," *Journal of Economic Behavior and Organization* 3 (1982): 367–88; and Hessel Oosterbeek, Randolph Sloof, and Gus Van de Kuilen, "Cultural Differences in Ultimatum Game Experiments: Evidence from a Meta-Analysis," *Experimental Economics* 7 (2004): 171–88.

156   **unique human sense of fairness:** Our cousin the chimpanzee does not appear
to share this human trait of evenhanded concern. In ultimatum studies designed
to explore whether chimps are willing to split unsolicited rewards, such as raisins
or chocolate, the predominant results suggest that their preference is to share little. While some ambiguity exists, it appears that in the chimp world, although
theft is quickly punished, the responder is insensitive to unfairness. Experiments
by Keith Jensen, Joseph Call, and other scientists at the Max Planck Institute for
Evolutionary Anthropology in Leipzig have shown that essentially when it comes
to raisins, chimpanzees are willing to accept just about any offer. Parenthetically,
it appears that it is not we humans who are the rational maximizers, as championed by neoclassical economists, seeking the greatest personal advantage in
every transaction, but rather our close cousins the chimpanzees. Keith Jensen,
Joseph Call, and Michael Tomasello, "Chimpanzees Are Rational Maximizers
in an Ultimatum Game," *Science* 318 (2007): 107–9; Keith Jensen, Joseph Call,
and Michael Tomasello, "Chimpanzees Are Vengeful But Not Spiteful," *Proceedings of the National Academy of Sciences* 104 (2007): 13046–50; and Ingrid Kai-
ser, Keith Jensen, Joseph Call, and Michael Tomasello, "Theft in an Ultimatum
Game: Chimpanzees and Bonobos Are Insensitive to Unfairness," *Royal Society of
Biology Letters* 10 (2012): 0519. A dissenting voice is that of Darby Proctor and her
colleagues of the Yerkes National Primate Center who reports that "humans and
chimpanzees show similar preferences in dividing rewards," Reply to Henrich and
Silk, *Proceedings of the National Academy of Sciences*, January 14, 2013.

157   **such habits help shape how we interpret:** Naomi Eisenberger and Matthew
Lieberman, "Why Rejection Hurts: A Common Neural Alarm System for Physical
and Social Pain," *Trends in Cognitive Sciences* 8 (2004): 294–300; and Matthew
D. Lieberman and Naomi I. Eisenberger, "Pains and Pleasures of Social Life," *Science* 323 (2009): 890–91. There is considerable overlap in the chemistry of pain
and pleasure. For example, the opiate morphine is used in medicine to reduce
physical pain, and genetically manipulating the brain's opioid reward system
reduces attachment behavior in blind, deaf, and hungry newborn mice. See Anna
Moles, Brigitte Kieffer, and Francesa D'Amato, "Deficit in Attachment Behavior
in Mice Lacking the μ-Opioid Receptor Gene," *Science* 304 (2004): 1983–86.

157   **the *emotional distress* of social rejection:** George Slavich et al., "Neural Sensitivity to Social Rejection Is Associated with Inflammatory Responses to Social
Stress," *Proceedings of the National Academy of Sciences* 107 (2010): 14817–22.

158   **In the Ultimatum Game, oxytocin . . . increases generous offers:** Paul J.
Zak, Angela A. Stanton, and Sheila Ahmadi, "Oxytocin Increases Generosity in
Humans," *PLoS ONE* 2 (2007).

158   **a diet low in tryptophan . . . decreases the acceptance rate of unfair
proposals:** Molly Crockett et al., "Serotonin Modulates Behavioral Reactions to
Unfairness," *Science* 320 (2008): 1739.

158   **The empathic virtues of fairness, patience, and compassion:** "Patience,
Fairness and the Human Condition," *Economist*, October 6, 2007.

160   **shaping social behavior . . . by mild and consistent rebuke:** Robert Boyd et
al., "The Evolution of Altruistic Punishment," *Proceedings of the National Academy of Sciences* 100 (2003): 3531–35.

160 **young children . . . make their wishes clear:** Lynne Murray and Liz Andrews, *The Social Baby: Understanding Babies' Communication from Birth* (UK: Children's Project, 2000). This book is a detailed and practical guide to understanding the first year of infant development and engaging with the newborn child.

160 **Substantial portions of the human brain . . . recognizing faces:** The discussion here is informed by these sources: Doris Tsao et al., "A Cortical Region Consisting Entirely of Face-Selective Cells," *Science* 311 (2006): 670–74; Andrew Meltzoff and Keith Moore, "Imitation of Facial and Manual Gestures by Human Neonates," *Science* 198 (1977): 75–78; "Your Mother's Smile," *Economist*, October 21, 2006; C. E. Parsons et al., "The Functional Neuroanatomy of the Evolving Parent-Infant Relationship," *Progress in Neurobiology* 91 (2010): 220–41; and Gill Peleg et al., "Hereditary Family Signature of Facial Expression," *Proceedings of the National Academy of Sciences* 103 (2006): 15921–26.

161 **mirror *neurons*:** For general summary, see, "A Mirror to the World: Empathy with Others Seems to Be Due to a Type of Brain Cell Called a Mirror Neuron," *Economist*, May 14, 2005; and Sandra Blakeslee, "Cells That Read Minds," *New York Times*, January 10, 2006. A key original study is G. Rizzolatti et al., "Premotor Cortex and the Recognition of Motor Actions," *Cognitive Brain Research* 3 (1996): 131–41. For a comprehensive scientific review, see Giacomo Rizzolatti and Liala Craighero, "The Motor-Neuron System," *Annual Review of Neuroscience* 27 (2004): 169–92; and Giacomo Rizzolatti, Maddalena Fabbri-Destro, and Luigi Cattaneo, "Motor Neurons and Their Clinical Relevance," *Nature Clinical Practice Neurology* 5 (2009): 24–34.

162 **the insula cortex helps modulate:** Laurie Carr et al., "Neural Mechanisms of Empathy in Humans: A Relay From Neural Systems of Imitation to Limbic Areas," *Proceedings of the National Academy of Sciences* 100 (2003): 5497–502.

164 **mirror neurons were relatively inactive in autistic children:** Mirella Dapretto et al., "Understanding Emotions in Others: Mirror Dysfunction in Children with Autism Spectrum Disorders," *Nature Neuroscience* 9 (2006): 28–30.

164 **it is through continuous social interaction that a child:** Leslie Brothers, *Friday's Footprint: How Society Shapes the Human Mind* (Oxford: Oxford University Press, 1997).

166 **risk-taking behaviors can rapidly escalate:** B. J. Casey, S. Getz, and A. Galvan, "The Adolescent Brain," *Developmental Review* 28 (2008): 62–77.

166 **meaningful family relationships can buffer adolescent risk-taking:** Eva Telzer et al., "Meaningful Family Relationships: Neurocognitive Buffers of Adolescent Risk Taking," *Journal of Cognitive Neuroscience* 25 (2013): 374–87. The development of strong family ties is independent of family income. Indeed there is some evidence that in high-earning families ($120,000 and above) the teenagers drink, smoke, and use more hard drugs than do typical high school students. Rates of anxiety and depression are particularly high in girls. See Suniya S. Luthar, "The Culture of Affluence: Psychological Costs of Material Wealth," *Child Development* 74 (2003): 1581–93. These and similar studies suggest that the key to adaptive development in the transition from latency to adolescence is the integration of the brain's orbitofrontal cortex and affective systems to effectively modulate emotion and behavior. J. H. Pfeifer et al., "Longitudinal Changes in Neural Responses to Emotional Expressions: Associations with Resistance to Peer influence and Risky Behavior During the Transition from Childhood to Adolescence," *Neuron* 69 (2011): 1029–36.

167   **an innovative classroom-based parenting program:** Mary Gordon, *Roots of Empathy: Changing the World Child by Child* (Toronto: Thomas Allen, 2005). For the original use of the term *moral imagination* in describing empathy, Gordon credits Thomas E. McCollough, *The Moral Imagination and Public Life* (Thousand Oaks, CA: CQ Press, 1991).

167   **as family structures fragment . . . consistency in human interaction is harder to find:** Jeanne Arnold et al., *Life at Home in the Twenty-First Century: 32 Families Open their Doors* (Los Angeles: Cotsen Institute Press, 2012).

168   **the computational demands of living in social groups:** Robin Dunbar, "Neocortex Size as a Constraint on Group Size in Primates," *Journal of Human Evolution* 20 (1992): 469–93.

169   **the new cortex . . . is 50 percent larger:** J. H. Stephan, H. Frahm, and G. Baron, "New and Revised Data on Volumes of Brain Structures in Insectivores and Primates," *Folia Primatologica* 35 (1981): 1–9.

169   **"Dunbar's number":** Robin Dunbar, "Co-evolution of Neocortex Size, Group Size and Language in Humans," *Behavioral and Brain Sciences* 16 (1993): 681–735.

170   **the larger the social network, the weaker are the ties:** Sam Roberts et al., "Exploring Variation in Active Network Size; Constraints and Ego Characteristics," *Social Networks* 31 (2009): 138–46; and Penelope Lewis et al., "Ventromedial Prefrontal Volume Predicts Understanding of Others and Social Network Size," *NeuroImage* 57 (2011): 1624–29.

172   **the gene FOXP2 in affected family members:** C. S. Lai et al., "A Forkhead-Domain Gene Is Mutated in a Severe Speech and Language Disorder," *Nature* 413 (2001): 519–23. FOXP2 is highly conserved in evolution; see W. Enard et al., "Molecular Evolution of FOXP2, a Gene Involved in Speech and Language," *Nature* 418 (2002): 869–72. There is a slight coding difference in humans that appears to have been shared with Neanderthals: Johannes Krause et al., "The Derived FOXP2 Variant of Modern Humans Was Shared with Neanderthals," *Current Biology* 17 (2007): 1–5; and "The Neanderthal Genome," *Economist*, May 8, 2010. But it was not shared with chimps: Genevieve Konopka, "Human-Specific Transcriptional Regulation of CNS Development Genes by FOXP2," *Nature* 462 (2009): 213–17.

173   **Chattering works well with many different chores:** "Chattering Classes: The Rules for Verbal Exchanges Are Surprisingly Enduring," *Economist*, December 23, 2006. Conversation is a sophisticated form of gossip. Honed to an art form in eighteenth-century France and in the coffeehouses of the Enlightenment in England, conversation is by definition an interaction. It is a game of language. Dale Carnegie with *How to Win Friends and Influence People* set down the ground rules: remember names, listen well, express genuine interest, smile, focus on the other individual not yourself, and make them feel important. For enthusiasts, conversation becomes one of the great pleasures of life and the basis for a civilized society.

173 **We call this new "grooming" behavior gossip:** Gregory Rodriguez, "A Community of Fans: Believe It or Not, Celebrity Gossip Can Be Good for You," *Los Angeles Times*, July 2, 2007. In July 2013 typing *Paris Hilton*, the name of the self-styled celebrity, into Google generated 199,800,000 hits in 0.21 seconds. Typing in the words *Queen Elizabeth* yielded 191,500,000 hits in 0.25 seconds, and that included both Elizabeth I and Elizabeth II. Is this a bad thing? Does a greater fascination with Paris Hilton, who has nothing but a hotel chain, money, and youth behind her, than with the Queens Elizabeth, who reflect the rich history of England, suggest that there is something sick about modern society? Not necessarily, argues Rodriguez: celebrity gossip may be good for us. In a survey of English schoolchildren, celebrity attachments appear to serve as pseudo-friends, discussions about whom served to strengthen interaction among real friends. For some young women the opportunity to indulge in celebrity gossip avoided otherwise awkward silences. Sports gossip seemed to play the same role for men.

173 **"little empirical evidence that women gossip more":** Eric K. Foster, "Research on Gossip: Taxonomy, Methods and Future Directions," *Review of General Psychology* 8 (2004): 78–99. This study, from the University of Pennsylvania, reminds me of the 1980s, when I too was teaching there. In those days the faculty club was a large and lively place—I'm sure it still is—and especially at lunchtime. The tables in the dining hall were round, some five feet across, and so closely packed that when the chatter in the room grew to its crescendo, it was impossible to hear the comments of those sitting across the same table. I remarked upon this one day, which brought much laughter from my senior colleagues. Professors, they explained, unlike psychiatrists, prefer to talk rather than listen. Thus it mattered little that the detail of the conversation at the table was lost in the cacophony, especially as the drift of the argument was usually clear. More important was the gossip of those persons sitting immediately behind one's chair, at a separate table. Thanks to the size and placement of the tables in the room, those discussions could be followed with ease, despite the noise. Eavesdropping at lunch was the perfect pastime for academics concerned with the gossip of the day.

173 **imagined, fixed systems of interrelationship:** Maurice Bloch, "Why Religion Is Nothing Special but Central," *Philosophical Transactions of the Royal Society: Biological Sciences* 363 (2008): 2055–61; and, Paul L. Harris, *The Work of the Imagination* (Hoboken, NJ: Wiley-Blackwell, 2000).

174 **"external" social conditions . . . "internal" biological processes:** George Slavich and Steven Cole, "The Emerging Field of Human Social Genomics," *Clinical Psychological Science* (January 2013), Cpx.sagepub.com.

Chapter 7: CHARACTER

176 **"A very young child has no self-command":** Adam Smith, *The Theory of Moral Sentiments* (1759; reprint edition Indianapolis: Liberty Classics, 1976), pt. 3, chap. 3.

176 **"A Clerk ther was of Oxenford":** Geoffrey Chaucer, *Canterbury Tales* (Norton Critical Edition, 2005), lines 287 and 310 of the General Prologue and the story of the Clerk. In modern English: "A clerk there was from Oxford who studied phi-losophy long ago . . . And gladly would he learn and gladly teach."

176   **"Now, what I want is facts":** Charles Dickens's *Hard Times* was first published in 1854 in serial form. Dickens's social criticism is focused on the utilitarian the-ory of Jeremy Bentham and James Mill—the greatest amount of happiness for the greatest number of people. Dickens believed this philosophy destroyed initiative, especially in working people oppressed by the Industrial Revolution.

178   **Organization for Economic Cooperation and Development (OECD):** For a review, see "The Great Schools Revolution: Dresden, New York and Wroclaw," *Economist*, September 17, 2011. While the United States as a whole performs comparatively poorly, there is considerable spread across individual states. For details of this performance and a discussion of the international rankings of *indi-vidual* states in the United States, see Catherine Gewertz, "In Math, Science, Most States Surpass the Global Average," *Education Week* 33 (2013): 6.

179   **the international consulting firm of McKinsey:** "How the World's Best Performing Schools Come Out on Top," *McKinsey on Society*, September 2007, http://bit.ly/1oJ18Hc. For a summary see "How to Be Top. What Works in Educa-tion: The Lessons According to Mckinsey," *Economist*, October 20, 2007.

179   **Finland . . . an exemplar:** Anu Partanen, "What Americans Keep Ignoring About Finland's School Success," *Atlantic*, December 2011.

180   **equitable distribution of opportunity for all students:** Pasi Sahlberg, *Finn-ish Lessons: What Can the World Learn From Educational Change in Finland?* (New York: Teachers College Press, 2011).

181   **decentralization, choice, and interschool competition:** National Assess-ment of Educational Progress, *America's Charter Schools: Results from the NAEP 2003 Pilot Study* (2006).

181   **student-to-teacher ratios:** Eric Hanushek, *The Evidence on Class Size* (Roch-ester, NY: W. Allen Wallis Institute of Political Economy, 1998); S. M. Shapson et al., "An Experimental Study on the Effects of Class Size," *American Educational Research Journal* (1980): 141–52; Karen Akerhielm, "Does Class Size Matter?" *Economics of Education Review* (1995): 229–41; and Alan B. Krueger, "Economic Considerations and Class Size," *Economics Journal* (2003): F34–F63.

183   **America's promotion of mass education:** Claudia Goldin, "Exploring the Present Through the Past: Claudia Goldin on Human Capital, Gender and the Lessons from History," *World Economics* 8 (2007): 61–124.

183   **"Education Slowdown Threatens US":** David Wessel and Stephanie Ban-chero, "Education Slowdown Threatens US," *Wall Street Journal*, April 26, 2012.

184   **the cost of college education in America:** "Higher Education: Not What It Used to Be," *Economist*, December 11, 2012; Tamar Lewin, "College May Become Unaffordable for Most in US," *New York Times*, December 3, 2008; "How to Make College Cheaper," *Economist*, July 9, 2011; "Student Loans: College on Credit," *Economist*, January 10, 2009; Jordan Weissmann, "How Colleges Are Selling Out the Poor to Court the Rich," *Atlantic*, May 2013.

184   **falling behind in the development of a . . . broadly educated citizenry:** J. H. Pryor et al., *The American Freshman: National Norms Fall 2012*, Higher Education Research Institute, UCLA, http://www.heri.ucla.edu; Lois Romano,

"Literacy of College Graduates Is on the Decline," *Washington Post*, December 25, 2005. For the complete report see *The Literacy of America's College Students*, American Institutes for Research, Report 636, 2006, http://bit.ly/1pNMsEh.

185 **"parents and students no longer choose the best education":** James Engell and Anthony Dangerfield, *Saving Higher Education in the Age of Money* (Charlottesville: University of Virginia Press, 2005). Not only in the United States is the cost of a university education rising rapidly. In an effort to contain costs Britain, a leader with America in higher education, has introduced market concepts in the evaluation of academic productivity and "top-up" fees for domestic students such that the cost of attending university will soon be comparable to that of the United States. See Simon Head, "The Grim Threat to British Universities," *New York Review of Books*, January 13, 2011; "Paying for University: Tinkering with the Ivories," *Economist*, July 2, 2011; and "Foreign University Students: Will They Come?" *Economist*, August 7, 2010.

186 **buying an education is different from buying a refrigerator:** Peter C. Whybrow, "My, My, Haven't We Grown?" *Times Higher Education*, January 6, 2006.

186 **the primary social role of the university:** John Maynard Keynes quoted in Keith Thomas, "What Are Universities For?" *Times Literary Supplement*, May 7, 2010.

190 **universal access to secondary education:** Daniel Tanner, "The Comprehensive High School in American Education," *Educational Leadership* (May 1982): 606–13.

191 **The physical learning environment also was changing:** *An Honor and an Ornament: Public School Buildings in Michigan*, Michigan Department of History, Arts and Libraries, September 2003.

192 **something was seriously amiss:** National Commission on Excellence in Education, *A Nation at Risk: The Imperative for Educational Reform* (1983), http://bit.ly/1fzyocj.

192 **Britain's effort toward comprehensive schooling:** OECD, *Equity and Quality in Education: Supporting Disadvantaged Students and Schools* (OECD Publishing, 2012), http://dx.doi.org/10.1787/9789264130852-en. See also Graeme Paton, "OECD: Fifth of British Teenagers 'Drop Out of School at 16,' " *Daily Telegraph*, February 9, 2012.

193 **privately schooled:** "Private Education: Is It Worth It?" *Economist*, March 1, 2008. See also "Staying on Board: In Both Britain and America Recession Has Done Little to Dent the Demand for Private Education," *Economist*, July 4, 2009.

193 **mobility between the social classes:** "Like Father, Not like Son: Measuring Social Mobility," *Economist*, October 13, 2012.

196 **The Pact:** Sampson Davis et al., *The Pact: Three Young Men Make a Promise and Fulfill a Dream* (New York: Riverhead Books, 2003).

197 **The Seven Habits:** Steven R. Covey, *The Seven Habits of Highly Effective People: Powerful Lessons in Personal Change,* rev. ed. (New York: Free Press, 2004).

198 **In Germany . . . more than 40 percent become apprentices:** Edward Luce, "Why the US Is Looking to Germany for Answers," *Financial Times*, April 15, 2013; and Eric Westervelt, "The Secret to Germany's Low Youth Unemployment," National Public Radio, April 4, 2012, http://n.pr/1lUu6hg.

199 **It's a lost opportunity:** Clive R. Belfield, Henry M. Levin, and Rachel Rosen, *The Economic Value of Opportunity Youth* (Civic Enterprises and W. K. Kellogg Foundation, 2012), http://bit.ly/XhmoIu.

199 **rolling the rock up the hill:** Albert Camus, *The Myth of Sisyphus* (1942; reprint edition New York: Penguin Modern Classics, 2000).

200 **"by factors determined by the age of 18":** James Heckman, "Schools, Skills and Synapses," *Economic Inquiry, Western Economic Association International* 46 (2008): 289–324.

200 **America's "testing mania":** "The Trouble with Testing Mania," *New York Times*, July 14, 2013. In 2001, in response to declining international performance on student testing, the U.S. Congress passed the No Child Left Behind Act, designed to hold schools accountable for yearly tests administered in exchange for federal aid to education. Previous studies had shown some acceleration and student performance especially when linked to teacher ability, but unfortunately the demand for testing in many instances drove schools away from good teaching to essentially focus upon teaching to the test and in some instances even committing fraud as in Atlanta. Michael Winerip, "Ex-schools Chief in Atlanta Is Indicted in Testing Scandal," *New York Times*, March 29, 2013. Also unfortunately the multiple choice tests employed do not test reasoning skills, which are much better determined by open-ended essays. Most of the high-ranking nations in the PISA surveys have not chosen to implement repeated standardized testing. In contrast, the United States has fallen victim to prescription formats that purport to provide fundamental rules for success. The facts are to the contrary: it is what we learn from each other—trust, curiosity, craft, and social skills—that is important in determining personal and economic achievement.

200 **the public school system . . . local property taxes:** "Editorial: Why Other Countries Teach Better," *New York Times*, December 17, 2013.

201 **The charter school movement:** Diane Ravitch, "The Myth of Charter Schools" (review of the film *Waiting for Superman* directed by Davis Guggenheim), *New York Review of Books*, November 11, 2010; "Charting a Better Course," *Economist*, July 7, 2012; U.S. Department of Education, National Center for Education Statistics, *The Condition of Education 2013*, NCES 2013–037, Charter School Enrollment.

201 **in Britain the recently championed "academies":** For general articles regarding changes in the British school system, see "Transforming British Schools: A Classroom Revolution," *Economist*, April 24, 2010; "Bagehot: Lessons from a Great School," *Economist*, February 4, 2012; Sian Griffiths, "Me and My 350 Schools," *Sunday Times* (London), February 21, 2010.

202 **Research into the achievements of the charter program is patchy:** See Center for Research on Education Outcomes (CREDO), *Multiple Choice: Charter School Performance in 16 States*, June 2009; and CREDO, *National Charter School Study, 2013*, 2013, http://credo.stanford.edu.

202 **the KIPP movement:** David Levin and Michael Feinberg established the nonprofit Knowledge is Power Program (KIPP) in 1994, in New York and Houston respectively. They were inspired by a two-year stint in the Federal program Teach for America. KIPP has now grown into America's largest nationwide charter program with (in 2013) 141 schools in twenty states and the District of Columbia, serving 50,000 students, 86 percent of whom come from low-income families. KIPP's website is http://kipp.org.

202 **the classic work on delayed gratification:** W. Mischel, Y. Shoda, and M. L. Rodriguez, "Delay of Gratification in Children," *Science* 244 (1989): 933–38. For a lucid and accessible update of Mischel's research over the years and its employment in the school setting, see Jonah Lehrer, "Don't!: The Secret of Self Control," *New Yorker*, May 18, 2009.

204 **brain regions mature differentially:** B. J. Casey, R. M. Jones, and T. A. Hare, "The Adolescent Brain," *Annals of the New York Academy of Sciences* 1124 (2008): 111–26; A. Galvan et al., "Earlier Development of the Accumbens Relative to Orbitofrontal Cortex Might Underlie Risk-Taking Behavior in Adolescents," *Journal of Neuroscience* 26 (2006): 6885–92; B. J. Casey et al., "Behavioral and Neural Correlates of Delay of Gratification 40 Years Later," *Proceedings of the National Academy of Sciences* 108 (2001): 14998–5003; and W. Mischel et al., "Willpower over the Life Span: Decomposing Self-Regulation," *Social Cognitive and Affective Neuroscience* 6 (2001): 252–56.

206 **experienced teachers have a significant "value-added":** Raj Chetty, John N. Friedman, and Jonah E. Rockoff, "The Long-Term Impacts of Teachers: Teacher Value-Added and Student Outcomes in Adulthood," National Bureau of Economic Research, Working Paper no. 17699, December 2011; and Chetty, Friedman, and Rockoff, "Measuring the Impacts of Teachers I: Evaluating Bias in Teacher Value-Added Estimates," NBER Working Paper no. 19423, September 2013. For a summary, see "Free Exchange: Knowledge for Earnings' Sake," *Economist*, October 12, 2013.

206 **character:** A useful, although simplistic, aid to memory—and a differentiation prevalent in the older psychology literature—is that *character* reflects acquired, predominantly intuitive behaviors. This is in contrast to *temperament*, which is considered an inherited emotional style already evident in infancy. The *personality* of an individual is then the sum of these two behavioral elements. For further explanation, see Peter C. Whybrow, Hagop S. Akiskal, and William T. McKinney, Jr., *Mood Disorders: Toward a New Psychobiology* (New York: Plenum Press, 1984), p. 185.

206 **intuitive *ethics*:** Jonathan Haidt and Selin Kesebir, "Morality," in S. Fiske, D. Gilbert, and G. Lindsey, eds., *Handbook of Social Psychology*, 5th ed. (Hoboken, NJ: Wiley and Sons, 2010), vol. 1.

207 **structural and cultural supports provided to young households:** Olga Khazan, "The Countries Where Women Have the Best Lives, in Charts," *Atlantic*, March 2013.

207 **the commercialization of children's lives:** Juliet Schor, "America's Most Wanted: Inside the World of Young Consumers," *Boston College Magazine*, Fall 2004; Juliet Schor, *Born to Buy* (New York: Scribner, 2004); L. M. Powell, J. L. Harris, and T. Fox, "Food Marketing Expenditures Aimed at Youth: Putting the Numbers in Context," *American Journal of Preventive Medicine* 45 (2013): 453–61; and Anup Shah, "Children as Consumers," Global Issues, 2010, http://bit.ly/1AdLyFN.

208 **we have been overindulging our children:** For a review of books focused on the dangers of overindulgence in childhood, see Elizabeth Kolbert, "Spoiled Rotten: Why Do Kids Rule the Roost?" *New Yorker*, July 12, 2012; and Judith Warner, "Kids Gone Wild," *New York Times*, November 27, 2005.

208 **the educational calendar:** "The Underworked American," *Economist*, June 15, 2009.

208 **material indulgence:** Suniya Luthar and Shawn Latendresse, "Children of Affluence: Challenges to Well-Being," *Current Directions in Psychological Science* 14 (2005): 49–53.

209 **social manners, patience, and self-control . . . rare American qualities:** Richard Reeves, "A Question of Character," *Prospect*, August 2008.

Chapter 8: HABITAT

210 **"The more living patterns there are":** Christopher Alexander, *The Timeless Way of Building* (New York: Oxford University Press, 1979), epigraphs to chaps. 1 and 7.

210 **The small Italian town of Sabbioneta:** Sabbioneta was designated a UNESCO World Heritage Site in 2008 as an exceptional testimony to Renaissance urban planning; http://whc.unesco.org/en/list/1287. Much has been written about the architecture of Sabbioneta, but a good beginning is the carefully prepared official guide, Umberto Maffezzoli, *Sabbioneta: guida alla visita della città* (Il Bulino: Edizioni d'arte, 1992). See also Andrew Mead, "Cracking the Code of the Ideal City," *Architectural Review*, September 21, 2011. For an offbeat but in-depth study of the city and the mind of its creator, Vespasiano Gonzaga, see James Madge, *Sabbioneta, Cryptic City* (London: Bibliotheque McLean, 2011).

211 **The Gonzaga family, known for their horse breeding:** The Gonzaga family and the city of Mantua played a significant role in the feuds and infighting that gripped Renaissance Italy for over two centuries. For an engaging read on the excesses and the cultural achievements of this era, see Kate Simon, *Renaissance Tapestry: The Gonzaga of Mantua* (New York: Harper & Row, 1988). The Gonzagas were essentially mercenaries or *condottieri*—literally "contractors"—who provided military services for a fee. The employment of private militia was the norm in Renaissance Italy. Venice in its long fight with the Ottoman Empire was one of the first city-states to engage a mercenary garrison, and several leaders of the Gonzagas provided military service to that city. The practice existed throughout Europe and particularly in northern Italy as the Habsburgs and other powerful groups sought to control the Italian peninsula. Vespasiano Gonzaga, from a minor branch of the Gonzaga family, was a classical example of someone who prospered as a mercenary. Educated in the Spanish royal court from the age of eleven, he benefited from military and diplomatic service to Philip II and later received contracts from the Habsburgs, which together with the land inherited and acquired by marriage led to his wealth. See David Parrott, *The Business of War: Military Enterprise and Military Revolution in Early Modern Europe* (Cambridge, UK: Cambridge University Press, 2012).

212   **the techniques of ancient Roman urban design:** Jan Pieper, *Sabbioneta: The Measuring Shape of an Ideal City* (2012), http://bit.ly/XhoWGx. In this fascinating report Pieper, from the faculty of architecture at the University of Aachen, analyzes the floor plan of Sabbioneta employing Roman techniques, which traditionally lay out the street map by working backward from the outer square or rectangle of walled city. The town plan is further oriented astronomically, along the axis of the sun's rising on the birthday of the founder, Vespasiano Gonzaga, which was December 6.

213   **the Venetian architect Andrea Palladio:** Bruce Boucher, *Andrea Palladio: The Architect in His Time* (New York: Abbeville Press, 1998).

216   **the old New Hampshire farmhouse:** Henry L. Williams and Ottalie K. Williams, *Old American Houses 1700–1850* (New York: Bonanza Books, 1967).

219   **Christopher Alexander, a celebrated architect:** Alexander is a maverick in the world of architecture. Born in Vienna in 1936, he grew up in England, studied mathematics at Trinity College Cambridge, and then migrated to the United States in 1958. After completing a Ph.D. in architecture at Harvard, he remained on the faculty working on cognition, then moved to Berkeley in 1963, where he taught for some thirty years. Fundamental to his work and writing is that people can and should design for themselves. This idea stems from Alexander's observation that most of the beautiful places in the world are not constructed by architects but have evolved from the day-to-day activity of the individuals living and working there. This truth applies not only to the buildings themselves but also to the details of their internal structure.

Take, for example, the design of a welcoming window seat. Close your eyes and concentrate on the images you remember. Make them live. The entering light, the shape of the window itself, the seat; use the power of imagination to call up scenes from memory. This provides the "pattern language." Keep it simple. Most important, instructs Alexander, is that once it is conceptualized in the mind, the window seat can be drawn, and if it can be drawn, it can be built. This is the "timeless way of building."

Alexander is best known for the trilogy based upon pattern language that was published by Oxford University Press in the 1970s: *A Pattern Language* (1977), *The Timeless Way of Building* (1979), and *The Oregon Experiment* (1975), which describes how Alexander and his colleagues at the Center for Environmental Structure at Berkeley developed and implemented a master plan for the University of Oregon.

220   **Jane Jacobs, the American-born Canadian activist:** Like Christopher Alexander, Jane Jacobs (1916–2006) believed in the power of people to create their own habitat. See Jacobs, "Downtown Is for People," *Fortune Magazine*, April 1958, and Jacobs, *The Life and Death of Great American Cities* (1961; reprint edition New York: Modern Library, 2011), in which she defends the organic growth of the city and offers a powerful critique of the urban renewal concepts of the 1950s. She was particularly opposed to downtown expressways that sliced through tightly knit neighborhoods and was influential in the cancellation of the Lower Manhattan Expressway in New York. When problems of suburban sprawl are considered in the context of urban planning, many of her arguments remain valid today. For a succinct review of Jacobs's influence, see Penny Lewis, "Salvation by Brick," in

Dave Clements et al., eds., *The Future of Community: Reports of a Death Greatly Exaggerated* (London: Pluto Press, 2008).

221 William Whyte, sociologist: Whyte (1917–99) believed in the sanctity and preservation of public space and was indirectly responsible for the establishment of the Project for Public Spaces, a "nonprofit planning, design and educational organization dedicated to helping people create and sustain public spaces that build stronger communities." The website is http://www.pps.org/. See William H. Whyte, *The Social Life of Small Urban Spaces* (1980; reprint edition Project for Public Spaces, 2001).

222 Los Angeles had the longest streetcar network: Robert C. Post, *Street Railways and the Growth of Los Angeles* (San Marino, CA: Golden West Books, 1989).

222 Los Angeles . . . totally dependent on the automobile: *Pavement Paradise: American Parking Space* (Culver City, CA: Center for Land Use Interpretation, 2007).

222 average commuting time on weekdays: Tom Tom, *North American Congestion Index 2012*. Tom Tom, a European company founded in 1991, focuses on developing software products for mobile devices including route planners and navigation devices. Its website is http://corporate.tomtom.com.

223 Victor Gruen, the architect who designed Valencia: For an interesting profile of Victor Gruen and his legacy, see Andy Logan and Brendan Gill, "Talk of the Town: New City," *New Yorker*, March 17, 1956; and Malcolm Gladwell, "Annals of Commerce: The Terrazzo Jungle," *New Yorker*, March 15, 2004.

223 Valencia has done well: See "America's Suburbs: An Age of Transformation," *Economist*, May 31, 2008; on housing market trends there in 2014, see the town's website, Valencia.com, as well as Trulia.com (accessed May 2014).

224 times are changing [in suburban America]: Christopher B. Leinberger, "The Next Slum: The Subprime Crisis Is Just the Tip of the Iceberg," *Atlantic*, March 2008; Hudson Sangree and Phillip Reese, "County Homeownership at Lowest Level Since '70s," *Sacramento Bee*, May 12, 2014.

224 areas that necessitate a long commute: "Median home prices across the nation continue to decline, but some experts are noting a link between falling house prices and commuting distances. Suburbs where commuters drive an hour or more to work are seeing some of the sharpest drops in prices." Kathleen Schalch, "Home Prices Drop Most in Areas with Long Commute," National Public Radio, April 21, 2008.

225 the shopping mall and suburban living: "Birth, Death and Shopping: The Rise and Fall of the Shopping Mall," *Economist*, December 22, 2007; and Christopher B. Leinberger, "Here Comes the Neighborhood," *Atlantic*, June 2010. Comparison statistics on retail space are from "Planet Money: Most Mall Space? That Would Be Us," National Public Radio, February 20, 2009; and "The United States Has Too Many Stores," Motley Fool, June 15, 2009, http://bit.ly/Y4LwCc.

225 for the automobile . . . the bloom is also off the rose: "Editorial: The Road Less Traveled: Car Use Is Peaking In the Rich World," and "Briefing: The Future of Driving. Seeing the Back of the Car," both in *Economist*, September 22, 2012. For a discussion of the shift in the purchasing preferences of twenty-to-thirty-year-old Americans, see Derek Thompson and Jordan Weissmann, "The Cheapest Generation: Why Millennials Aren't Buying Cars or Houses and What That Means for the Economy," *Atlantic*, September 2012.

226   **the technological challenges to achieving a sustainable . . . future:** These data are taken from a report from the Siemens Company, "Smarter Neighborhoods, Smarter City," 2012, http://bit.ly/1usgZM0.

226   **Portland, Oregon, is the poster child:** "The New Model: Portland and 'Elite Cities,' " *Economist*, April 15, 2010.

230   **La Fromagerie:** As Patricia Michelson tells the story, she first became enamored of cheese while on a skiing holiday in France. Subsequently, selling Beaufort Chalet d'Alpage and other cheeses out of her garden shed in Highbury, London, she found that the neighbors were also enthusiastic. The next step was to open a cheese shop, in 1992. Teaching herself the fine art of cheese husbandry, Patricia began selling carefully sourced artisan cheeses from around Europe and from England and Wales. But more than that she became interested in the subtle skill of maturing and caring for cheeses, including rare and unusual varieties. Ten years later there was a second store in Marylebone. Her prize-winning books, *The Cheese Room* (2001) and *Cheese* (2010), have secured her reputation as a leading aficionado. See her website http://www.lafromagerie.co.uk.

230   **Howard de Walden Estates:** Three hundred years ago London was essentially what is now Westminster, and it was crowded. After the plague of 1666 and the Great Fire a year later, there was pressure for expansion. Aristocratic property owners began developing their farmland estates around the capital through a leasehold mechanism whereby they leased their land to builders and speculators for ninety-nine years. The leaseholder collected the rents on the properties that they built, but the family estate retained the title to the land and had oversight regarding the style and function of the buildings constructed on it. That system remains in place and, politics aside, has provided unusual stability, character, and consistency to the development of the several districts that in aggregate are now considered "central" London.

231   **a sustainability that is timeless:** Tony McGuirk, "My Kind of Town: Marylebone, London," *Architecture Today*, July 2, 2008.

233   **obesity epidemic [in UK]:** "NHS Choices: Latest Obesity Stats for England Are Alarming" (2013), Child and Maternal Health Intelligence Network, Public Health England, http://bit.ly/1AdTGpG.

233   **an urban environment that encourages physical activity:** Thomas Eitler, Edward McMahon, and Theodore Thoerig, *Ten Principles for Building Healthy Places* (Washington, DC: Urban Land Institute, 2013). For the Piano Staircase, see http://www.thefuntheory.com/piano-staircase.

233   **revitalizing our relationship with the food we eat and where it comes from:** See Karen Franck, ed., *Food and the City* (Fletcher, NC: Academy Press, 2005).

234   **the Natural Kitchen is the partnership:** The Natural Kitchen is located at 77-78 Marylebone High Street, London, W1U 5JX.

Chapter 9: FOOD

235 **"Husbandry is, with great justice, placed":** *The Complete Farmer, or a General Dictionary of Husbandry in All Its Branches,* was published in London in 1777 by "a society of gentlemen" devoted to the "encouragement of arts, manufacturers and commerce." The quotation is taken from the preface, entitled the "advertisement" of the book. This extraordinary compendium is a dictionary of agricultural practice in the late eighteenth century "delivered in the plainest and most intelligent manner, and enriched with all the discoveries hitherto made in any part of Europe." It stands as an unusual reminder of what was once common practice, but is now largely beyond public awareness, in "the art of tilling, manuring, and cultivating the earth, in order to render it fertile" within the natural cycle of the seasons.

235 **"Agriculture is surely the most important":** Colin Tudge is a British science writer and broadcaster. This quotation is from Tudge's review of Paul McMahon's *Feeding Frenzy: The New Politics of Food* (London: Profile Books, 2013). See also Colin Tudge, *So Shall We Reap: What's Gone Wrong with the World's Food—And How to Fix It* (London: Penguin Books, 2004).

236 **it is in *the cooking of food* that we are truly distinct:** Richard Wrangham, *Catching Fire: How Cooking Made Us Human* (New York: Basic Books, 2010); and "What's Cooking?" *Economist,* February 21, 2009. Cooking is a uniquely human attribute. No society is without it. Indeed, it can be argued that the human brain, consuming as it does 25 percent of the body's energy, would be difficult to keep supplied without cooking to provide nutrients in easily digestible form.

236 **"Food is culture":** Massimo Montanari, *Food Is Culture,* trans. Albert Sonnenfeld (New York: Columbia University Press, 2006).

237 **Food production . . . has become industrialized:** Barbara Farfan, "World's Largest Supermarkets and Groceries, 2013," About.com, http://abt.cm/1nPmjkl. In 2013 global food retail sales were more than $4 trillion annually, according to the U.S. Department of Agriculture. See also Stephen Leeb, "Wal-Mart Fattens Up on Poor America with 25% of U.S. Grocery Sales," *Forbes,* May 20, 2013, http://onforb.es/1yw3U21.

237 **divorced from the natural ecology:** Paul Levy, "Good Enough for the Welsh," *Times Literary Supplement,* November 9, 2007 (a review of Joan Thirsk's *Food in Early Modern England, Phases, Fads, Fashions 1500–1760*).

238 **"ushered a new creature onto the world stage":** Michael Pollan, *In Defense of Food: An Eater's Manifesto* (New York: Penguin Books, 2008); Jason Epstein, "A New Way to Think About Eating," *New York Review of Books,* March 20, 2008; and Michael Pollan, "Farmer in Chief: What the Next President Can and Should Do to Remake the Way We Grow and Eat Our Food," *New York Times Magazine,* October 12, 2008.

238 **Americans have taken a renewed interest in what they are eating:** C. M. Hasler, "The Changing Face of Functional Foods," *Journal of the American College of Nutrition* 19, supp. 5 (2000): 499–506.

239 **cooking of food has become . . . popular sport:** "Does a trend signify a movement, even a revolution?" asks Jane Handel, the editor of *Edible Ojai,* one

of a network of magazines "to celebrate local foods, season by season." See "Editor's Note," *Edible Ojai*, Spring 2008, http://bit.ly/1l38PHf. Edward Behr's maverick quarterly publication *The Art of Eating* has achieved a similarly vaunted reputation. See Joshua Chaffin, "No Artificial Sweeteners," *Financial Times Weekend*, January 11, 2009. Over the same decade a flood of popular books extolled good food; see Joline Godfrey, "Armchair Feast: A Celebration of Books, Articles and Stories About Food and Agriculture," *Edible Ojai*, Spring 2008. Among the celebrity chefs, Britain's Jamie Oliver (of the *Naked Chef* book and television series) has been one of the more provocative, striving to improve unhealthy diets in the U.K. and the United States.

239 the Slow Food movement: In 2008 the Slow Food Movement had 85,000 interconnected member groups in 132 countries. See its website at http://www.slowfood.com.

240 the color and taste of fruits: H. Martin Schaefer, K. McGraw, and C. Catoni, "Birds Use Fruit Color as Honest Signal of Dietary Antioxidant Rewards," *Functional Ecology* 22 (2008): 303–10.

241 diet . . . combating the recurrence of illness: P. Greenwald, C. K. Clifford, and J. A. Milner, "Diet and Cancer Prevention," *European Journal of Cancer* 37 (2001): 948–65. There are large international differences in the incidence of many cancers, and epidemiological studies suggest that diet plays its part. The exact molecular mechanisms through which protection or vulnerability is induced, however, have yet to be specifically defined in human studies. See Marjorie L. McCoullough and Edward L Giovannucci, "Diet and Cancer Prevention," *Oncogene* 23 (2004): 6349–64; and D. W. Dawson et al., "High-Calorie, High-Fat Diet Promotes Pancreatic Neoplasia in the Conditional KrasG12D Mouse Model," *Cancer Prevention Research* 6 (2013): 1064–73.

241 agriculture . . . ushered in profound changes in what we eat: Tom Standage, *An Edible History of Humanity* (New York: Walker & Co., 2009).

242 the story of lactose: Nabil Sabri Enattah et al., "Identification of a Variant Associated with Adult-Type Hypolactasia," *Nature Genetics* 30 (2002): 233–37. The findings support the theory that originally all humans, beyond infancy, were lactose intolerant and that the ability to drink milk as an adult is related to a genetic variation that permits continued production of the lactase enzyme. Without this specific enzyme, the lactose in milk passes through the stomach undigested and is acted upon by bacteria in the large intestine, producing the bloating and gaseous sensation well known to those who are lactose intolerant.

243 our postindustrial diet: Loren Cordain et al., "Origins and Evolution of the Western Diet: Health Implications for the 21st Century," *American Journal of Clinical Nutrition* 81 (2005): 341–54. Growing evidence suggests that high-fructose corn syrup, which is prominent in soft drinks and in processed foods, may play a significant role in the development of obesity and type 2 diabetes, in that the body metabolizes it differently from glucose and may lead to fat accumulation in the liver and ultimately greater blood lipid levels. See Costas Lyssiotis and Lewis Cantley, "F Stands for Fructose and Fat," *Nature* 502 (2013): 181–82.

243 links between the growth patterns of a city and how it eats: Carolyn Steel, *Hungry City: How Food Shapes Our Lives* (London: Random House UK, 2009). In this fascinating history Steel covers the birth of agriculture in the Fertile Crescent and the development of domesticated grains before turning to the contrast between the city-based civilization of Rome and the invading Gothic hordes. The lesson to be learned from this clash of cultures is that historically there are different ways of securing a food supply. In Athens many owned farms beyond the gates of the city, and similarly in Rome the cultivated land surrounding the densely populated areas were considered equally important to the city itself. But away from the Mediterranean, Europe was still covered in dense forest. The Germanic tribes lived by hunting and fishing and pasturing horses, cows, and pigs in the forest. The greater part of their diet consisted of milk, cheese, and flesh—a life that seemed uncivilized to the organized Roman mind.

But in its time Rome became an aberration, a city of perhaps a million people heavily dependent on grain supplies from conquered territories. After Rome's fall, urban civilization declined, and hunting cultures restored the concept of forest as privileged territory. It was the beginning of feudalism, where typically the lands around the villages and towns were owned by a feudal lord and worked by peasants. Urban civilization began to make a comeback during the Renaissance. Self-sufficient communities with protective walls and market gardens became the template for a new type of city. Such fortified communities developed in Europe and still can be seen in parts of Tuscany with city and country in harmony. As Steel comments, "Look after your countryside, and it will look after you." For a concise overview of her work and thinking, see her TEDxDanubia 2011 talk at http://www.youtube.com/watch?v=aLOHsc86Ikc.

244 **"The great commerce of every civilized society":** Adam Smith, *The Wealth of Nations* (1776; reprint edition New York: Random House, Modern Library, 1994), bk. 3, chap. 1.

246 **pioneering contributions to agricultural science:** For general discussion, see Felipe Fernandez-Armesto, *Near a Thousand Tables: A History of Food* (New York: Free Press, 2002), particularly chap. 8; V. Smil, *Enriching the Earth: Fritz Haber, Carl Bosch and the Transformation of World Food Production* (Cambridge, MA: MIT Press, 2001); and Jan Willem Erisman et al., "How a Century of Ammonia Synthesis Changed the World," *Nature Geoscience* 1 (2008): 636–39.

246 **an American agronomist:** Norman Borlaug (1914–2009) was born into a Norwegian farming family in Iowa. As a young man during the Depression, he visited Minneapolis where he was disturbed by the soup kitchens and the hunger he witnessed. First devoting himself to a better understanding of plant disease, he began breeding new seed varieties to achieve higher yields, first in Mexico and later across the world. He died in 2009 at ninety-five. See his obituary, "Norman Borlaug, Feeder of the World," *Economist*, September 19, 2009.

247 **Lady Eve Balfour here in Britain:** Eve B. Balfour, *The Living Soil* (London: Faber & Faber, 1943). Eve Balfour (1899–1990) was a key figure in creating the organic gardening and farming movement and one of the founders of Britain's Soil Association. In a classic experiment, she divided the land of her estate at Haughley in Suffolk, England, into two sections: one was farmed "organically" and the other "conventionally" with chemical fertilizers. *The Living Soil* records the results and her insights regarding the Haughley experiment. "The health of soil, plant, animal and man is one and indivisible," she asserted. Throughout her life she practiced what she preached and died at ninety-one.

247   the destructive use of DDT: Rachel Carson, *Silent Spring* (Boston: Houghton Mifflin, 1962). Rachel Carson (1907–64) was an aquatic biologist who turned her attention to environmental conservation and to the dangers of synthetic pesticides in the 1950s. Many of these chemicals had been developed during World War II and had come into common use in the postwar period as weed control agents, particularly DDT. Carson spent several years documenting the environmental damage of these products and their potential danger to human health and to the food chain. Although initially bitterly opposed by the chemical industry, Carson's work ultimately led in 1970 to the establishment of the U.S. Environmental Protection Agency.

248   the Punjab, the cradle of India's "green" revolution: "Punjab Heading for Water Crisis," *Times of India*, June 20, 2012.

248   the Great High Plains Aquifer: Michael Wines, "Wells Dry, Fertile Plains Turn to Dust," *New York Times*, May 19, 2013; and Dan Charles, "Kansas Farmers Commit to Taking Less Water from the Ground," National Public Radio, October 21, 2013. China has an even worse challenge; see "Water: All Dried Up," *Economist*, October 12, 2013. In response farmers are beginning to consider ancient grains untouched by factory agricultural practice, including sorghum: this staple crop in the dry lands of Africa demands less water but is hardy and nutritious. L. Dykes and Lloyd W. Rooney, "Sorghum and Millet Phenols and Antioxidants," *Journal of Cereal Science* 44 (2006): 236–51.

249   a system both expensive and wasteful: There is massive confusion in the pricing of food, with a market distorted in part by government subsidy and other inducements. For a window into that confusion, see "The End of Cheap Food," *Economist*, December 8, 2007. See also Tristram Stuart, "No Appetite for Waste," *Financial Times Magazine*, July 4–5, 2009. An English writer, environmentalist, and campaigner, Stuart writes about waste in Britain. In the United States it is estimated that 8 to 10 percent of "perishable" goods are discarded, which means that each year retailers dump food worth about $20 billion: another $28 billion worth is thrown out by American households and restaurants. See "Shrink Rapped: America's Food Retailers Should Wage a Tougher War on Waste," *Economist*, May 17, 2008.

250   What is needed is a third way: "The 9 Billion-People Question: A Special Report on Feeding the World," *Economist*, February 26, 2011; and Sarah Murray, "Business and Food Sustainability: How to Feed People and Save the Planet," *Financial Times Special Report*, January 27, 2010.

251   a new documentary: *Ground Operations: Battlefields to Farmfields* (2012), a film produced by Dulanie Ellis, www.facebook.com/GroundOperations.

252   Farmer Veteran Coalition: Casey Simons, "Helping Veterans, Helping Farmers: Michael O'Gorman's Farmer-Veteran Project," *Food First: Institute for Food and Development Policy*, July 23, 2012, www.foodfirst.org.

253   Production is increasingly concentrated in the industrialized sector: U.S. Environmental Protection Agency, "Ag 101: Demographics," www.epa.gov/agriculture/ag101/demographics.html.

254   **the aggressive promotion of novel farming practices:** "Lexington: Farming as Rocket Science," *Economist*, September 7, 2013.

255   **30 percent of shoppers will . . . purchase local products:** Cynthia Pansing et al., *Changing Tastes: Urban Sustainability Directors Network* (Arlington, VA: Wallace Center at Winrock International, 2013); Jerry Hirsch, "Natural Selection Among Grocers," *Los Angeles Times*, November 3, 2007; Jerry Hirsch, "Grocery Stores Down Size to Better Fit Local Needs," *Los Angeles Times*, May 17, 2008; and Corby Kummer, "The Great Grocery Smackdown," *Atlantic*, March 1, 2010.

256   **Desert Rain Café:** Ted Robbins, "Arizona Café Makes Healthy Fare for Native Americans," National Public Radio, June 19, 2009. For the café's website, see www.desertraincafe.com.

257   **the challenge in remaking a viable fresh-food system is formidable:** Don Shaffer, "Remaking the Food System," *Stanford Social Innovation Review*, September 30, 2013, http://bit.ly/1sCCSrE.

258   **the Food Commons:** Larry Yee, "The Food Commons 2.0: Imagine, Design, Build . . . ," October 2011, http://bit.ly/1p6ngcI.

258   **the Philadelphia-based Common Market:** For details of Common Market programs, see Commonmarketphila.org. See also Dianna Marder, "Philadelphia's Common Market Wins $1.1 Million Grant," *Inquirer*, Philly.com, June 30, 2011; and "Common Market Boosts Urban Access to Fresh Food, Helps Local Farms Thrive," *RSF Social Finance*, September 6, 2012, http://bit.ly/1oMOuFS.

259   **"What we eat and drink":** Peter Forbes, *The Great Remembering: Further Thoughts on Land, Soul, and Society* (San Francisco: Trust for Public Land, 2001). Peter Forbes, photographer, writer, and conservationist was for a decade the leader of the conservation efforts undertaken in New England for the Trust for Public Lands. In 2001, with Helen Whybrow, he cofounded the Center for Whole Communities, a land-based leadership development and learning center based at Knoll Farm in Fayston, Vermont; see its website, www.knollfarm.org.

263   **World War II . . . "victory" garden:** Mary MacVean, "Echoes of Victory," *Los Angeles Times*, January 10, 2009. In Los Angeles in 2013, there were 1,261 registered urban agriculture sites—school gardens, community gardens, and commercial sites. Urban farmers travel, on average, 13.9 miles to deliver their produce. Data from UCLA's Luskin School of Public Affairs, August 15, 2013, Cultivate losangeles.org.

Chapter 10: IMAGINATION

264   **"My shaping spirit of imagination":** Samuel Taylor Coleridge, "Dejection: An Ode" (1802). Coleridge, depressed about his marriage, addicted to opiates, and in love with Sara Hutchinson (the sister of Wordsworth's future wife), fears that his poetic powers are waning: "afflictions bow me down to earth . . . rob me of my mirth . . . [and] what nature gave me at my birth, my shaping spirit of Imagination."

264   **"I am enough of an artist":** Quoted in George Sylvester Viereck, "What Life Means to Einstein: An Interview," *Saturday Evening Post*, October 26, 1929.

264 **The Museum of Jurassic Technology:** Lawrence Weschler, *Mr. Wilson's Cabinet of Wonder* (New York: Random House, 1995). The MJT gained a certain notoriety that was not entirely welcomed by its founder, David Wilson. See Jeanne Scheper, "Feasting on Technologies of Recycling in the Jurassic," *Other Voices* 3 (May 2007), http://bit.ly/1BeotUK; and Gemma Cubero, *Mr. Wilson's Ways of Knowing*, October 2011, http://bit.ly/1pNZyBm. For a virtual visit, see *Inhaling the Spore: A Journey Through the Museum of Jurassic Technology*, a film directed by Leonard Feinstein, 2006. A jubilee catalogue, *The Museum of Jurassic Technology*, was published in 2002 by McNaughton and Gunn.

267 **Comparing the early intellectual development of . . . the great apes, with that of the human infant:** Data taken from Giada Cordoni and Elizabeth Palagi, "Ontogenetic Trajectories of Chimpanzee Social Play: Similarities with Humans," *PLoS ONE*, November 16, 2011; Felix Warneken and Michael Tomasello, "Altruistic Helping in Human Infants and Young Chimpanzees," *Science* 311 (2006): 1301–3; Victoria Wobbler et al., "Differences in the Early Cognitive Development of Children and Great Apes," *Developmental Psychobiology* 56 (2014): 547–73.

269 **children weave together:** Paul L. Harris, *The Work of the Imagination* (Oxford: Oxford University Press, 2000); and Harris, *Trusting What You're Told: How Children Learn from Others* (Cambridge, MA: Harvard University Press, 2012). Harris is the Victor S. Thomas Professor at the Harvard Graduate School of Education.

271 **music can evoke definitive . . . responses:** Leonard B. Meyer, *Emotion and Meaning in Music* (Chicago: University of Chicago Press, 1956).

271 **"making heaven descend upon earth":** Charles Darwin, *The Descent of Man* (1871; reprint edition London: John Murray 1890), pt. 3, chap. 19, p. 569.

271 **"music expresses itself through sound":** Daniel Barenboim, *Everything Is Connected: The Power of Music* (London: Orion Books, 2007).

272 **employing pleasant and unpleasant music to evoke emotion:** Stefan Koelsch et al., "Investigating Emotion with Music: An fMRI Study," *Human Brain Mapping* 27 (2006): 239–50. For a discussion of the beat in music and activation of the basal ganglia, see Jessica Grahn, "The Neurosciences and Music III: Disorders and Plasticity," *Annals of the New York Academy of Sciences* 1169 (2009): 35–45.

273 **When the imagination is at work, . . . the whole brain:** Vincent Costa et al., "Emotional Imagery: Assessing Pleasure and Arousal in the Brain's Reward Circuitry," *Human Brain Mapping* 31 (2010): 1446–57.

273 **"when, from the sight of a man":** Thomas Hobbes, *Leviathan* (1651), chap. 2.

274 **the brain's "mental workspace":** Alexander Schlegel et al., "Network Structure and Dynamics of the Mental Workspace," *Proceedings of the National Academy of Sciences* 110 (2013): 16277–282.

275 **both David Hume and Adam Smith recognized the essential nature of imagination:** Robin Downie, "Science and the Imagination in the Age of Reason," *Journal of Medical Ethics: Medical Humanities* 27 (2001): 58–63.

276 **"It is not simply that there is more connectivity":** Peter Tse, "Symbolic Thought and the Evolution of Human Morality," in Walter Sinnott-Armstrong, ed., *Moral Psychology*, vol. 1, *The Evolution of Morality: Adaptations and Innateness* (Cambridge, MA: MIT Press, 2007).

276 **"the burgeoning of unequivocal art":** Richard Klein, "Out of Africa and the Evolution of Human Behavior," *Evolutionary Anthropology* 17 (2008): 267–81.

276 **the ancient cave paintings of France and Spain:** Jean Clottes, *Cave Art* (London: Phaidon Press, 2008). Clottes is the historian who assembled the team that explored the Chauvet caves (named after Jean-Marie Chauvet, who discovered them in 1994) in the Ardèche region of south-central France. For background to that find and for the debate surrounding the significance of European Paleolithic cave painting see, Judith Thurman, "First Impressions: What Does the World's Oldest Art Say About Us?" *New Yorker*, June 23, 2008.

276 **close proximity with the Neanderthals:** "Cross breeding may have given modern humans genes useful for coping with climates colder than Africa's, but the hybrid offspring probably suffered from infertility." Ewen Callaway, "Modern Human Genomes Reveal Our Inner Neanderthal," *Nature News*, January 29, 2014.

278 **communication with the gods of the underworld:** Gregory Curtis, *The Cave Painters: Probing the Mysteries of the World's First Artists* (New York: Anchor, 2007).

278 **"Religious-like phenomena":** Maurice Bloch, "Why Religion Is Nothing Special but Is Central," *Philosophical Transactions of the Royal Society* 363 (2008): 2055–61.

280 **"technopoly":** Neil Postman, *Technopoly: The Surrender of Culture to Technology* (New York: Vintage Books, 1993).

280 **sat down with IBM's Deep Blue:** Garry Kasparov, "The Chess Master and the Computer," *New York Review of Books*, February 11, 2010; and Garry Kasparov, *How Life Imitates Chess* (UK: Arrow Books, 2008).

283 **the tsunami of information:** Barrett Sheridan, "Is Cue the Cure for Information Overload?" *Bloomberg BusinessWeek*, June 19, 2012.

284 **the statistics for other industrialized nations are comparable:** "Mobile Technology Fact Sheet," Pew Research Center's Internet and American Life Project, http://www.pewinternet.org/fact-sheets/mobile-technology-fact-sheet.

284 **the work-management theories of Frederick Taylor:** Sonia Taneja, Mildred Pryor, and Leslie Toombs, "Frederick W. Taylor's Scientific Management Principles: Relevance and Validity," *Journal of Applied Management and Entrepreneurship* 16, no. 3 (2011).

284 **enhancing human muscle power . . . different from helping humans think:** James Fallows, "The 50 Greatest Breakthroughs Since the Wheel," *Atlantic*, November 2013.

285 **privacy . . . shopping online:** Alice Marwick, "How Your Data Are Being Deeply Mined," *New York Review of Books*, January 9, 2014.

285 **four intensely competitive and wealthy companies:** "Another Game of Thrones," *Economist*, December 1, 2012.

286 **"chipping away [at the] capacity for concentration":** Nicholas Carr, *The Shallows: What the Internet is Doing to Our Brains* (New York: Norton, 2010).

287 **a powerful temptation during lectures:** Faria Sana, Tina Weston, and Nicholas Cepeda, "Laptop Multitasking Hinders Classroom Learning for Both Users and Nearby Peers," *Computers and Education* 62 (2013): 24–31.

287 **"Information only *appears* to be free on the Internet":** Michael Saler, "The Hidden Cost: How the Internet Is Using Us All" (a review of *Who Owns the Future* by Jaron Lanier), *Times Literary Supplement*, May 24, 2013.

287 **the "digital exhaust" of Web searches:** Tim Harford, "Big Data: Are We Making a Big Mistake?" *Financial Times Magazine*, March 29–30, 2014.

289 **such skilled practice provides an anchor:** Richard Sennett, *The Craftsman* (New Haven, CT: Yale University Press, 2008).

289 **Being skillful in body and mind builds . . . a sense of mastery:** Daniel Charny, *Power of Making: The Importance of Being Skilled* (London: Victoria and Albert Museum, 2011); and the exhibition catalog *Design and the Elastic Mind* (New York: Museum of Modern Art, 2008).

Reprise: WISDOM

293 **"Mankind achieved civilization by developing":** F. W. Hayek, *The Fatal Conceit: The Errors of Socialism* (Chicago: University of Chicago Press, 1988).

293 **"Gross National Product does not allow":** Robert F. Kennedy, speech delivered at the University of Kansas, March 18, 1968, http://bit.ly/1l6CSMy.

294 **the Mont Pèlerin Society:** The MPS was established by a group of scholars, mainly economists, who sought to strengthen the values of Western democracy and classical liberalism in the post–World War II period. Convened in April 1947 by Friedrich von Hayek, the society is named after the place of its first meeting, Mont Pèlerin, near Montreux, Switzerland.

294 **the HMS *Beagle*:** Originally constructed as a frigate and launched in 1820, the *Beagle* was soon refitted as a survey vessel, making three voyages between 1826 and 1843. Charles Darwin, at twenty-two, was chosen as the "gentleman naturalist" to accompany Capt. Robert Fitzroy on the second expedition, which made extensive surveys of South America before moving on to the Galápagos. The voyage (eventually a circumnavigation of the globe) took five years. See Alan Moorehead, *Darwin and the Beagle* (New York: Harper & Row, 1969), for a friendly, well-illustrated read about the epic expedition. For Darwin's original descriptions and insights, see Charles Darwin, *The Voyage of the Beagle: Charles Darwin's Journal of Researches*, ed. Janet Browne and Michael Neve (New York: Penguin Classics, 1989). The quotations employed here are from chapter 17, which describes Darwin's visit to the Galápagos Islands. For a list of Darwin's complete publications, see http://darwin-online.org.uk/.

295 **the Galápagos finches:** From their seed-eating ancestors in South America, some finch species, while preserving their seed-eating preferences, are distinct for having evolved into cactus dwellers, with a longer, thinner beak, or in becoming seed-eating tree dwellers. More than half of the defined species of the Galápagos are now tree-dwelling insect eaters. See Jonathan Weiner, *Beak of the Finch*, (New York: Vintage Books, 1995).

297 **"as the first who succeeded in elaborating":** Friedrich A. Hayek, *The Fatal Conceit: The Errors of Socialism*. Quotations and references to Darwin's diaries are taken from *The Collected Works of F. A. Hayek*, ed. W. W. Bartley (Chicago: University of Chicago Press, 1988), vol. 1, chap. 1. I am also indebted here to Larry Arnhart for his essay, "The Evolution of Darwinian Liberalism," presented at the Mont Pèlerin Society meeting, June 22–29, 2013. For an introduction to

Hayek, his philosophy, and his writings, see John Cassidy, "The Price Prophet," *New Yorker*, February 7, 2000.

297 **"designs of extraordinary complexity":** John Kay, "Darwin's Humbling Lesson for Business," *Financial Times*, July 3, 2013.

298 **it is "tradition" . . . that holds the social order together:** Hayek, *Fatal Conceit*, vol. 1, p. 21; and Mark Pagel, *Wired for Culture: Origins of the Human Social Mind* (New York: Norton, 2012). Pagel, an evolutionary biologist, employs the concept of social learning rather than tradition in his argument, but he essentially comes to the same conclusion—that social learning acts on societies and sculpts them.

299 **the idea of progress:** This short history draws upon J. B. Bury, *The Idea of Progress: An Inquiry into Its Origins and Growth* (1932; reprint edition New York: Cosimo, 2008). John Bagnell Bury (1861–1927) was an Irish historian and classical scholar who for the last twenty-five years of his life was the Regius Professor of Modern History at the University of Cambridge.

300 **gross domestic product (GDP):** The original variant of the GDP, the gross national product (GNP), first formulated in the 1930s, was the brainchild of Simon Kuznets, the Russian-born American economist who received the Nobel Prize for his work in 1971. Both measures (they differ only slightly), in addition to tracking the internal dynamics of a nation's goods and services, enable the important comparison of aggregate economic activity across nations and across time. But as Kuznets emphasized, the measures were not intended to provide a sensitive index of well-being, except as it may be inferred from material consumption. See Robert Fogel et al., *Political Arithmetic: Simon Kuznets and the Empirical Tradition in Economics* (Chicago: University of Chicago Press, 2013).

300 **well-being will improve with money:** This is a complex and debated area of investigation, although most national-level comparisons find that wealthier countries tend to be happier. See E. Deiner and E. M. Suh, "National Differences in Subjective Well-Being," in E. Kahnemann, E. Diener, and N. Schwartz, eds., *Well-being: The Foundations of Hedonic Psychology* (New York: Russell Sage Foundation, 1999), pp. 434–50. But evident from World Bank data is that after GNP per capita reaches around $9,500, the correlation with well-being weakens, and further increases in GNP have a diminishing impact on happiness scores. See D. G. Meyers, "The Funds, Friends and Faith of Happy People," *American Psychologist* 55 (2000): 55–67; and Zakri Abdul Hamid and Anantha Duraiappah, "The Growing Disconnect Between GDP and Well-Being," World Economic Forum blog, May 16, 2014, http://forumblog.org/2014/05/growing-disconnect-gdp-wellbeing/. For a balanced review and analysis of the continued value of GDP, see Jan Delhey and Christian Kroll, "A Happiness Test for the New Measures of National Well-Being: How Much better than GDP are They?" in H. Brockmann and J. Dehey, eds., *Human Happiness and the Pursuit of Maximization: Is More Always Better?* (Dordrecht: Springer, 2013), pp. 191–210.

300 **in 2013 the GDP of the United States was $15,800 trillion:** The data presented here are from About.com: *US Economy*, prepared by Kimberly Amadeo. Gross national product (GNP) includes economic output by all persons and businesses considered American, regardless of their location. Gross domestic product

(GDP) includes all products made and sold in the United States, regardless of the national ownership of the manufacturer.

300 **gross domestic product (GDP):** GDP has four main components. The first is personal consumption, which in 2013 accounted for 70 percent of what the United States produces. This category is subdivided into durable goods—cars, refrigerators, furniture, et cetera—and nondurable goods, such as food and energy, and services that are consumed. The latter accounts for 48 percent of U.S. consumption, a significant rise since World War II. The other three categories are business investment, government spending, and the net exports of goods and services.

300 **In America shopping is a tradition:** Shopping also drives indebtedness. By the early 1990s annual personal savings, which were 8 to 10 percent of income between 1946 and 1980, had fallen below personal indebtedness to credit card companies. In 2007, just before the global financial crash, household indebtedness in the United States reached 132 percent of disposable income. Statistics quoted will be found in the following sources: "Dropping the Shopping," *Economist*, July 25, 2009; Paul Starr, "A Different Road to a Fair Society," *New York Review of Books*, May 22, 2014; David Leonhardt, "All for the 1 Percent, 1 Percent for All," *New York Times Magazine*, May 4, 2014; and Annie Lowrey, "Recovery Has Created Far More Low-Wage Jobs than Better-Paid Ones," *New York Times*, April 28, 2014.

300 **"What happened to our country's stride and spirit":** Frank Bruni, "America the Shrunken," *New York Times*, May 4, 2014.

301 **no distinction between the quantity and quality of growth:** Roger Boyd, "Economic Growth: A Social Pathology," *Resilience*, November 2013, http://www.resilience.org/stories/2013-11-07/economic-growth-a-social-pathology.

302 **the United States now consumes approximately 25 percent of the world's resources:** Randy Scheer and Doug Moss, "Use It and Lose It: The Outsize Effect of US Consumption on the Environment," *Scientific American*, September 14, 2012.

303 **we are again losing species at a rapid rate:** Elizabeth Kolbert, *The Sixth Extinction: An Unnatural History* (New York: Henry Holt, 2014); S. L. Pimm et al., "The Biodiversity of Species and Their Rates of Extinction, Distribution and Protection," *Science Magazine*, May 30, 2014.

303 **"Progress might have been all right once":** Douglas Parker and Dana Gioia, *Ogden Nash: The Life and Work of America's Laureate of Light Verse* (Chicago: Ivan R. Dee, 2005).

303 **If human progress is to be made rational and sustainable:** James G. Speth, *The Bridge at the Edge of the World: Capitalism, the Environment, and Crossing from Crisis to Sustainability* (New Haven, CT: Yale University Press, 2009).

304 **Nor will that balance be fostered:** Philip K. Howard, *The Rule of Nobody: Saving America from Dead Laws and Broken Government* (New York: Norton, 2014).

304 **the creativity of resilient, knowledgeable, and innovative individuals:** Brian Walker, David Salt, and Walter Reid, *Resilience Thinking: Sustaining Ecosystems and People in a Changing World* (Washington, DC: Island Press, 2006).

305   **public sentiment for change is apparent:** See Dan Ariely, "Americans Want to Live in a Much More Equal Country [They Just Don't Realize It]," *Atlantic*, August 2012. U.S. society is far more uneven in terms of wealth than Americans believe it to be. Furthermore Americans want much more equality than both what they have and what they think they have. These are Ariely's conclusions from a survey of 5,522 people interviewed about wealth in America. Those surveyed guessed that around 9 percent of wealth was owned by the bottom two quintiles (40 percent) of the U.S. population and 59 percent by the top quintile (20 percent), while in reality the bottom 40 percent had only 0.3 percent of wealth, and the top quintile 84 percent. John Rawls, *A Theory of Justice* (1971; Cambridge, MA: Belknap Press, 1999), defines a just society as one that an individual is willing to enter, with knowledge of the conditions, at any social level; using that definition, then the preference of the respondents was for a society more equal than any other in the world, with 32 percent of the wealth belonging to the wealthiest quintile, and 11 percent to the poorest. Political persuasion made little difference in the preferred distribution.

305   **Industry . . . has begun to pay attention:** "The Cost of Doing Nothing: Climate Change and the Economy," *Economist*, June 28, 2014; Coral Davenport, "Industry Awakens to the Threat of Climate Change," *International New York Times*, January 23, 2014; Paul Brown, "Coca-Cola in India Accused of Leaving Farms Parched and Land Poisoned," *Guardian*, July 23, 2003; and "Indian Officials Order Coca-Cola Plant to Close for Using Too Much Water," *Guardian*, June18, 2014.

306   **the World Economic Forum:** The forum is a Swiss nonprofit foundation "committed to improving the state of the world," founded in 1971 by Klaus Schwab. Funded by one thousand member companies, it is based in Geneva and has an annual budget of around $5 billion. See its website, http://www.weforum.org.

306   **a sustainable, "circular" economy . . . Walter Stahel:** The circular economy seeks to decouple wealth from resource consumption through the practical application of systems theory and dynamic feedback. For a concise introduction, see Michael Braungart and Bill McDonough, *Cradle to Cradle: Remaking the Way We Make Things* (New York: North Point Press, 2002).

306   **Dame Ellen MacArthur:** "Navigating the Circular Economy: A Conversation with Dame Ellen MacArthur," McKinsey and Company, February 2014, http://bit.ly/1bNilUJ.

307   **pollution . . . has taken its toll on marine life:** Daniel Pauly, *5 Easy Pieces: The Impact of Fisheries on Marine Ecosystems (The State of the World's Oceans)* (Washington, DC: Island Press, 2010); Jonathan Leake, "Fish Stocks Eaten to Extinction by 2050," *Sunday Times* (London), July 11, 2010; and Greg Stone, "The Five Biggest Threats to Our Oceans," World Economic Forum, June 5, 2014, http://forumblog.org/2014/06/challenges-worlds-oceans/.

308   **[marine] reserve . . . in the Galápagos islands:** Data from Galapagos Conservancy, http://www.galapagos.org/conservation/marine-conservation.

309   **incentive-based systems:** R. Quenton Grafton et al., "Incentive-based Approaches to Sustainable Fisheries," *Canadian Journal of Fisheries and Aquatic Science* 63 (2006): 699–710.

309 **Ayana Elizabeth Johnson, a marine biologist:** Ayana Elizabeth Johnson and
     Daniel Kaiser Saunders, "Time Preferences and the Management of Coral Reef
     Fisheries," *Ecological Economics* (April 2014): 130–39; and Svati Kirsten Narula,
     "How the Famous Marshmallow Study Explains Environmental Conservation,"
     Atlantic, March 2014.

310 **destructive consequences of selfishness:** Garrett Hardin, "The Tragedy of
     the Commons," *Science* 162 (1968): 1243–48.

310 **Elinor Ostrom . . . common resource management:** The most comprehen-
     sive guide to Ostrom's work is Amy Poteele, Marco Janssen, and Elinor Ostrom,
     *Working Together: Collective Action, the Commons, and Multiple Methods in Prac-
     tice* (Princeton: Princeton University Press, 2010). She died in 2012 at the age of
     eighty-eight.

311 **collectively we can acquire that wisdom:** Cross-cultural studies have pro-
     posed definitions of wisdom that share common elements. These include: rational
     decision making based on general knowledge of life; prosocial behaviors involving
     empathy, compassion, and altruism; emotional stability; insight or self-reflection;
     decisiveness in the face of uncertainty; and tolerance of divergent value systems.
     See Dilipe Jeste and James Harris, "Wisdom—A Neuroscience Perspective," *Jour-
     nal of the American Medical Association* 304 (2010): 1602.

Index